Series Editors:
Steven F. Warren, Ph.D.
Joe Reichle, Ph.D.

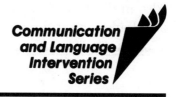

**Communication
and Language
Intervention
Series**

Volume 8

Exploring the
Speech–Language Connection

Also in the Communication
and Language Intervention Series:

Communication
and Language
Intervention
Series

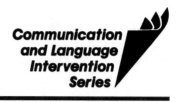

Volume 8

Exploring the Speech–Language Connection

Edited by

Rhea Paul, Ph.D.
Professor
Department of Communication Disorders
Southern Connecticut State University
Lecturer
Yale Child Study Center
New Haven

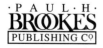

·P A U L·H·
BROOKES
PUBLISHING Cº

Baltimore • London • Toronto • Sydney

Paul H. Brookes Publishing Co.
Post Office Box 10624
Baltimore, Maryland 21285-0624

www.pbrookes.com

Typeset by Maryland Composition Company, Inc., Glen Burnie, Maryland.
Manufactured in the United States of America by
Thomson-Shore, Inc., Dexter, Michigan.

The case studies discussed in Chapter 5 are based on real people and circumstances, but names have been changed to protect identities.

Library of Congress Cataloging-in-Publication Data

Exploring the speech–language connection / edited by Rhea Paul.
    p.   cm.—(Communication and language intervention series ; 8)
    Includes bibliographical references and index.
    ISBN 1-55766-325-4
    1. Communicative disorders.   2. Language acquisition.   3. Speech.
  I. Paul, Rhea.   II. Series.
  RC423.E98   1998   97-29523
  616.85′5—dc21   CIP

British Library Cataloguing in Publication data are available from the British Library.

Contents

Series Preface

THE PURPOSE OF THE *Communication and Language Intervention Series* is to provide meaningful foundations for the application of sound intervention designs to enhance the development of communication skills across the life span. We are endeavoring to achieve this purpose by providing readers with presentations of state-of-the-art theory, research, and practice.

In selecting topics, editors, and authors, we are not attempting to limit the contents of this series to those viewpoints with which we agree or that we find most promising. We are assisted in our efforts to develop the series by an editorial advisory board consisting of prominent scholars representative of the range of issues and perspectives to be incorporated in the series.

We trust that the careful reader will find much that is provocative and controversial in this and other volumes. This will be necessarily so to the extent that the work reported is truly on the so-called cutting edge, a mythical place where no sacred cows exist. This point is demonstrated time and again throughout this volume as the conventional wisdom is challenged (and occasionally confirmed) by various authors.

Readers of this and other volumes are encouraged to proceed with healthy skepticism. In order to achieve our purpose, we take on some difficult and controversial issues. Errors and misinterpretations inevitably are made. This is normal in the development of any field and should be welcomed as evidence that the field is moving forward and tackling difficult and weighty issues.

Well-conceived theory and research on development of both children with and children without disabilities are vitally important for researchers, educators, and clinicians committed to the development of optimal approaches to communication and language intervention. For this reason, each volume in this series includes chapters pertaining to both development and intervention.

The content of each volume reflects our view of the symbiotic relationship between intervention and research: Demonstrations of what may work in intervention should lead to analyses of promising discoveries and insights from developmental work that may in turn fuel further refinement by intervention researchers.

An inherent goal of this series is to enhance the long-term development of the field by systematically furthering the dissemination of theoretically and empirically based scholarship and research. We promise the reader an opportunity to participate in the development of this field through the debates and discussions that occur throughout the pages of the *Communication and Language Intervention Series.*

Editorial Advisory Board

Volume Preface

ALTHOUGH THE PROFESSIONAL TITLE for those of us who work with individuals with communication disorders is *speech-language pathologist,* the two aspects of the profession and the science that underlies them are too often viewed as separate enterprises conducted in isolation from each other. Whereas speech and language are obviously related in communication situations, they are too often treated as distinct in the clinical and developmental literature. In addition, though there are certainly disorders that affect speech without affecting language and vice versa, it is often the case that individuals, particularly developing children, experience difficulties in both realms. Research on disorders of communication frequently focuses exclusively on issues concerning articulation, ignoring the effects of higher-level processes on pronunciation. However, the processes involved in the formulation and comprehension of language are too often studied without regard to the effects of—or on—the output channel. Intervention programs aimed at improving communication skills in children frequently address either speech or language goals, with no attempt to develop an integrated program even in children whose needs clearly overlap both areas.

This volume represents an attempt to begin to integrate knowledge and practice around these topics. The aim of the volume is to focus attention on the ways in which speech and language support each other, interact, and create synergies in development and to explore the ways in which the two converge and diverge in communication disorders. In order to achieve this goal, the volume explores speech–language connections both in normal acquisition and in a variety of communication disorders in which the connection appears to have particular relevance. These disorders include specific language impairment, severe motor and physical speech impairments, hearing impairments, Down syndrome, and dysfluency. By examining the ways in which speech and language function and exert mutual influences in these aspects of development and disorders, the hope is that a more general theory about their connection can begin to be formed, which would lead to hypotheses that could be tested in typical development and would have implications for remediating disorders. The goal of this volume, then, is to raise questions rather than to answer them, to bring together what little is known about the ways in which speech and language influence each other, to define what is known and to identify what is not. By staking out this unknown territory, researchers will be in a stronger position to develop studies that will help to map its features and ultimately to use it to cultivate intervention programs that address in a more integrated way the full range of communicative needs that so many individuals present.

The volume begins by addressing issues of the connections between speech and language in typical early development. In Chapter 1, Oller and colleagues examine the ways in which infant sound production evolves toward meaningful speech. Stoel-Gammon, in Chapter 2, looks at the relationships between phonological and lexical acquisition in the first stages of language development. In the latter chapters, contributors discuss various communication disorders as case studies in the interactions of speech and language.

In Chapter 3, Locke discusses some theoretical approaches to understanding how speech–language interactions in typical development can contribute to our understanding of specific language disorders in children. Shriberg and Austin, co-authors of Chapter 4, look at comorbidity of speech and language disorders in order to identify distinct patterns of communication impairments. They raise important questions about the genetic bases of the development of each of these aspects of communication. In Chapter 5, Bleile explores the relationships between speech and language development in the fascinating case of children temporarily deprived of vocal abilities at an early stage of language acquisition as a result of tracheostomy. Paul, in Chapter 6, examines the development of language in children with severe limitations in vocal expressive ability due to speech motor impairments and looks for clues to the effects on language development of the inaccessibility of speech as the primary channel for expression.

Miller and Leddy, co-authors of Chapter 7, take on the speech–language connection in children with Down syndrome, who have both physical and cognitive problems that affect their acquisition of both abilities. In Chapter 8, Nelson and Welsh look at speech–language relationships in children with the opposite problem: intact motor speech ability for expression but limited capacity for processing input because of hearing impairment. In Chapter 9, Tetnowski infers speech–language connections by looking at linguistic effects on disfluency in people who stutter. Swank and Larrivee explore in Chapter 10 the issue of the way in which phonological development and its progeny, phonological awareness, contribute to the development of skill in written language. Finally, in Chapter 11, Camarata brings together the information presented in the rest of the volume and from it draws conclusions for developing intervention programs for children with speech and language disorders.

It is hoped that readers find this volume provocative and that it provides an impetus to find ways to integrate into their own thinking and practice the various processes that compose the complex phenomenon of human communication. We have far to go before we achieve fully developed descriptions of this phenomenon that interweave processes that we are used to thinking of in isolation. If readers of this volume find themselves beginning to frame questions in their everyday work with communication disorders about how speech and language issues can be integrated, our aim will have been attained. What is more, we may begin to move toward the ability to develop the rich descriptions needed to fully comprehend human communication and to develop holistic programs to remediate its disorders.

Contributors

The Editor

Rhea Paul, Ph.D., Professor, Department of Communication Disorders, Southern Connecticut State University, 501 Crescent Street, New Haven, Connecticut 06515-1555; and Lecturer, Yale Child Study Center. Dr. Paul has published more than 50 research articles on children's language development and disorders, is author of *Pragmatic Activities for Language Intervention* (Communication Skill Builders, 1992) and *Language Disorders from Birth Through Adolescence: Assessment and Intervention* (Mosby–Year Book, 1995), and is co-author with Jon F. Miller of *The Clinical Assessment of Language Comprehension* (Paul H. Brookes Publishing Co., 1995). She is a fellow of the American Speech-Language-Hearing Association and won the 1996 Editor's Award from the *American Journal of Speech-Language Pathology.*

The Chapter Authors

Diane Austin, B.Mus., Associate Research Specialist, Waisman Center on Mental Retardation and Human Development, University of Wisconsin–Madison, 1500 Highland Avenue, Room 447, Madison, Wisconsin 53705-2280. Ms. Austin is an associate research specialist with the Phonology Project at the Waisman Center on Mental Retardation and Human Development at the University of Wisconsin–Madison and a student in biostatistics. Her research interests include measurement in conversational speech and computer-assisted classification of speech disorders.

Ken M. Bleile, M.D., Associate Professor and Head, Department of Communicative Disorders, University of Northern Iowa, 238 Communication Arts Center, Cedar Falls, Iowa 50614-0356. Dr. Bleile's research interests lie in the areas of child phonology, language disorders in children, pediatric head injury, and multicultural issues. He is the author of *Manual of Articulation and Phonological Disorders* (Singular Publishing Group, 1995) and *Articulation and Phonological Disorders: A Book of Exercises* (Singular Publishing Group, 1996). Along with John Folkins, Dr. Bleile received the 1990 Editor's Choice Award from the *Journal of Speech and Hearing Disorders.* His research has been featured in *Pediatric News* and *Advance.*

Stephen M. Camarata, Ph.D., Associate Professor of Hearing and Speech Sciences, The Vanderbilt University School of Medicine; Associate Professor of Special Education, Peabody College, and Investigator, John F. Kennedy Center for Research in Human Development, Vanderbilt University; Director, Scottish Rite Child Language Disorders Center, Bill Wilkerson Hearing and Speech Center, 1114 19th Avenue South, Nashville, Tennessee 37212. Dr. Camarata's areas of research interest include the treatment of speech and language disorders in children. He is also quite involved in studying child development in the home, particularly among the seven offspring sharing his residence.

Alan B. Cobo-Lewis, Ph.D., Research Assistant Professor, Departments of Psychology and Pediatrics, University of Miami, Psychology Annex, Post Office Box 249229, Coral Gables, Florida 33124-0721. Dr. Cobo-Lewis received his doctoral degree from the University of Wisconsin, where he studied perception. His research interests are communicative development and visual perception and the construction of mathematical and statistical methods for psychology.

Rebecca E. Eilers, Ph.D., Dean, College of Liberal Arts and Sciences, University of Maine, 5774 Stevens Hall, Room 105, Orono, Maine 04469-5774. Dr. Eilers is a developmental psychologist with research interests in language and speech development in infants and children, both those who are typically developing and those who are atypically developing.

Linda S. Larrivee, Ph.D., Assistant Professor, Department of Communication Science and Disorders, University of Missouri–Columbia, 303 Lewis Hall, Columbia, Missouri 65211. Dr. Larrivee's teaching and research interests include language and reading disabilities in school-age children and adolescents. She has extensive clinical experience in promoting the language and reading skills of children and adolescents with language-learning disabilities.

Mark Leddy, Ph.D., CCC-SLP, Assistant Professor, Department of Communicative Disorders, University of Wisconsin–Whitewater, 800 West Main Street, Whitewater, Wisconsin 53190. Dr. Leddy is a speech-language pathologist who has worked extensively with adults who have Down syndrome. He has made presentations at various state, national, and international meetings about the communication characteristics of adults with Down syndrome. In addition to his position as an assistant professor at the University of Wisconsin–Whitewater, Dr. Leddy is a fellow at the Waisman Center on Mental Retardation and Human Development at the University of Wisconsin–Madison.

Sharyse L. Levine, M.A., M.S., Doctoral Student, Department of Pediatrics, Mailman Center for Child Development, University of Miami, Post Office Box 248185, Coral Gables, Florida 33124. Ms. Levine is a doctoral candidate in clinical psychology at the University of Miami, where she specializes in children and families. She received her master's degree in developmental and educational psychology from Teachers College, Columbia University, New York City.

John L. Locke, Ph.D., Professor and Head of Department, Department of Human Communication Sciences, University of Sheffield, 18 Claremont Crescent, Sheffield S10 2TA, ENGLAND. Dr. Locke holds a chair in the Department of Human Communication Sciences at the University of Sheffield, England. He believes that human language is in the first instance a deeply biological capability with a range of interesting cultural consequences. Dr. Locke is the author of nearly 100 journal articles and book chapters and is the author of three books: *Phonological Acquisition and Change* (Academic Press, 1983), *The Child's Path to Spoken Language* (Harvard University Press, 1993), and *The De-Voicing of Society: Why We Don't Talk to Each Other Anymore* (Simon & Schuster, 1998). He serves on a number of editorial boards and edits the journal *Applied Psycholinguistics*.

Jon F. Miller, Ph.D., Professor and Chair, Department of Communicative Disorders, University of Wisconsin–Madison, 1975 Willow Drive, Madison, Wisconsin 53706. Dr. Miller has published extensively on language development and disorders and is completing a series of longitudinal research projects on early language development in children with Down syndrome.

Keith E. Nelson, Ph.D., Professor, Department of Psychology, Pennsylvania State University, 414 Moore Building, University Park, Pennsylvania 16802. Dr. Nelson continues to explore the nature of children's learning, as he has since 1972. By crossing domains of learning—children's speech, sign, art, and text—of children with and children without disabilities, new empirical and theoretical patterns are revealed.

D. Kimbrough Oller, Ph.D., Professor and Chair, Department of Communication Disorders, University of Maine, 5754 North Stevens Hall L-5, Orono, Maine 04469. Dr. Oller received his doctoral degree from the University of Texas in 1971. His research has been published widely in journals of speech and hearing, psycholinguistics, and developmental psychology. His work focuses heavily on vocal development in children at risk for communication disorders.

Barbara Zurer Pearson, Ph.D., Research Assistant Professor, Departments of English and Psychology, Bilingualism Study Group, University of Miami, 221 Psychology Annex, 5665 Ponce de Leon Boulevard, Coral Gables, Florida 33124-0721. Dr. Pearson majored in French as an undergraduate at Middlebury College in Vermont as well as at the Sorbonne in Paris, where she first became fascinated with her own and others' abilities to speak and think in two languages. She has since pursued that fascination in Miami, Florida, in her work toward receiving two graduate degrees and in her programmatic research on first language acquisition and bilingual development with the University of Miami Language Project.

Lawrence D. Shriberg, Ph.D., Professor, Department of Communicative Disorders, Waisman Center on Mental Retardation and Human Development, University of Wisconsin–Madison, 1975 Willow Drive, Madison, Wisconsin 53706. Dr. Shriberg is a professor in the Department of Communicative Disorders and a principal investigator at the Waisman Center on Mental Retardation and Human Development at the University of Wisconsin–Madison. His research focuses on the origins and treatment of child speech disorders.

Carol Stoel-Gammon, Ph.D., Professor, Department of Speech and Hearing Sciences, University of Washington, 251 Eagleston Hall JG-15, 1417 N.E. 42nd Street, Seattle, Washington 98105-6246. Dr. Stoel-Gammon received her doctoral degree in linguistics from Stanford University in Palo Alto, California. Her teaching and research interests are children with typical phonological development and children with phonological development disorders. She is particularly interested in the relationship between babbling and speech and in early identification of toddlers with speech and language disorders.

Linda K. Swank, Ph.D., Assistant Professor, Communication Disorders Program, Speech-Language-Hearing Center, University of Virginia, Colony Plaza, 2205 Fontaine Avenue, Suite 202, Charlottesville, Virginia 22903. Dr. Swank's teaching and research interests include early identification and treatment of language-based reading disorders. She co-authored the Phonological Awareness and Literacy Screening (PALS) (University of Virginia, 1997), the first-ever statewide assessment of phonological awareness and early literacy skills conducted in Virginia. The emphasis of her work is on research to practice in the area of language impairments in children and adolescents as these impairments affect academic performance.

John A. Tetnowski, Ph.D., Assistant Professor, Speech and Hearing Sciences Program, Department of Speech Communication, Portland State University, 75 Neuberger Hall, Post Office Box 751, Portland, Oregon 97207-0751. Dr. Tetnowski's research and clinical interests include the evaluation and treatment of fluency disorders, objective measurement of voice disorders, and the use of technology in clinical and educational environments. He is Vice President for Scientific and Educational Affairs of the Oregon Speech-Language and Hearing Association and is Oregon's representative to the Special Interest Division on Fluency and Fluency Disorders of the American Speech-Language-Hearing Association.

Janet A. Welsh, Ph.D., Project Associate, Fast Track Project, Pennsylvania State University, Sally Building, 2053 Cato Avenue, University Park, Pennsylvania 16801. Dr. Welsh has major interests in children's language and social development and the way in which these developmental domains interact and influence one another. Her current work includes the development of interventions that promote social skills acquisition and early literacy in young children.

Acknowledgments

THE SEED FOR THIS VOLUME was planted by Robin Chapman. She provided me with a first chance to think about relationships between speech and language in a chapter she gave me the opportunity to write for her book on processes of language acquisition and disorders. I also owe thanks to Lawrence D. Shriberg, for his indulgence of my early attempts to connect the two in clinical practice and for his continuing encouragement to integrate their disparate literatures. I am deeply grateful to the contributors to this volume, who worked with short deadlines and graciously endeavored to shape their thinking about the issues they addressed to the theme I had identified. My colleagues at Portland State University—Candace Gordon, Mary Gordon-Brannan, Steve Kosokoff, Joan McMahon, and Ellen Reuler—did everything possible to be helpful in allowing me to complete this project in the midst of a busy schedule of teaching and administrative duties. Finally, I want to express my appreciation to Melissa A. Behm, Elaine Niefeld, and everyone at Paul H. Brookes Publishing Co. for their patience, encouragement, and support throughout the book's preparation.

To the memory of my beloved husband, Charles Isenberg, whose gentle soul and generous spirit brought him to know, so much better than I, that

> *The race is not to the swift, . . .*
> *nor the battle to the strong . . .;*
> *but time and chance happeneth to them all.*

(Ecclesiastes 9:11–12)

The light of his mind still shines in my heart, as it does in the hearts of all who knew him.

Exploring the
Speech–Language Connection

1

Vocal Precursors to Linguistic Communication

How Babbling Is Connected to Meaningful Speech

D. Kimbrough Oller, Sharyse L. Levine,
Alan B. Cobo-Lewis, Rebecca E. Eilers,
and Barbara Zurer Pearson

W ITHOUT ANY OBVIOUS INSTRUCTION, we know certain things about how to communicate with infants, and they likewise with us. They look at us, and we look back, smiling and talking in tones of voice we do not use, for example, with people who sit next to us on airplanes (Fernald et al., 1989; Papoušek, Papoušek, & Symmes, 1991). When infants cry, we react, assuming that they may be in discomfort or may be hungry (Lester et al., 1994). When they cough or sputter, we pick them up and pat their backs, assuming that they may be in respiratory distress. When they make what have been called comfort sounds, even in the first days of life (Stark, 1980), we come close and look intently at them, smiling, talking to them, perhaps imitating the sounds of infancy, perhaps producing full sentences (Beebe, Stern, & Jaffe, 1979; Kaye & Fogel, 1980; Stern, Jaffe, Beebe, & Bennett, 1975; Vietze, Abernathy, Ashe, & Faulstich, 1978), even though the infants surely do not understand the words or syntax of our utterances. However, the infants, when they engage in these interchanges, seem to understand something else, something emotional, something about connections among people, perhaps something about their own identities as human beings.

We do not assume that when we speak to infants we are wasting our breath, nor do we generally spend much effort reflecting on the possibility that the sounds infants produce are disconnected from the capacity for linguistic communication. On the contrary, we quite naturally assume that the vocalizations of infants that sound like speech are precursors to speech and that the

This chapter was supported by Grant R01 DC00484 from the National Institute on Deafness and Other Communication Disorders and by philanthropic support from Austin Weeks.

actions of vocalization, gesture, and gaze that transpire between adults and infants are significant if not meaningful (Papoušek & Papoušek, 1979; Papoušek, Papoušek, & Bornstein, 1985). We intuitively launch ourselves into a mode of communication that seems appropriate, feels right, and gives us some fundamental pleasure.

Given these facts about the nature of communication between adults and infants, it is remarkable that for many years linguists and psychologists made the assumption that early vocalizations of infancy were unrelated to later speech. This was a major concern during the 1960s and early 1970s, when the field of child language studies began to expand, because there was little interest in infant vocalizations at that time. Jakobson (1941) had convinced most of those who might have otherwise been interested that there was no point in studying infant sounds: He said that babbling and speech were unrelated. In particular, he said that there was no phonetic relationship between babbling and speech and that babbling was a conglomeration of all the sounds of all the world's languages produced at random.

He could hardly have been more mistaken. In fact, babbling sounds are drawn from essentially the same very limited repertoire as the sounds of early speech (Cruttenden, 1970; Menyuk, 1968; Oller, Wieman, Doyle, & Ross, 1975; Rees, 1972). They include predominantly consonant–vowel (CV) syllables that appear to be composed of stop, nasal, and glide consonants (primarily labials and alveolars), and a small number of vowels. It is surely no accident that the very same repertoire is universal or nearly universal in the spoken languages of the world. Conspicuously absent from the babbling of the great majority of infants are the rare sounds of languages: the retroflex consonants, the ejectives, the aspirated fricatives, the implosives, and so forth.

The similarity of babbling and early speech sounds and their similarity with the universal sounds of natural languages seem to demand a conclusion: Babbling is part and parcel of the capacity for language (see Locke, 1983). Babbling is a manifestation of an emerging linguistic capacity in its form and in its use as a medium of transmission of emotional content between infants and other people. However, there is more to the connection between babbling and meaningful speech than the general conclusion that a connection exists, and there is much more that needs to be done empirically to make the understanding of the relationship between babbling and speech more theoretically and practically useful.

This chapter focuses on a key question about the details of the relationship between babbling and speech. At a general level, what we want to know is whether the act of babbling (i.e., of entering key stages of babbling, of practicing babbling) is a prerequisite to later meaningful speech (i.e., whether the occurrence of concrete acts of babbling encourages or accelerates the onset of meaningful speech). Empirically speaking, these are large questions, and answering them appears to require data sets that are both larger than the existing ones and, in some ways, more difficult to acquire.

We begin with a smaller aspect of the larger questions, one that is more manageable from the standpoint of data acquisition and more compatible with existing investigative efforts. We seek to assess the temporal relationship of the most salient early event in speech-like vocalizations, the onset of canonical babbling in infants we have followed longitudinally, and the occurrence of the first identifiable words in the speech of the same children. However, before this study is described, some background is necessary.

FRAMEWORK FOR DESCRIPTION

What is canonical babbling, and why is it so important? *Canonical babbling* has been defined in our work to include well-formed syllables, exemplified in common babbled utterances that might be transcribed as [ba], [iba], [baba], [dIdI], [ɛnɛ], or [wœwœ]. These well-formed or canonical syllables consist of at least one well-formed, vowel-like element and at least one well-formed, articulated consonant-like element, and the two must be connected by a quick transition (corresponding to a well-formed movement of the vocal tract) (Oller, 1986). The requirement of a well-formed transition rules out glottal consonants (e.g., [h], glottal stop) as the consonantal elements of canonical syllables because glottal syllables require no formant transition.

There are some additional definitional requirements, but it is not necessary to know them to acquire a sense of what is meant by the term *canonical babbling*. Human listeners recognize canonical syllables when they hear them because such syllables sound like speech. Vocalizations that are noncanonical sound less like speech. Coughing, sneezing, and crying, for example, are easily distinguished from speech because they lack well-formed consonants and vowels and include vocal qualities that differ from those of speech. Other examples include moaning, which does not typically include consonants, and squealing and growling, which involve vocal qualities that are identifiably nonspeech. Isolated vowels (e.g., [e], [o]) or sequences of vowels only (e.g., [auaiɛoɛ]) do have a speechlike character, but their lack of consonants makes them seem less speechlike than canonical syllables.

The intuitive nature of the recognition of canonical babbling has been verified in a variety of studies of concordance between judgments regarding the onset of the canonical stage by parents of infants in our longitudinal studies and judgments made by extensively trained laboratory staff. The studies showed that parents operating on little more than definitions recited to them by staff and a few examples presented on audiotape are capable of recognizing canonical babbling in their own infants (Eilers et al., 1993). The concordance between laboratory staff and parental judgments is so high that it justifies our relying heavily on parent report in some aspects of our studies where extensive laboratory observation is not practicable.

Study of Babbling

The presumed importance of canonical babbling is based in part on circumstantial evidence. Babbling and speech are phonetically similar. The similarity is so great that scientists are drawn to conclude that they must come from the same source. However, we cannot be absolutely sure, because we cannot observe the presumed source directly and thus can only infer its nature. So, does babbling cause speech? Is it one of several causes? Is babbling required for speech to occur? Or are babbling and speech just accidentally similar, having no fundamental connection?

Because we cannot be absolutely sure, we proceed on the basis of apparent probabilities. It seems increasingly unlikely that babbling and speech are *not* related, although there are still fundamental questions. Could it be that babbling is produced by the same mechanisms that will later constitute the foundations of speech, but that the actual performance of babbling, the act of practicing the pronunciation of canonical syllables, is unnecessary to the development of speech? If so, then one might expect to find some infants who never perform babbling, never enter a canonical stage, and yet proceed to speaking typically. The study of infants with tracheostomies who are incapable of vocalizing during the period when babbling typically occurs and who begin to talk fairly soon after decannulation (see, e.g., Locke & Pearson, 1990) provides useful evidence on this issue, although the evidence is only partial and leaves open several interpretive possibilities. Infants with tracheostomies are inhibited from vocalizing but are not prevented entirely from exercising the vocal tract (e.g., by opening and closing the mouth, by moving the tongue around) and in many cases are not prevented from producing voiced sounds; that is, they can sometimes cover the external tube with a finger, forcing air to pass through the vocal tract, and thus are sometimes able to vocalize. Furthermore, although infants with tracheostomies have been reported to begin speaking soon after decannulation, they typically show some lag before speaking meaningfully, and months or years later they may have delays in talking when compared with their age peers (Ross, 1983; Simon, Fowler, & Handler, 1983).

Thus, to find out how babbling influences early speech, additional evidence is needed. One kind of evidence that is important concerns the temporal relationship of onset for canonical babbling and speech in typically developing children, a relationship that has not been studied systematically.

The Question of Logical Limitations

Is it logically possible for a person to speak without first babbling? In our investigation, we presume the logical possibility that speech could occur in the absence of babbling. A child or other person could, in the abstract, produce no babbling at all before saying words composed of canonical syllables. Some meaningful speech acts are composed of noncanonical syllables. For example, children sometimes use onomatopoetic "words" such as a meowing sound (with no consonant at all) to mean *kitty* or a barking sound (again with no consonant) to mean *dog*. Quay (1993) reported that an early first word for one individual she studied was pronounced "mm" and meant, loosely, *animal*. In adults or children, *yes* can be pronounced "mhm," and *uh-oh* is pronounced with no articulated consonants. Children can also *mispronounce* real words, leaving out the consonants. Thus, even though the great majority of real words are composed of canonical syllables, there are a number of ways that non-canonical pronunciations can be used as words, especially in the very early speech of children.

It would be difficult, if not impossible, to create a large vocabulary without consonants and consonant-to-vowel transitions, and presumably that is why languages are composed of canonical syllables and segmental units. However, when children begin speaking meaningfully, their vocabulary requirements are minimal. They may recognize only a few words, and their spoken vocabularies may begin with a single item that persists as the only identifiable meaningful word for months. Thus, from the standpoint of communication, children do not necessarily need canonical syllables at the very beginning of their speech development.

The question we evaluate in researching the temporal relationship of babbling and speech, therefore, does not have a logically predetermined answer. Infants *might* start speech communication before they start canonical babbling, although our reading of studies and our experience in longitudinal research suggests that this is very unlikely (e.g., Oller & Eilers, 1988; Velten, 1943; Vihman, Ferguson, & Elbert, 1986). Other than the study of infants with tracheostomies, the literature provides no systematic effort to determine whether some infants may start speaking before producing canonical babbling, and it provides no quantitative information on the length of the typical time lags between onset of canonical babbling and first words.

METHODS

This section focuses on speech development research in the laboratories at the University of Miami, which is based primarily on longitudinal studies of both typical infants and those with linguistic disabilities. It describes the methods and procedures used in this research.

Subjects

For the purposes of this chapter, the focus is on infants in four subgroups: 15 full-term infants from homes of middle socioeconomic status (SES), 12 full-term infants from homes of low SES, 8 preterm infants from homes of middle SES, and 7 preterm infants from homes of low SES. For all of these infants, a carefully verified date for the onset of canonical babbling was obtained. Also obtained was the date on which each of the children reached a vocabulary of five words and, for most of the children (13 full-term middle SES, 5 full-term low SES, 8 preterm middle SES, and 7 preterm low SES), the date on which the children began to use a single meaningful word. At 24 months of age, a mean length of utterance (MLU) for all of the full-term infants and for most of the preterm infants (at corrected age, six preterm middle SES and six preterm low SES) was also obtained. These data represent the primary evidentiary focus in this chapter. The larger groups from which these infants were drawn have been described in Eilers et al. (1993). For the purposes of this chapter, we selected all of the infants for whom we obtained data on the onset of canonical babbling, the first word, fifth word, and MLU.

The subjects in all of the groups were drawn from the Dade County, Florida, community through mail solicitation. Parents were informed that, if they wished to participate in the longitudinal research, they would be required to bring their infant to the laboratory at the university at least once monthly through the first year of life and once every 2 months for the second year. During the visits, tape recordings would be made of the infants vocalizing and interacting with both parents and laboratory staff. In addition, parents would keep a diary of developmental progress of the infants to be reviewed and updated at each laboratory session with the assistance of laboratory staff. Questionnaires would be administered during each session to ensure that parents kept their diaries current and to obtain additional information.

The assessment of SES was based on a combination of questionnaire items drawn from Hollingshead (1978) and Nam and Powers (1983). In general, parents of the middle SES infants were white-collar workers with at least some college education, and the families included two parents living at home. Parents of low SES infants were blue-collar workers with little or no college education, and family stability was typically lower than that of middle SES families. The low SES families were from Categories 3 and 4 in the five-level system of Hollingshead (for more details, see Eilers et al., 1993). The low SES families were not wealthy; but they were also not illiterate, unemployed, or on welfare. The families from the middle SES category were all designated as being of higher SES than the low SES families. Most were from Category 2 in the system. Thus, the distinction between middle and low SES in this study is not the maximum distinction that could be obtained. In an attempt to evaluate groups in which the distinction between SES groups was greater, Oller, Eilers, Basinger, Steffens, and Urbano (1995) recruited a group of infants from the fifth (lowest) category of Hollingshead; however, there were major difficulties with subject attrition and reliability during this semilongitudinal study. Useful data were obtained while the infants were in the laboratory, but it was not possible to obtain an adequate body of reliable data on the onset of canonical babbling or first words in infants from Category 5 because of the very wide sampling interval used to maintain the participation of families. The problem of obtaining reliable data on onset of babbling and speech in very low SES families was due *not* to the inability of the parents to recognize or report their infants' behavior but rather to our inability to maintain regular contact with the families.

The distinction between full-term and preterm infants in this study also was not the maximum that could be used, but in this case the reason was not based on inability to obtain data from infants in more widely discrepant groups. Rather, the reason was based on our interest in evaluating infants of differing gestational ages without confounding that factor with differences in general health or traumatic history. We sought healthy preterm infants, avoiding recruitment of infants with known disabilities. Consequently, we enrolled infants only if they had had uneventful perinatal histories, with the exception of prematurity (including Apgar scores of 8 or greater). Birth weights for the preterm infants were 1,400–2,100 grams (mean = 1,932), and gestational ages at birth averaged 32.8 weeks, with no preterm infant having a gestational age greater than 36 weeks. Mean birth weight for the full-term infants was 3,543 grams. All infants had periodic hearing evaluations using visual reinforcement audiometry during the second half of their first year of life. No sensorineural hearing impairments were detected. When conductive losses were detected, infants were referred immediately for further evaluation and treatment.

Procedures to Determine Onset of Canonical Babbling

The study relied heavily on parent report in determining when infant vocal patterns changed in important ways. This reliance appears to have been well justified based on independent empirical evidence. A background on the nature of early vocalizations may help explain both the process of determination of age of onset and its justification.

From the first month of life, infants produce vocalizations. Many of these are vegetative in origin (e.g., burps, coughs, sneezes, hiccups), and others have specific signaling value even though they are produced without apparent intent on the part of infants. For instance, crying in particular appears to be produced by infants reflexively in response to pain, startle, or hunger (Lester et al., 1994). Crying in the first days of life appears to have only the most distant relationship with speech, partly because it includes special sound qualities that differ from those of speech and partly because even if crying indicates an infant's state, it does not appear to be produced voluntarily (at least not during the first weeks of life). Sounds that appear to be more related to an emerging speech capacity begin to occur soon after birth, including a variety of precursors to canonical babbling that develop during the first months of life. Vocalizing during this period appears to be exploratory in nature (Zlatin, 1975), and although infants do not appear to have control of canonical babbling (i.e., they do not produce it repetitively), occasional canonical syllables do occur, even in the first 3 months of life. These occurrences of isolated canonical syllables are apparently the accidental result of exploratory vocalization.

When the canonical stage begins (usually between 5 and 8 months of age), there is a discernible change in production of speechlike sounds. Parents notice that the infant seems to be producing wordlike utterances of one syllable or more with the intention to do so (Oller, 1980; Papoušek, 1992). One manifestation of control is repetitive production, typically seen in reduplicated sequences of well-formed syllables, such as [bababa]. The key point is that parents as well as other people notice this change in the infant without any instruction. In our studies, we present the term *canonical syllable* to parents and provide them with examples from real infants on tape recordings. We contrast canonical syllables with precanonical utterances such as quasivowels, isolated full vowels, and marginal babbles (which have overly slow transitions from consonant-like to vowel-like elements).

It has become increasingly clear that adults have a natural, biologically determined capability to recognize speech and speechlike utterances. Three facts support this presumption: 1) Humans of speaking age are able to recognize speech even when it is produced in languages that they have never heard before (e.g., they do not confuse foreign languages with coughing, sneezing, moaning, or some other kind of vocalization), and, consequently, they must be able to recognize speechlike quality in vocalizations; 2) if humans could not recognize the speechlike utterances of their infants, they could not make stage-appropriate adjustments in how they speak to the infants to encourage communicative growth; and 3) parents do appear to make such adjustments (i.e., by attempting to attribute meaning to the infant's canonical utterances) around the time that infants begin canonical babbling (Papoušek, 1992). Furthermore, it is important to reemphasize that parents' observations regarding canonical babbling in their infants are highly concordant with observations of trained laboratory staff.

The determination of onset of canonical babbling in our research with the infants in the longitudinal study involved two parts. First, parents (who had all been instructed on what canonical babbling is) reported by telephone that their infants had entered the canonical stage on the day on which they believed the stage had begun. Second, laboratory staff scheduled five appointments to see the infants as soon after the telephone report as possible. The appointments were ideally to occur on the 5 consecutive days immediately following the call, but in practice the five appointments were spread over a period as long as 2 weeks. During these laboratory sessions, the laboratory staff verified that the infants were indeed in the canonical stage. After verification, dates for onset of canonical babbling were assumed to be the dates provided by the parents.

Of the families in this study, there were only two cases (reported in Eilers et al., 1993) for which the date of the first parent report of canonical babbling had to be revised, and both of these cases were anomalous: The infant had produced a single-day "blip" of canonical babbling, at which point the parent had called and after which the infant had stopped babbling as noted by the parents *before* the first laboratory appointment, wherein laboratory staff verified that the infant was not yet in the canonical stage. Later telephone reports of stable onsets for canonical babbling and subsequent 5-day verifications were required in those two cases. Thus, the only cases of discordance between laboratory and parent observations appeared to be based on real vacillation on the part of the infants, not on the failure of accurate observation by the parents. Consequently, to our knowledge, all of the parents in the study were correct in their observations of onset of canonical babbling.

Because parents were able to make reliable judgments, it was possible for us to obtain data on onset of canonical babbling that were of much higher temporal resolution than would have been possible otherwise. Sampling at monthly intervals leaves room for error on the order of weeks in determination of onset. Lynch, Oller, Steffens, Levine, and Basinger (1995), based on work with typical infants and those with Down syndrome, found that reliance entirely on a criterion level of quantitative performance of canonical babbling from infants in the laboratory (specifically, a $\geq .15$ canonical-babbling ratio) at monthly sessions of 20–30 minutes duration entailed obtaining an onset of canonical babbling that was almost 2 months *later* than that obtained based on the combination of parent report and laboratory verification. This discrepancy of assigned onset dates based on different methods calls for an explanation.

Evaluations of infant quantitative performance in the laboratory show tremendous session-to-session variability within infants (see Oller, Eilers, Steffens, Lynch, & Urbano, 1994; Steffens, Oller, Lynch, & Urbano, 1992). This is not surprising, because infant state and interests were extremely varied from day to day. Furthermore, the samples obtained on audiotape in the laboratory were based on a very narrow window of observation, typically a 20- to 30-minute session of recording. The samples on which parents based their judgments, in contrast, were from various points of every day, a procedure that provides a broad window of observation.

Samples of infant sounds used as a basis for judgment of vocal stages by laboratory staff were also typically larger than those available on audiotape. At each appointment, laboratory personnel met parents and infants in a reception area; exchanged greetings and information about how the day's session would be conducted; and took the family to the laboratory, where there was often a waiting period while another infant's recording session was completed. There were additional periods of conversation with parents and interaction with infants after recording sessions were completed. During these times, often 20 minutes or more in length, laboratory staff had the opportunity to observe the infant vocalizing. Parents often would bring audiotape recordings that had been made at home (with dates and times of day) to illustrate infant performance for staff. There were even notable occasions on which parents would call from home to say the infant was producing canonical syllables and would have the laboratory staff listen to the infant's sounds over the telephone. Considering all of these opportunities to observe infant vocal performance, staff judgments about vocal stage of infants were typically based on much more than laboratory-recorded samples.

Because there was often clear evidence based on the many opportunities of observation to confirm that infants were in the canonical stage well before they produced criterion-level samples in the laboratory sessions, the dates obtained in the laboratory quantitative evaluations by Lynch et al. (1995) provide overestimates of actual onset of canonical babbling. For our study, reliable, high-resolution dates of onset were necessary; consequently, the combination of parent report and laboratory verification was deemed the most appropriate and practical approach.

Procedures for Establishing Date of Onset of First Words

At the beginning of meaningful speech, parents and infants negotiate the nature of communication units. Because infants produce a variety of sounds in the course of a day, some that may be words and some babbling (Braunwald, 1978), the judgment of what is a word is an active task for the caregiver. This is not a short-lived problem, as babbling persists for months after the onset of meaningful speech (Elbers, 1982; Vihman & Miller, 1988). In our study, babbling was present in the majority of the samples from the children, even at 24 months of age.

Parents were instructed to provide diary information and dates of the infant's first words, with indications of the very first usages that they noticed. They were asked to consider all cases in which the infant used a sound consistently and spontaneously, not merely imitatively, in relation to particular objects or situations. Thus, the infant's consistent pronunciations were treated as words if they were based on adult pronunciations of real English words or if they were phonetically consistent forms that were made up and utilized as parents and infants negotiated their communicative units and were used with consistent meaning or illocutionary force (Dore, Franklin, Miller, & Ramer, 1976).

In addition to the diary information, parents in many cases also provided data on their infant's word comprehension and usage by filling out the MacArthur Communicative Development Inventories (CDI) for Infants (Fenson et al., 1993) on an approximately bimonthly basis when the infants were between 8 and 16 months of age. The CDI was used to monitor the infants' levels of receptive vocabulary in the early months and later their productive vocabulary as well. After 16 months of age, the CDI for Toddlers was administered, providing a basis for evaluating newly acquired, spontaneously produced (not imitated) words. However, the CDI data were not obtained for all of the infants or for many of the bimonthly intervals, because the evaluation did not become available until the longitudinal study was well under way. Consequently, for this study's purposes, the CDI data were not available in many cases. Those data that were available were used only to help enhance the diary information regarding word usage provided by parents and confirmed in the laboratory. In general, parents filled out the questionnaires at home; but the questionnaires were discussed at each laboratory visit with staff, who made a concerted effort to ensure careful and consistent responses by the parents.

The occurrence of the first word, as reported by parents, was documented and verified in the laboratory at scheduled visits and, when possible, was reevaluated during CDI discussions. Staff questioned the parents regarding the consistency and specificity of the sound–meaning pairing in the infant's usage and periodically reminded parents that, by themselves, imitative productions of sounds that might be merely babbling were not to be considered words. For an utterance to be counted as a word, it was required that the item be produced by the infant in the laboratory during one of the recording sessions monitored by laboratory personnel during the 2–3 months after the parents first noted the occurrence of the word at home. Assuming that the infant produced the word attributed to him or her by the parent in the laboratory, and assuming that its usage fit the criteria previously indicated, the age at which the infant began using this word according to the parents was recorded in the data files as the date of the child's first word spoken. A parallel evaluation procedure was used to determine the age at which infants had reached five words, and, again, assuming that all of the criteria were met, the parents' designated date was used as the date on which the infant reached five words.

Mean Length of Utterance

To provide a more general assessment of language skills in the children, MLU was also assessed at 24 months of age (plus or minus 1 month). The language sample was obtained as part of a broader evaluation, the Sequenced Inventory of Communicative Development (Hedrick, Prather, & Tobin, 1984), according to procedures suggested by Miller (1981), which were an adaptation of procedures recommended by Brown (1973). We sought to record at least 50 utterances during the procedure, and we succeeded in the majority of cases. Four of the children in the study did not have MLU values available for the 24-month age level; thus, their data were not included in the present report.

RESULTS

This section describes the results of the study whose methods were previously discussed. These results include the connection between canonical babbling and talking and the possible effects of SES.

The Lag Between Canonical Babbling and Talking

The 42 children in the study began canonical babbling at (corrected) ages ranging from 17.6 to 36.8 weeks (mean = 26.4, standard deviation [SD] = 4.69).

Their first words appeared at ages ranging from 42.6 to 71.2 weeks (mean = 54.4, SD = 6.7), and their fifth words appeared from ages 45.0 to 80.8 weeks (mean = 62.0, SD = 7.3). All of the children in all of the groups began the canonical babbling stage many weeks before they began to speak meaningfully. Figure 1 shows the ages of onset for canonical babbling and for the first word for each of the children for whom both data points were obtained. The shortest lag among these 33 infants was 8.1 weeks, and the longest was 46.6 weeks (mean = 27.9, SD = 7.5).

Data on the fifth word were somewhat more plentiful, especially in the full-term low SES group. Figure 2 shows the ages of onset for canonical babbling relative to the fifth word of meaningful speech for the 42 children for whom both data points were obtained. The shortest lag was 18.1 weeks, and the longest was 56.2 weeks (mean = 35.6, SD = 8.7).

The data indicate that in these infants talking always began substantially after canonical babbling had been established. However, despite having gone through the canonical stage of babbling and consequently having the capacity to produce canonical syllables for many weeks, several of the children did show first words of noncanonical form, for example, the word *hi* pronounced either with a vowel alone or with the noncanonical consonant [h], which does not include supraglottal articulation as required by the definition of canonical syllables. Other early noncanonical words included, for example, onomatopoetic usages.

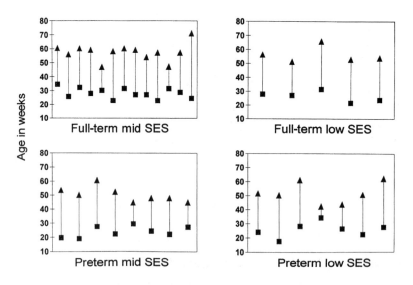

Figure 1.   Canonical babbling (CB) onset versus first-word onset. Each child is represented by a square (representing age of onset of CB) connected to a triangle (representing age of onset of the first word).

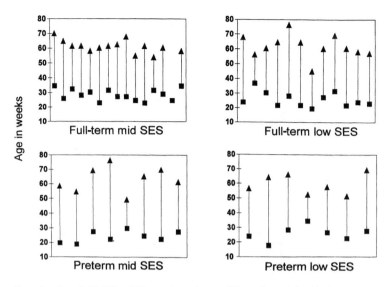

Figure 2. Canonical babbling (CB) onset (square) versus fifth-word onset (triangle).

Correlation of Canonical Babbling Onset with First Words and MLU

Data presented in Figure 3 indicate that age of canonical babbling onset did not strongly predict the age at which children began to use either their first word or their first five words. Neither of the low correlations (.12 and −.005) was statistically reliable, suggesting a notable independence of age of canonical babbling and age of early word use. In contrast, the age of first word usage did correlate reliably ($p < .00015$) with the age at which five words were attained ($r = .61$). Children who reached the stage of a first word relatively early also reached a fifth word relatively early.

Data on MLU at 24 months of age for the 39 children who provided such data showed a range from 1.00 to 3.74 morphemes per utterance (mean = 1.58, $SD = .52$). These MLU values were not strongly predicted by any of the other measures. Age of onset of canonical babbling, first word, and fifth word all showed low correlations with MLU (.13, −.08, and −.17, respectively), correlations that were not statistically reliable.

Effects of Prematurity and SES

Although our effort was primarily focused on the general relationship of canonical babbling and early speech, possible effects of prematurity or SES have also been considered. The original design was intended to address the possible effects of biological (preterm) and social (low SES) risk in the development of speech and its precursors. Figure 4 provides a summary of the data

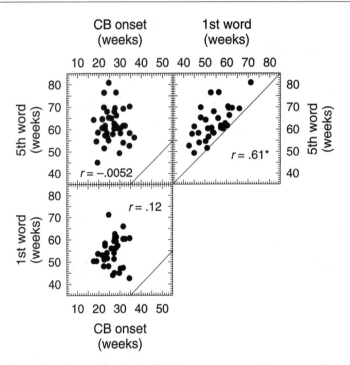

Figure 3.   Correlations of canonical babbling (CB), first-word, and fifth-word onsets.
(*, statistically reliable.)

and indicates that preterm infants (at corrected ages) did *not* show important delays in any of the possible comparisons. On the contrary, in cases in which notable advantages occurred, they favored the preterm infants. For example, as has been reported based on a broader sample from the same longitudinal study (Eilers et al., 1993), preterm infants began canonical babbling a little earlier (by 2.4 weeks in these particular infants) than their full-term peers (though this tendency was seen only in the middle SES group). Onset of the first word was also proved to occur earlier in the corrected-age preterm infants than in their full-term peers (at 51.1–57.2 weeks), a difference that was statistically reliable ($t = 2.84, p < .01$). By the onset of five words, the difference between the preterm and full-term groups had diminished and was no longer statistically reliable (ages 61.54–62.24 weeks; $t = .28$), although the trend toward an advantage for the preterm infants remained notable in the low SES group.

Additional surprises were found in the analysis of presumed social risk. Low SES infants did not show later onset of canonical babbling than their middle SES counterparts but showed a 1.2-week advantage (not statistically reliable). In addition, low SES infants did not trail their middle SES counterparts in onset of the first word or in the onset of five words but showed slightly earlier ages of onset for meaningful words (by ages 53.6–54.8 weeks for the first

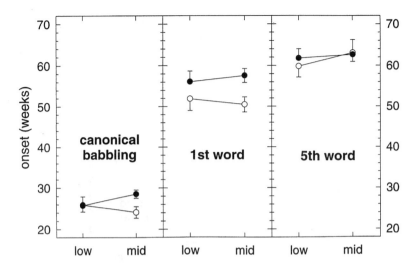

Figure 4.   Canonical babbling (CB), first-word, and fifth-word onset as a function of SES and prematurity. (●, full term; ○, preterm.)

word and by ages 61.0–62.8 weeks for the fifth word; both t's unreliable). Only in MLU did the middle SES infants show a reliable advantage ($t = 2.29$, $p < .03$) over their low-SES peers (means of 1.74 and 1.40 morphemes per utterance). The data, displayed in Figure 5, show that the full-term infants also had slightly, though not statistically reliable, higher MLUs than their preterm counterparts (1.63–1.48, respectively).

DISCUSSION

From a learning theory perspective, language acquisition clearly involves much more than merely learning to control the vocal musculature; from a maturational perspective, language acquisition clearly involves more than the mere unfolding of the phonological capacity (Bates, Benigni, Bretherton, Camaioni, & Volterra, 1979; Bruner & Sherwood, 1983; Greenfield & Smith, 1976; Mundy, Kasari, & Sigman, 1992; Mundy, Sigman, & Kasari, 1990; Tomasello & Farrar, 1986). From either perspective, there is much about language learning that is not phonological. Such areas as recognition of objects and events, categorization of objects and events into classes, and establishment of joint reference to classes all involve quite different types of cognition from those required for vocalizing in a speechlike manner. However, it is clear that no person can learn to speak a language effectively without a phonological system and, in particular, without control over canonical syllables. Well-formed syllabic units are an essential aspect of the infrastructure of phonology. Considering these facts, it may seem predictable that all 42 infants in the study

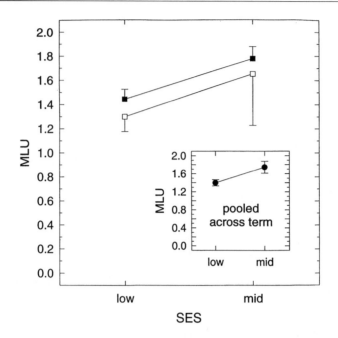

Figure 5. MLU (mean length of utterance at age 2) as a function of socioeconomic status (SES) and prematurity. (■, full term; □, preterm.)

discussed in this chapter began canonical babbling many weeks before they began to talk.

The shortest lag found between canonical babbling and first words in this study occurred in an infant who was hospitalized during the period when most of the infants entered the canonical stage. Shortly after the illness, she began babbling; and 8.1 weeks after that, her first word appeared. In the context of her illness and hospitalization, the relatively short lag (87% shorter than the next shortest lag found in the study) suggests that this particular child may have presented a pattern influenced by less-than-optimal general health. The longest lag found in the study was more than 10 months, a duration that does not appear to be particularly remarkable, given that almost half of the children (16 of 33) for whom first-word data were obtained showed lags of more than 7 months.

These data might suggest that canonical babbling is an empirical prerequisite for any word usage. Such a conclusion would be overturned by the discovery of a single child who might speak before the stage of canonical babbling. This is not an impossibility, because, as noted previously in this chapter, it is possible to produce *some* words that are composed of noncanonical syllables, and some early words of children are indeed noncanonical. It therefore remains logically possible for *some* child to begin speaking before canonical babbling, and, as a result, the case for babbling as a prerequisite to speech cannot be made airtight by any amount of empirical evidence.

The age of onset of canonical babbling does not appear to predict either the age of first word or the age of first five words strongly. The correlation is very low and not statistically reliable, accounting for a miniscule proportion ($<$ 2% for first words, $<$ 1% for first five words) of variance. Confidence interval evaluation indicates that the first five words' correlation, in particular, is so miniscule that, even if the study were rerun with new groups of similar size, it would be highly unlikely ($p < .05$) that the obtained correlation would account for as much as 10% of variance.

The very low predicted variance may be a result of the onset of canonical babbling being only one of many factors that influence the onset of speaking. For a person to talk, he or she must understand much about the world and about social relationships; be able to pronounce syllables and to associate particular syllables with particular situations, objects, or events; and be able to retrieve those associations at appropriate times. Because the ability to produce well-formed syllables is just one of these many capabilities, it may be that it simply does not play a particularly large role in the total picture of learning to produce first words and thus does not influence variance prediction significantly.

Other studies have reported somewhat more encouraging data on relationships between early vocal capabilities and early talking (see Bates et al., 1979; Menyuk, Liebergott, & Schultz, 1986; Murphy, Menyuk, Liebergott, & Schultz, 1983). Methodological differences between those studies and the one discussed in this chapter make it difficult to interpret the differing outcomes; in particular, none of the studies cited used the infraphonological framework (consequently, the onset of canonical babbling, as defined in this chapter, was not a factor in any of them), and none sought to address the issue of early meaningful speech. However, it is important to note that correlations between vocal development and speech development might prove to be much higher if they were based on a different approach. One possibility suggested by P. Mundy (personal communication, April 1996) is that predictability of first words might be highly related to onset of consolidated control over canonical babbling rather than to initial onset. This suggestion is based on the idea that babbling may begin with some degree of instability and that within a few weeks it might stabilize in a measurable way, just as walking tends to develop through an early stage of instability and a later stage of consolidated control. It remains to be seen whether consolidated control can be reliably measured (perhaps by considering consistency of production of canonical syllables or variety of types of such syllables produced), but the philosophical issue remains worthy of consideration, as we may have selected an infelicitous point in the development of babbling for purposes of predicting later speech development.

The data from the present study offer information that needs to be explained, but they do not stringently limit the possible interpretations of the relationship of babbling and speech. The role of practice in babbling is hard to assess, given present evidence; that is, there is very little information about how much babbling infants do in a variety of settings, and there are no existing studies on the relationship of the amount of babbling practice that occurs and either the quantity or quality of early speech in individual children. Yet infants certainly seem to be exercising when they babble, and it is hard to imagine that such exercise is entirely wasteful.

Biological Nature of Babbling

Babbling may occur in part because people are constituted to perform the parts of the linguistic enterprise on a schedule that is suited to acquisition, but that schedule may also have idiosyncrasies resulting more from evolutionary history than from ontogenetic practicality. The stages of infant vocal development may to some extent recapitulate stages of hominid development toward a full linguistic capability. Our very distant ancestors may have acquired the ability to produce syllables first, perhaps in the service of pragmatically limited, prereferential signals, and the ability to use syllables in the service of pragmatically diverse, referential linguistic functions at a later point in evolution. The importance of syllables and the need in referential communication to be able to produce any particular type of syllable at will (and under extremely diverse circumstances, as in cases where syllabic words are used to refer to events that are not in the "here and now") may have encouraged the diversification of uses and circumstances of syllable production, and, in that process, early hominids may have acquired a tendency to produce syllables for pure pleasure or interest (with no signal value or meaning); in short, they may have acquired a tendency to babble. If so, the modern human infant may carry a tendency to babble that reflects our early history of producing syllables in the absence of linguistic meaning. That tendency to babble may have been solidified as a biologically canalized system (a system difficult to deflect from its preordained course) as syllables came to play an increasingly important role in survival.

That canonical babbling is a canalized ability is consonant with the many results that have shown robustness of the babbling tendency in the face of presumed obstacles: Multiple languages in the home, prematurity, low SES— even very low SES—or even Down syndrome do not seem to produce long delays in the onset of canonical babbling (Eilers et al., 1993; Lynch et al., 1995; Oller, 1995; Oller et al., 1995). It may not be absolutely necessary that people babble; but almost all do it, and apparently on schedule, unless there is a severe illness that disrupts the schedule.

The biological nature of babbling can be placed in further perspective by considering its relationship with other motoric developments. In Eilers et al.

(1993), it was found that a series of motoric milestones (i.e., canonical babbling, rhythmic hand banging, sitting unsupported, crawling on hands and knees) tended to occur within a few months of each other, and all had mean ages of onset at about 6 months. Rhythmic hand banging especially was found to be specifically related to canonical babbling (which might also be viewed as a repetitive rhythmic activity, at least insofar as reduplicated canonical sequences are concerned). Both canonical babbling and rhythmic hand banging showed accelerated development in preterm infants, although sitting and crawling did not, and both canonical babbling and rhythmic hand banging showed relatively mild delays of a few weeks in infants with Down syndrome, although sitting and crawling were delayed by many months in infants with Down syndrome compared with typically developing infants. There also is clear evidence of delays in a variety of motoric areas, including canonical babbling, in infants born with cerebral palsy (Eilers, Neal, & Oller, 1996).

To say that the development of a capability is biologically significant and canalized is not to say that experience plays no role in its appearance. It is known that babbling *is* affected by experience because deaf infants are delayed (often by many months) in onset of babbling (Oller & Eilers, 1988), and preterm infants (at gestationally corrected ages) tend to begin babbling a few weeks earlier than their full-term counterparts (Eilers et al., 1993). These facts suggest that some critical amount of experience is needed to trigger the onset of the very robust phenomenon of canonical babbling. The experience appears to be accumulated slowly in deaf children, and it appears to be accumulated early in the case of preterm infants compared with their full-term counterparts.

The Role of Experience

The role of experience in how much babbling is performed is also important to consider. Eilers et al. (1993) and Oller et al. (1995) found that the amount of babbling per unit time was less in low SES infants (or very low SES) than in middle SES infants. This finding may represent a precursor to the finding reported in the present study that MLU was greater in middle SES than in low SES infants at 24 months of age. The results in both cases suggest that there are fundamental structural properties of language development (e.g., the infraphonological form of syllables, the connection between words and meanings) that are relatively robust and canalized and that there are operational properties of language development (e.g., amount of use, practical application of capabilities) that may differ notably in children growing up in differing social circumstances. In other studies addressing language capabilities in young children, the practical knowledge of vocabulary and ability to use language effectively have been found in a number of ways to be subpar in low SES children (Harris, Barrett, Jones, & Brookes, 1988; Hart & Risley, 1981).

The results of the study presented in this chapter may also be taken to suggest that the onset of first words is canalized; every infant in the study began to talk by 15 months of age. At the same time, the development of words is clearly experience based in part; after all, the children in this study learned English and Spanish, not Farsi and Swahili. The study did not evaluate in detail the children's later development of syntactic capabilities; but it is clear that these too can be viewed as representing both a canalized human faculty, because most human children gain control of the syntax of their language over a relatively brief period of childhood, and as a phenomenon that is distinctly dependent on experience, because children learn different syntactic systems for different languages. For example, the children in the present study learning English or Spanish had to learn different syntactic patterns (word orders) to express noun–adjective relations in the two languages. Language is a phenomenon where all its fundamental aspects, including phonological production capabilities as manifest in babbling, lexical capabilities as manifest in early word use, and syntactic capabilities as manifest in early word combinations, are both canalized and learned. This paradox illustrates a key aspect of the task of research in child language acquisition: to differentiate the characteristics of development that resist deflection from their biologically preordained course and to determine what the critical experiences are that enable the natural, preordained development.

CONCLUSIONS

To summarize what is known about the relationship between babbling and language development, it would be appropriate to say that the ability to produce canonical syllables is a necessary but not a sufficient condition for the acquisition of elaborate spoken language abilities. Canonical babbling certainly occurs before the onset of speaking in most infants, but it is not clear that it has to occur before the onset of speaking in all infants. Although canonical babbling is biologically significant and to some extent biologically predetermined, experience with the sounds of the voice is necessary to instigate canonical babbling. This required experience appears to be obtainable in a variety of circumstances, and SES appears to play no role in the onset of canonical babbling. Little is known directly about how important it may be to practice babbling, but indirectly it is clear that the amount of babbling that infants do and the subsequent length of their word combinations (at 2 years of age) are affected by SES. That SES is related to effectiveness of language use later in life provides a broad hint that early practice with babbling and early application of word and primitive syntactic knowledge in the speech of 2-year-olds may lay foundations that are of great practical import.

The results of the study presented in this chapter add only a small piece to a puzzle. There now exists quantified information on the lag between the onset of canonical babbling and speech. However, there are many questions that remain about the relationship. No single study will answer such questions, but converging evidence from a variety of studies is gradually helping to establish an understanding of the ways that early vocalizations of infants function as precursors to the linguistic capacity.

REFERENCES

Bates, E., Benigni, L., Bretherton, I., Camaioni, L., & Volterra, V. (1979). *The emergence of symbols: Cognition and communication in infancy.* New York: Academic Press.

Beebe, B., Stern, D., & Jaffe, J. (1979). The kinetic rhythms of mother–infant interactions. In A.W. Siegman & S. Feldstein (Eds.), *Of speech and time* (pp. 23–34). Hillsdale, NJ: Lawrence Erlbaum Associates.

Braunwald, S.R. (1978). Context, word, and meaning: Toward a communicational analysis of lexical acquisition. In A. Lock (Ed.), *Action, gesture and symbol: The emergence of language* (pp. 485–527). New York: Academic Press.

Brown, R. (1973). *A first language.* Cambridge, MA: Harvard University Press.

Bruner, J., & Sherwood, V. (1983). Thought, language and interaction in infancy. In J. Call, R. Galenson, & L. Tyson (Eds.), *Frontiers of infant psychiatry* (pp. 38–55). New York: Basic Books.

Cruttenden, A. (1970). A phonetic study of babbling. *British Journal of Disorders of Communication, 5,* 110–118.

Dore, J., Franklin, M.B., Miller, R.T., & Ramer, A.L.H. (1976). Transitional phenomena in early language acquisition. *Journal of Child Language, 3,* 13–28.

Eilers, R.E., Neal, A.R., & Oller, D.K. (1996, April). *Late onset babbling as an early marker of abnormal development.* Paper presented at the International Conference on Infant Studies, Providence, RI.

Eilers, R.E., Oller, D.K., Levine, S., Basinger, D., Lynch, M.P., & Urbano, R. (1993). The role of prematurity and socioeconomic status in the onset of canonical babbling in infants. *Infant Behavioral Development, 16,* 297–315.

Elbers, L. (1982). Operating principles in repetitive babbling: A cognitive continuity approach. *Cognition, 12,* 45–63.

Fenson, L., Dale, P., Reznick, J.S., Thal, D., Bates, E., Hartung, J., Pethcik, S., & Reilly, J. (1993). *MacArthur Communicative Development Inventories (CDI).* San Diego: Singular Publishing Group.

Fernald, A., Taeschner, T., Dunn, J., Papoušek, M., Boysson-Bardies, B., & Fukui, I. (1989). A cross-language study of prosodic modifications in mothers' and fathers' speech to preverbal infants. *Journal of Child Language, 16,* 477–501.

Greenfield, P.M., & Smith, J.H. (1976). *The structure of communication in early language development.* New York: Academic Press.

Harris, M., Barrett, M., Jones, D., & Brookes, S. (1988). Linguistic input and early word meaning. *Journal of Child Language, 15,* 77–94.

Hart, B., & Risley, T.R. (1981). Grammatical and conceptual growth in the language of psychologically disadvantaged children: Assessment and intervention. In M.J. Begab, H. Garber, & H.C. Hayward (Eds.), *Psychosocial influences in retarded performance: Vol. 2. Strategies for improving competence* (pp. 181–198). Baltimore: University Park Press.

Hedrick, D.L., Prather, E.M., & Tobin, A.R. (1984). *Sequenced Inventory of Communication Development (SICD) Test manual.* Seattle: University of Washington Press.

Hollingshead, A.B. (1978). *Two-factor Index of Social Status.* Unpublished manuscript, Yale University, New Haven, CT.

Jakobson, R. (1941). *Kindersprache, Aphasie, und allgemeine Lautgesetze* [*Child language, aphasia, and phonological universals*]. Uppsala, Sweden: Almqvist and Wiksell.

Kaye, K., & Fogel, A. (1980). The temporal structure of face-to-face between mothers and infants. *Developmental Psychology, 16,* 454–464.

Lester, B.M., Boukydis, C.F.Z., Garcia-Coll, C.T., Peucker, M., McGrath, M.M., Vohr, B.R., Brem, S., & Oh, W. (1994). Developmental outcome as a function of the goodness of fit between the infant's cry characteristics and the mother's perception of her infant's cry. *Pediatrics, 95*(4), 516–521.

Locke, J.L. (1983). *Phonological acquisition and change.* New York: Academic Press.

Locke, J.L., & Pearson, D. (1990). Linguistic significance of babbling: Evidence from a tracheostomized infant. *Journal of Child Language, 17,* 1–16.

Lynch, M.P., Oller, D.K., Steffens, M.L., Levine, S.L., & Basinger, D.L. (1995). Development of speech-like vocalizations in infants with Down syndrome. *American Journal on Mental Retardation, 100*(1), 68–86.

Menyuk, P. (1968). The role of distinctive features in children's acquisition of phonology. *Journal of Speech and Hearing Research, 11,* 138–146.

Menyuk, P., Liebergott, J., & Schultz, M. (1986). Predicting phonological development. In B. Lindblom & R. Zetterstrom (Eds.), *Precursors of early speech* (pp. 79–93). New York: Stockton Press.

Miller, J. (1981). *Assessing language production in children: Experimental procedures.* Baltimore: University Park Press.

Mundy, P., Kasari, C., & Sigman, M. (1992). Joint attention, affective sharing, and intersubjectivity. *Infant Behavior Development, 15,* 377–381.

Mundy, P., Sigman, M., & Kasari, C. (1990). A longitudinal study of joint attention and language development in autistic children. *Journal of Autism and Developmental Disorders, 20,* 115–128.

Murphy, R., Menyuk, P., Liebergott, J., & Schultz, M. (1983, April). *Predicting the rate of lexical acquisition.* Paper presented at the Biennial Meeting of the Society for Research in Child Development, Detroit, MI.

Nam, C.V., & Powers, N.G. (1983). *Socioeconomic approach to status measurement.* Houston, TX: Cap & Gown Press.

Oller, D.K. (1980). The emergence of the sounds of speech in infancy. In G. Yeni-Komshian, J. Kavanagh, & C. Ferguson (Eds.), *Child phonology: Vol. 1. Production* (pp. 93–112). New York: Academic Press.

Oller, D.K. (1986). Metaphonology and infant vocalizations. In B. Lindblom & R. Zetterstrom (Eds.), *Precursors of early speech* (pp. 21–33). New York: Stockton Press.

Oller, D.K. (1995, February). *Early speech and word learning in bilingual and monolingual children.* Paper presented at the American Association for the Advancement of Science, Atlanta, GA.

Oller, D.K., & Eilers, R.E. (1988). The role of audition in infant babbling. *Child Development, 59,* 441–449.

Oller, D.K., Eilers, R.E., Basinger, D., Steffens, M.L., & Urbano, R. (1995). Extreme poverty and the development of precursors to the speech capacity. *First Language, 15,* 167–188.

Oller, D.K., Eilers, R.E., Steffens, M.L., Lynch, M.P., & Urbano, R. (1994). Speech-like vocalizations of infancy: An evaluation of potential risk factors. *Journal of Child Language, 21,* 33–58.

Oller, D.K., Wieman, L., Doyle, W., & Ross, C. (1975). Infant babbling and speech. *Journal of Child Language, 3,* 1–11.

Papoušek, H., & Papoušek, M. (1979). The infant's fundamental adaptive response system in social interaction. In E. Thoman (Ed.), *Origins of the infant's social responsiveness* (pp. 175–208). Hillsdale, NJ: Lawrence Erlbaum Associates.

Papoušek, M. (1992, May). *Melodic gestures in maternal speech to preverbal infants: Similarities and differences across species.* Paper presented at the Eighth International Conference on Infant Studies, Miami Beach, FL.

Papoušek, M., Papoušek, H., & Bornstein, M.H. (1985). The naturalistic vocal environment of young infants: On the significance of homogeneity and variability in parental speech. In T. Field & N. Fos (Eds.), *Social perception in infants* (pp. 219–297). Norwood, NJ: Ablex.

Papoušek, M., Papoušek, H., & Symmes, D. (1991). The meanings of melodies in motherese in tone and stress languages. *Infant Behavior Development, 14,* 414–440.

Quay, S. (1993). *Language choice in early bilingual development.* Unpublished doctoral dissertation, Cambridge University, England.

Rees, N. (1972). The role of babbling in the child's acquisition of language. *British Journal of Disorders of Communication, 7,* 17–23.

Ross, G.S. (1983). Language functioning and speech development of six children receiving tracheostomy in infancy. *Journal of Communication Disorders, 15,* 95–111.

Simon, B.M., Fowler, S.M., & Handler, S.D. (1983). Communication development in young children with long-term tracheostomies: A preliminary report. *International Journal of Pediatric Otorhinolaryngology, 6,* 37–50.

Stark, R.E. (1980). Stages of speech development in the first year of life. In G. Yeni-Komshian, J. Kavanagh, & C. Ferguson (Eds.), *Child phonology: Vol. 1. Production* (pp. 73–92). New York: Academic Press.

Steffens, M.L., Oller, D.K., Lynch, M.P., & Urbano, R. (1992). Vocal development in infants with Down syndrome and infants who are developing normally. *American Journal on Mental Retardation, 97,* 235–246.

Stern, D.N., Jaffe, J., Beebe, B., & Bennett, S.L. (1975). Vocalizing in unison and in alternation: Two modes of communication within the mother–infant dyad. In D. Aaronson & R. Rieber (Eds.), *Developmental psycholinguistics and communication disorders* (pp. 89–100). New York: New York Academy of Sciences.

Tomasello, M., & Farrar, J. (1986). Joint attention and early language. *Child Development, 57,* 1454–1463.

Velten, H.V. (1943). The growth of phonemic and lexical patterns in infant language. *Language, 19,* 281–292.

Vietze, P.M., Abernathy, S.R., Ashe, M.L., & Faulstich, G. (1978). Contingent interaction between mothers and their developmentally delayed infants. In G.P. Sackett (Ed.), *Observing behavior: Vol. I. Theory and applications in mental retardation* (pp. 115–132). Baltimore: University Park Press.

Vihman, M.M., Ferguson, C.A., & Elbert, M. (1986). Phonological development from babbling to speech: Common tendencies and individual differences. *Applied Psychology, 7,* 3–40.

Vihman, M.M., & Miller, R. (1988). Words and babble at the threshold of language. In N. Smith & J. Locke (Eds.), *The emergent lexicon* (pp. 151–183). New York: Academic Press.

Zlatin, M. (1975). *Preliminary descriptive model of infant vocalization during the first 24 weeks: Primitive syllabification and phonetic exploratory behavior* (Final Report, Project No 3-4014, NE-G-00-3-0077). Unpublished report, Purdue University, Department of Audiology and Speech Sciences, West Lafayette, IN.

2

Sounds and Words
in Early Language Acquisition
The Relationship Between Lexical
and Phonological Development

Carol Stoel-Gammon

W ORDS HAVE TWO ESSENTIAL COMPONENTS, sound and meaning; the link between the two is arbitrary, varying from one language to another. Thus, the
word for a small domesticated feline is *cat* in English, *gato* in Spanish, *neko* in
Japanese, and *paka* in Swahili. One of the major tasks facing children learning
to talk is figuring out the sound–meaning relationships of the words in their
ambient language. Most studies of lexical acquisition assume that the abstract,
cognitive demands of word meaning represent the foremost task in acquiring
a word and the physical aspects of articulating that word play a secondary role.
Research on speech and language development in young children, however,
raises questions about this view, suggesting that, at least in the early period of
word learning, factors associated with the production of speech may be as important as the cognitive factors.

To acquire a word, a child must become aware that a particular sequence
of sounds is linked to a particular meaning—for example, that the
consonant–vowel sequence [ʃu] refers to something that can be worn on the
foot. Production of the word *shoe* requires more than recognition of the
sound–meaning link involved; the child must also learn the articulatory movements needed to make the voiceless fricative [ʃ] (or something close to it)
followed by the vowel [u]. Accurate pronunciation of *shoe* is not easy, and
children's early attempts at producing it often sound more like [du] or [su]
than [ʃu]. In contrast, some words are pronounced relatively accurately from
their earliest appearance. The words *mommy* and *daddy* are good examples,

This chapter was supported in part by Grant R01-HD32065-NICHD from the National Institute of Child Health and Human Development.
Throughout this chapter, the consonant [h] is classified as a glide; classification as a fricative
would alter statements regarding the occurrence of fricative and glide manner classes.

even though production of these words involves coordination of various aspects of the vocal apparatus. The first syllable of *mommy*, for example, requires that the vocal cords be vibrating while the lips are closed and the velopharyngeal port is open for the [m], followed by closure of the velopharyngeal port and opening of the jaw for the vowel [a]. Pronunciation of the first syllable of *daddy*, in contrast, requires that the tongue apex be touching the alveolar ridge while the velopharyngeal port is closed; vocal fold vibration must occur during closure or begin immediately after release of closure and continue into the vowel as the tongue is pulled from the alveolar ridge. Despite these seemingly complex sequences of articulatory movements, 1-year-olds are capable of producing the syllables [ma] and [dæ] with apparent ease but struggle with the articulation of *shoe*.

Why might this happen? Learning to pronounce a word is facilitated (or hindered) by a number of perceptual, cognitive, and articulatory factors, including its semantic complexity, its social or emotional significance for the child, the number of times the child hears the word, and its articulatory complexity. Each of these factors contributes to the observed patterns of word learning. This chapter focuses on issues related to the last two variables, frequency of input and ease of articulation, by examining the relationship between early phonological and lexical acquisition. The first section summarizes research on the relationship between phonetic aspects of prelinguistic vocalizations and early meaningful speech. The second section discusses phonological aspects of children's first words, noting the presence of common tendencies as well as individual differences in children with typical and atypical language development. The third section examines phonological and lexical patterns beyond the first-word period, providing an in-depth analysis of the phonological characteristics of children's early vocabularies. Taken together, the research indicates that the relationship between phonological and lexical development changes over time, with phonology influencing lexical development in the earliest stages of learning to talk and the lexicon influencing phonological development later.

BABBLE AND ITS RELATIONSHIP TO SPEECH

Infants are exposed to two types of vocal input in the prelinguistic period: the speech of others and their own productions. Both are crucial for the acquisition of adult language. Adult input provides the basis for learning the sound–meaning associations that underlie word meaning. This aspect is important because children who cannot hear words of the ambient language do not learn to produce them. Hearing their own vocal output is also important for children's subsequent production of words. Children must recognize the links between their own oral-motor movements and the resulting acoustic signal. Thus, the 6-month-old who frequently produces [ba] becomes aware of the tie between the tactual and kinesthetic sensations associated with this syllable and the auditory signal that occurs. Once this step is accomplished, infants must learn that their production of [ba] resembles the adult words *ball, bottle,* and *Bob.* When these two types of learning have occurred, the prelinguistic form [ba] can serve as a basis for production of words from the target language.

Speech has a skill component, and, as with any skilled activity, practice increases the control and precision with which a movement is performed. Thus, the more often a baby produces the movements that shape the vocal tract to produce particular sounds and sound sequences, the more automatic those movements become and ultimately the easier it is to execute them in producing meaningful speech. In an investigation of the transition from babble to speech, Vihman (1992) identified a set of frequently occurring consonant–vowel (CV) syllables ("practiced" syllables) produced by each individual in the prelinguistic period and reported that, for most individuals, early words were "primarily drawn from the repertoire of practiced syllables" (p. 406) from their prespeech vocalizations. Given this finding, it could be predicted that infants who have a large stock of practiced syllables have an advantage in early word acquisition because they have a larger repertoire of phonetic forms to which meaning can be attached. However, some infants do not use their practiced syllables when acquiring a lexicon. For example, Vihman (1992) reported that individuals who evidenced slower vocabulary acquisition were those who failed to use their practiced syllables in meaningful speech production, and Stoel-Gammon (1989) reported that one of the two late talkers (i.e., children with a limited vocabulary at ages 21–24 months) she studied produced many CV syllables in his nonmeaningful productions but did not use these forms in his attempts at real words.

There is a good deal of overlap in the phonetic form of babble and speech. The canonical CV syllable occurs frequently in both. Furthermore, the consonants that occur most often in canonical babbling—stops, nasals, and glides—are those that typically appear in early word productions; consonant classes that are infrequent in babble—liquids, fricatives, and affricates—are precisely those that appear later in meaningful speech (Robb & Bleile, 1994; Stoel-Gammon, 1985). A child's first words co-occur with the production of CV babbles, and meaningful and nonmeaningful vocalizations coexist for nearly a year. Robb, Bauer, and Tyler (1994) reported that when children have a productive vocabulary of about 10 words, their vocal output consists of almost equal proportions of meaningful and nonmeaningful utterances with minimal distinction in phonetic form. By the time the lexicon has increased to about 50 words, meaningful utterances occur approximately three times more frequently than nonmeaningful utterances.

FIRST WORDS AND SOUNDS

The first word generally appears around the child's first birthday, and the productive lexicon grows to 50–60 words by 18 months, rising to 250–350 words by 24 months. As noted previously, word production requires an awareness of the link between a particular sequence of speech sounds and a particular meaning and the knowledge of the articulatory movements needed to articulate the sequence of sounds that resembles the target. For some words, the sequence of speech sounds may already be present in the child's babble, as in the case of the nonmeaningful [ba] used subsequently for the word *ball*. In contrast, acquisition of a word like *shoe* involves learning not only the link between sound and meaning but also a set of unfamiliar articulatory movements. The disparity in the amount of learning involved in acquiring the words *ball* and *shoe* leads to the prediction that, all other things being equal, target words with phonetic properties that mirror a child's prelinguistic vocalizations will be acquired earlier than words with features (e.g., speech sounds, syllable shapes) that are not present in the prespeech repertoire.

Support for this prediction comes from longitudinal investigations of the transition from babble to speech showing that phonetic features of an infant's prelinguistic vocalizations (i.e., individual differences in place and manner of articulation of consonants, syllable shape, and vocalization length) are often carried forward to the first words (Stoel-Gammon & Cooper, 1984; Vihman, Ferguson, & Elbert, 1987). Further evidence comes from an experimental study of the acquisition of nonsense words. Messick (1984) examined children's phonetic inventories in babbling and then taught the children nonsense words that were either phonetically similar or dissimilar to their own babbled forms. After 10 sessions of exposure to the two types of words, the children produced a significantly greater number of words that were phonetically similar to their babble, although they showed no differences in their ability to understand the two types of nonsense forms.

In examining the babble–speech link in a larger time frame, we find a growing body of evidence linking prelinguistic vocal development with general speech and language skills throughout early childhood (Stoel-Gammon, 1992, 1998). Longitudinal studies have shown correlations between the following pairs of factors: the age of onset of canonical babble and the age of onset of meaningful speech (Stoel-Gammon, 1989), the amount of vocalization at age 3 months and vocabulary size at age 27 months (Kagan, 1971), the number of CV syllables at age 12 months and age at use of first words (Menyuk, Liebergott, & Schultz, 1986), use of consonants at age 12 months and phonological skills at age 3 years (Vihman & Greenlee, 1987), and diversity of syllable and sound types at ages 6–14 months and performance on speech and language tests at age 5 years (Jensen, Boggild-Andersen, Schmidt, Ankerhus, & Hansen, 1988). In each case, infants who produced more in the prelinguistic period (i.e., more vocalizations at age 3 months, more CV syllables at age 12 months) had superior performance on subsequent speech and language measures during childhood. These correlations further support the view that babbling serves as a foundation for the acquisition of speech and language. Infants who produce a greater number of prelinguistic vocalizations, particularly a greater number of canonical utterances with a variety of consonants and vowels, have acquired a greater arsenal of "building blocks" that can be recruited for the production of words. The closer the tie between the phonetics of babble and the phonological properties of a word, the greater the chance that the word will be acquired early. The acquisition of words such as *mommy* and *daddy* serves as a clear illustration of the link.

Learning to Say "Mommy": The Role of Phonology

In 1960, the renowned linguist Roman Jakobson noted that many languages use simple reduplicated forms for parental names. In some cases, the language has two forms of the same word, a standard form and a "nursery" form used primarily in speech to children. For example, in English, the words *mother* [mʌðɚ] and *father* [faðɚ] represent the standard terms, and the words *mama, mommy, papa,* and *daddy* are nursery forms. Phonologically, the standard terms contain phonemes that pose articulatory difficulties for young children (e.g., interdental fricatives, *r*-colored vowels), whereas the nursery forms are characterized by simple reduplicated CV syllables with oral or nasal stops.

Early acquisition of the nursery forms can be attributed in part to two interacting factors. First, children recognize the similarity between their own babbled forms (e.g., [mama], [baba], [dædæ]) and the nursery names for *mother* and *father*. Second, adults recognize that a baby's babbled productions resemble words like *mommy* and *daddy*. When a 7-month-old infant produces a vocalization that sounds like [mama] or [dædæ], English-speaking parents are likely to respond with glee, repeating the form and thus providing the infant the context needed to relate sound and meaning. As a consequence of these interactions, the nonmeaningful productions [mama] and [dædæ] have a good chance of entering the child's lexicon, becoming the words *mommy* and *daddy*.

Locke (1985) hypothesized that phonological factors contribute not only to the early acquisition of parental terms, but also to the widely documented finding that, across languages, the nursery word for the male parent (e.g., *daddy, papa*) is usually acquired before the word for the female parent. This finding seems somewhat puzzling given that, in most cases, the infant spends more time with the female parent and thus is likely to be exposed to the word for *mother* more often than the word for *father*. Arguing for the role of phonetic factors to explain the documented difference in order of acquisition, Locke noted that, across languages, terms for *father* are likely to contain oral stops, either bilabial (e.g., *papa*) or dental/alveolars (e.g., *daddy*), whereas words for *mother* are more likely to contain nasal consonants, usually /m/. Because oral stops occur more frequently than nasals in babbled utterances, infants produce forms like [baba] or [dada] more often than forms like [mama]. The close match between the babbled form and the nursery word for the male parent would thus make it more likely that the child would incorporate the words *daddy* or *papa* into the productive vocabulary before the word *mama*.

Individual Differences in Early Lexical and Phonological Development

Children's early vocabularies display both common trends and individual differences. Studies analyzing vocabulary growth beyond the first few words suggest that, in addition to pragmatic factors, individual phonological preferences influence the composition of a child's vocabulary during the first-50–word period. For example, in their study of three young children, Ferguson and Farwell (1975) reported that one child had a disproportionate number of words with the sibilant consonants [s, z, ʃ, tʃ, ʤ] such as *cereal, shoes, cheese, juice, see, eyes, ice,* and *sit,* which were largely absent from the vocabularies of the two other children. Stoel-Gammon and Cooper (1984) also traced the early vocabulary development of three children: Daniel, Will, and Sarah. In their study, Daniel had a clear preference for words ending in velar stops with forms such as *quack, rock, clock, sock, whack, milk, frog, yuk, block,* and *walk* in his lexicon. Of his first 50 words, 22% ended in a velar stop compared with 8% (Sarah) and 4% (Will) of velar-final words for the other two children. Will favored fully reduplicated forms like *quack-quack, oink-oink, yack-yack,* and *bye-bye.* Words of this type accounted for 26% of his first 50 words but for only 8% of Daniel's words and 4% of Sarah's. The third child in the study, Sarah, did not display any individual phonological preferences in her vocabulary, showing nearly equal distributions in terms of sound types and syllable structures. A shared characteristic of all three children was the high proportion of target words beginning with labials. Of the first 50 words for each subject, 28% of Sarah's words and 30% of words in the vocabularies of Daniel and Will began with a labial consonant. As noted in the following section, frequent use of labial stops, particularly initial /b/, is a characteristic of the early vocabularies of almost all children acquiring English.

The presence of individual differences in lexical acquisition leads to the question of why one child acquires many words with sibilants, but another acquires few words with fricatives and many with velars. Ferguson and Farwell (1975) hypothesized that the individual patterns of word selection resulted from differences in their subjects' production capabilities, specifically in their ability to produce consonants of particular place and manner classes. On the basis of their analyses of early lexical acquisition, they proposed that children attempt to say words with sounds and syllable structures they can accurately produce and avoid words that are difficult for them phonologically. Since the publication of their study, other researchers have reported similar findings for children with typical speech and language development and for those with atypical developmental patterns. There are no reports of a lexical selection pattern in which the critical feature was not a part of the child's productive repertoire.

Clear instances of avoidance of words on the basis of their phonology are more difficult to document because there are many reasons why particular words may be lacking in a child's early lexicon. Menn (1976) provided an example of avoidance in her longitudinal study of Jacob. The early vocabularies of most children contain a number of words beginning with /b/, including *baby, ball, bottle, balloon, bye-bye*, and others. In contrast, the only /b/-initial word Jacob tried to produce before the age of 19 months was *bye-bye*, which he pronounced as [daɪdaɪ], with a [d] rather than a [b]. At 19 months, he added the word *box* to his vocabulary (pronouncing it with an initial [b]), followed shortly by five other words beginning with /b/. Words with initial /p/ did not appear in Jacob's vocabulary until he was 20 months old.

After Ferguson and Farwell's (1975) seminal study, several researchers raised the possibility that the observed individual patterns could result from differences in input frequency rather than phonological preferences. That is, perhaps the child who acquires words ending in velar stops is simply exposed to more words of this type. To exclude input frequency as a critical factor, the amount of exposure to various phonological forms would have to be controlled, a situation that is not possible in a naturalistic setting. Using an experimental paradigm involving the teaching of nonsense words, Schwartz and Leonard (1982) controlled both phonological composition of the target words and their input frequency. In their experiment, spontaneous speech samples from the children were analyzed to determine the inventory of consonants and syllable structures that occurred. The researchers then created an individualized set of nonsense words for each subject; half of the words in the set were characterized by consonants and syllable structures that were "in" the child's repertoire (IN words), and the other half contained consonants "outside" the productive repertoire (OUT words). The words in each set were then presented to the child an equal number of times in a playlike format. Analysis of production and comprehension patterns for subjects with productive vocabularies of fewer than 75 words yielded two consistent findings: 1) The children produced more IN words than OUT words, and 2) there were no differences in the comprehension of IN words and OUT words. Thus, Schwartz and Leonard were able to confirm a phonological bias in the acquisition of a productive vocabulary.

Lexical selection in some children involves creation of a template (sometimes referred to as a *word recipe*) that is applied to the pronunciation of words sharing certain phonetic properties. Waterson (1971) reported that her son produced the words *Randall, window, finger*, and *another* as [ɲaɲo], [ɲeːɲeː], [ɲiːɲu], and [ɲaɲa], respectively. Although the target words vary segmentally, they all share the features of penultimate stress and presence of a nasal consonant, both of which are reproduced in the child's pronunciation. Based on this finding, Waterson hypothesized that children attend to and subsequently attempt to reproduce the most salient features of a target word. In so doing, they modify adult targets to conform to articulatory routines that the children are capable of producing.

In some cases, a child's production template yields forms that bear little resemblance to the target words. Leonard and McGregor (1991) described a child who developed a template that required fricative elements of the target word to appear in final position. Thus, the child pronounced *zoo* as [uz], *fine* as [amf], *soap* as [ops], *Snoopy* as [nupis], and *stop* as [taps]. In cases like this, the apparent idiosyncratic productions can be seen as systematic once the template becomes evident. Further discussion and examples of templates can be found in Macken (1996), Velleman (1996), and Vihman (1996).

Speech in Children with Atypical Development

Relatively few studies have examined the relationship of babble and speech among children who exhibit delays in lexical acquisition, although this topic is crucial to understanding early speech and language disorders. The findings from three investigations are summarized in this section. The first two are based on single individuals who participated in larger studies, and the third involves a group of children with specific expressive language delay. In the first study, Stoel-Gammon (1989) noted that one child's premeaningful vocalizations from ages 9 to 21 months differed from those of her 33 peers in that she produced almost no utterances with CV syllables. Thus, she had few practiced syllables (Vihman, 1992) to use for the production of real words. This child was the slowest of the group to enter the stage of meaningful speech (defined as the production of 10 different adult-based words in a 60-minute speech sample). Even at age 24 months, her speech sample contained fewer than 10 adult-based words.

The second case study describes Johnny, who displayed typical babbling patterns at age 9 months but was slow to acquire words (Stoel-Gammon & Stone, 1991). Johnny's mother reported a productive vocabulary of 10 words at age 19 months, 3 weeks, an age at which most children have a lexicon of 50–100 words. At age 22 months, Johnny's productive vocabulary was only 15 words, and he exhibited a very strong lexical selection pattern, characterized by a marked preference for words with labial consonants. His first 15 words, in order of acquisition, were *mama, balloon, book, ball, airplane, bye-bye, bottle, hot, bus, apple, bath, peekaboo, uh-oh, all gone*, and *bad boy*. Johnny's nonmeaningful productions at age 22 months were also characterized by a preference for labial consonants. The only supraglottal consonants produced in a sample of 125 utterances (meaningful and nonmeaningful) were labials, primarily the voiced stop [b]; the only other consonants occurring in the sample were a few glottal stops and a harsh glottal fricative that occurred in utterance-final position. During a clinical assessment at age 23 months, Johnny's phonetic repertoire remained limited to labial and glottal consonants, and attempts at eliciting CV syllables with nonlabial consonants were unsuccessful. This case, although limited to a single child, raises several issues regarding babble and speech. First, Johnny's babbling was typical at age 9 months, with labial, alveolar, and velar consonants produced as part of CV syllables. Why, then, was his repertoire so limited 10 months later? Second, to what extent can Johnny's rate of vocabulary acquisition be attributed to his severely limited phonetic repertoire of late babbling? to his lexical selection pattern? to his experiencing multiple ear infections between ages 9 months and 22 months?

Finally, Whitehurst, Smith, Fischel, Arnold, and Lonigan (1991) analyzed speech samples from 37 individuals with specific expressive language delay when the children were, on average, 28 and 33 months of age. At the first data collection session, the subjects' speech samples displayed characteristics usually associated with younger, typically developing children: Nonmeaningful utterances occurred more than twice as often as utterances with identifiable words, and 63% of nonmeaningful utterances were categorized as vowel babble, that is, vocalizations lacking consonants. Two variables from the samples were strongly related to expressive language scores 5 months later: 1) Rates of word use were positively correlated, and 2) rates of word use at the second session was negatively correlated with rate of vowel babble at the first session. The authors concluded that consonantal babble (i.e., use of CV syllables) facilitates expressive language for subjects with specific expressive language delay, whereas vowel babble competes with expressive language in this population.

Summary and Implications

The material presented thus far in this chapter supports the view that prelinguistic vocal development influences both lexical and phonological development in the subsequent period of meaningful speech. Prespeech vocalizations provide infants with practice in articulating sounds and syllables needed for the production of words and, through auditory and kinesthetic feedback, allow them to recognize the similarities between their own vocalizations and the adult models. Infants with a large stock of babbled vocalizations begin to talk earlier and acquire a productive vocabulary more rapidly than their peers with limited babble. This finding has implications for early identification of children with atypical speech and language development. A limited phonetic repertoire during the prespeech period may be an indicator of delays in phonological and lexical acquisition.

BEYOND THE FIRST WORDS: PHONOLOGICAL ACQUISITION

The influence of lexical selection on vocabulary acquisition declines beyond the first-50–word period as the child's articulatory capabilities increase; by age 24 months, the typically developing child has acquired a productive vocabulary of 250–350 words and can produce multiword sentences. Although the phonological system is far from complete at this age, the basic syllable shapes and sound classes are present, and about half of what a 2-year-old says can be understood by a stranger (Coplan & Gleason, 1988). On average, a 2-year-old has a phonetic inventory containing voiced and voiceless labial, alveolar, and (usually) velar stop consonants; labial and alveolar nasals; glides [w] and [h]; and some fricatives, usually [f] and [s] (Paynter & Petty, 1974; Prather, Hedrick, & Kern, 1975; Stoel-Gammon, 1985, 1987). In terms of syllable and word shapes, the repertoire includes open and closed syllables that can combine to form disyllabic words. In addition, the typical 2-year-old can produce some words with consonant clusters in initial and final position (Stoel-Gammon, 1987).

By age 36 months, the phonetic inventory of the typically developing child has expanded considerably to include exemplars of all place, manner, and voice classes and a variety of syllable and word shapes. Although the phonological system is not yet adultlike, the basic elements of the adult system are present; approximately 75% of a 3-year-old's speech is intelligible to a stranger (Coplan & Gleason, 1988). In their study of children ages 2–4 years, Prather et al. (1975) reported that all phonemes except /v, z, ð, ʤ, ʒ/ were customarily used at age 36 months, meaning they were produced correctly by at least half of the children in at least one of the word positions tested. The phonemes that were mastered by 36-month-olds in the study (i.e., those that were produced correctly in initial and final position by 75% of the children) included all the stop, nasal, and glide phonemes and the fricative /f/. In addition, the average child at age 36 months produced some consonant clusters in word-initial and word-final position (Templin, 1957).

Phonological and Lexical Development

In previous sections of this chapter, it is argued that a child's developing phonological system exerts strong influences on acquisition of the lexicon, specifically that children tend to acquire words with phonological features that they can produce and avoid words with features that are difficult for them. Although this lexical selection strategy may be advantageous at the outset of lexical acquisition, children must eventually attempt to produce words with phonetic features beyond their capabilities if they are to acquire new words. As children acquire larger productive vocabularies, the nature of the relationship between phonological and lexical development shifts. In the early period, phonological patterns influence lexical acquisition; later, the influence becomes bidirectional between lexicon and phonology. This section examines the developing vocabularies of children acquiring English, with a focus on the phonological composition of the words in the vocabularies of children between ages 12 and 30 months. The phonological features of these words are then compared with documented patterns of early phonological acquisition of children acquiring English to test the hypothesis that phonological features found frequently in the target lexicon will be acquired earlier than features that occur infrequently.

Phonological Characteristics of the Target Lexicon

Stoel-Gammon (1995) examined general phonological characteristics of children's early vocabulary by analyzing words from the MacArthur Communicative Development Inventories (CDI), a parent report form that assesses productive vocabulary by means of a checklist of commonly used words and phrases (Fenson et al., 1993). In previous analyses, Dale and Fenson (1993, 1996) examined responses to the CDI and assigned an age of acquisition to each word on the list, defined as the age at which the word appeared in the vocabularies of at least half the children in a particular age group. Using this metric, the age of acquisition for the words *daddy* (the first word to meet the criterion), *sleepy*, and *tomorrow* were ages 11.5 months, 25.35 months, and 29.25 months, respectively. Stoel-Gammon's phonological analysis of the CDI was based on all words that met the criterion for age of acquisition by 30 months, a total of 598 words. The figure of 598 words does not mean that the average child has a vocabulary of 598 words at age 30 months; this number refers only to words that were present in the vocabularies of half the 30-month-old children. In addition to this set of shared words, individual children acquire a unique set of proper names, including their own name and the names of siblings, relatives, and pets; the names of places they often visit; and special toys they own. Names such as these could not be included in the analysis, because their phonological forms vary from one child to another. For the same reason, animal sounds (though typically acquired early) were not included, because they too vary in terms of their phonological makeup.

The goal of the analysis was to characterize the shared vocabulary in terms of phonetic properties so that comparisons between the phonological characteristics of words acquired early and those acquired late could be made. General trends in the phonological composition of the words acquired by age 30 months are summarized in Figures 1–3. Figure 1 shows that of the 598 words in the data set, 356 (60%) are monosyllables and 203 (34%) are disyllables; 32 words are formed of three syllables; and only 7 have more than three syllables. The longest word in the sample, *refrigerator*, has five syllables. The most common word shapes in terms of CV structure, in descending order of frequency, are CVC (30%), CVCV (9%), CCVC (8%), CVCC (7%), and CV (6%). Consonant clusters are relatively rare, occurring in 19% of the words in initial position and 13% in final position. Stress placement (not shown in the figure) is extremely uniform across the sample. Of the 242 words of more than one syllable, 218 (90%) have stress on the first syllable. If monosyllabic words are classified as having stress on the first syllable, then we can say that 96% of the words have stress on the first syllable.

Figures 2 and 3 present analyses of initial and final segments in the 598 words. Manner of articulation for consonants is displayed in Figure 2 and place of articulation in Figure 3. In both figures, vowel targets are combined and shown as a single group. Stop consonants constitute the most frequent manner

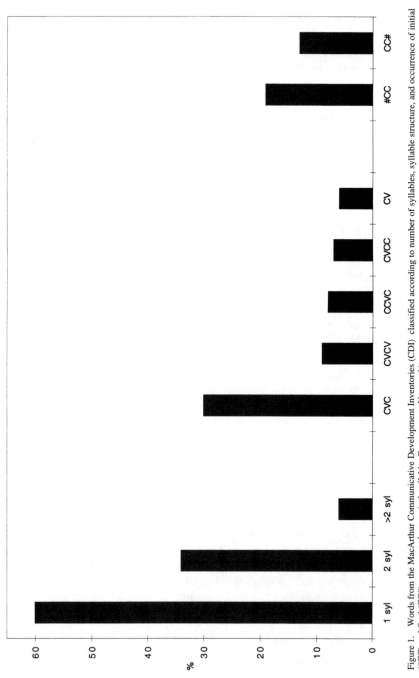

Figure 1. Words from the MacArthur Communicative Development Inventories (CDI) classified according to number of syllables, syllable structure, and occurrence of initial (#CC) and final (CC#) consonant clusters. (syl, syllable; C, consonant; V, vowel.)

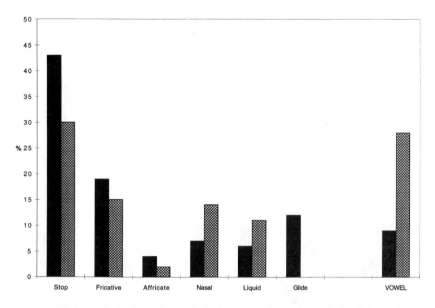

Figure 2.   Words from the MacArthur Communicative Development Inventories (CDI) classified according to manner of articulation of initial and final consonants. (■, initial consonants; ▓, final consonants.)

class, accounting for 43% of segments in initial position and 30% in final position (see Figure 2). Fricatives are the next most frequent manner class in both word positions, followed by glides (initial position only), nasals, and liquids. (As stated previously, the phoneme /h/ is classified as a glide throughout these analyses.) Positional differences are apparent: In word-initial position, obstruents (i.e., stops, fricatives, affricates) predominate, occurring at the onset of 66% of the words; only 9% of the words begin with a vowel. By comparison, 28% of the words end with a vowel, and 47% have word-final obstruents.

In terms of place of articulation (Figure 3), two trends are quite apparent: 1) Bilabial and alveolar consonants occur most frequently in word-initial position, and 2) alveolars predominate word-final position. The difference in the proportion of word-initial and word-final labial consonants (bilabial and labiodental) is striking: 33% of words begin with a labial phoneme (/p, b, m, w, f, v/), but only 10% end with a labial.

The Role of Frequency of Occurrence

The previous analyses can be used to test the hypothesis that phonological features that occur frequently in the target lexicon are acquired early by children and that features that are less frequent are more prone to error. In all analyses presented in this chapter, frequency of occurrence data are based on numbers

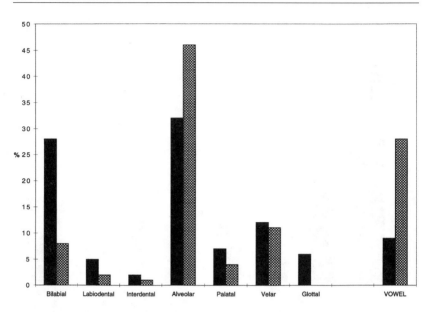

Figure 3.   Words from the MacArthur Communicative Development Inventories (CDI) classified according to place of articulation of initial and final consonants. (■, initial consonants; ▨, final consonants.)

of word types (i.e., different words) rather than tokens. Thus, although the fricative /ð/ occurs in the words *this, that, these,* and *those* and consequently may be frequent in an analysis based on tokens, it appears at the onset of only six words in the CDI list, yielding an extremely low frequency of occurrence in terms of word types.

The following parallels between frequency of occurrence of phonological features and acquisition error data can be viewed as support for the hypothesis:

- *Syllable Number*   The lexical analysis shows that one- and two-syllable words occur most frequently. Phonological acquisition data show that words of more than two syllables are often reduced to disyllables (weak syllable deletion).
- *Syllable Shape*   The lexical analysis shows that target words with singleton consonants in initial and final position are more frequent than targets with consonant clusters. Phonological acquisition data show that consonant clusters are late to be acquired and are often reduced to singleton consonants (cluster reduction).
- *Stress*   The lexical analysis shows that the majority of words with more than one syllable have stress on the first syllable. Phonological acquisition data show that unstressed syllables are omitted more frequently in word-initial position than in final position.

- *Manner of Articulation*   The lexical analysis shows that stop consonants constitute the most frequent manner class in both initial and final position. Phonological acquisition data show that stops are acquired early in phonological acquisition and often serve as substitutes for target fricatives and affricates (stopping).
- *Place of Articulation*   The lexical analysis shows that bilabial and alveolar consonants occur more frequently than velars. Phonological acquisition data show that bilabials and alveolars are acquired earlier and that alveolars often serve as substitutes for velars (velar fronting).

The match between frequency of occurrence in the target lexicon and acquisition data is not perfect, however. In particular, fricatives are the second most frequent class of consonants, accounting for approximately 18% of target phonemes in initial position and 15% in final position (see Figure 2). In contrast, the acquisition data show that, with the exception of [s] and [f], the class of fricatives is acquired relatively late, particularly the voiced targets /v, ð, z, ʒ/. In this case, data on frequency of occurrence are not supported by data on phonological acquisition. In addition, Figure 2 shows that glides and nasals occur less frequently than fricatives, yet they tend to be acquired earlier.

Developmental Trends in the Early Lexicon

The proposed hypothesis should also be examined by looking at developmental trends in the early lexicon to see how frequency of occurrence of phonological patterns changes over time. This analysis was performed by comparing phonological features of words from the CDI that reached age of acquisition by 19 months (100 words) with words whose age of acquisition was between 20 and 30 months (498 words). Comparisons of syllable number, syllable structure, and stress placement are presented in Table 1. The primary developmental change emerging from these comparisons involves consonant clusters. The proportion of initial clusters increases from 12% to 20% and the proportion of final clusters from 5% to 15%, reflecting an increase in the use of words that are phonetically more complex. Little to no change occurs in other aspects of syllable structure and stress placement.

Table 2 presents a comparison of place and manner features occurring in the target forms from ages 11 months to 19 months and from ages 20 months to 30 months. The most notable change for manner of articulation is the decrease in the proportion of stop consonants in word-initial position with a concomitant increase in the proportions of fricatives and liquids. For place of articulation, there is a decrease in the proportion of bilabial consonants in word-initial position and an increase in the proportional occurrence of bilabials in word-final position. The proportion of words ending in a vowel also decreases. Given that fricatives and liquids are acquired later than stops and that closed syllables are acquired later than open syllables, the observed changes

Table 1.   Developmental comparison of syllable and stress features

	Ages 11–19 months (%)	Ages 20–30 months (%)
Syllable structure		
CVC	37	28
CVCV	9	8
CV	6	6
CCVC	6	9
CVCC	4	7
CVCVC	3	3
Consonant clusters		
CC(C)–	12	20
–VCC(C)	5	15
Number of syllables		
1	63	59
2	32	34
3	4	6
>3	1	1
Stress placement[a]		
First syllable	98	96

[a]Monosyllabic forms are classified as having first-syllable stress.
C, consonant; V, vowel

suggest a developmental trend toward words that are phonetically more diffi-cult.

Developmental changes in frequency of occurrence of particular phonemes can also be examined in light of the proposed hypothesis. Figures 4 and 5 present a comparison of segments in word-initial and word-final posi-tion across three data sets: 1) words from the CDI acquired by age 19 months ($n = 100$); 2) words acquired between ages 20 and 30 months ($n = 498$); and 3) 20,000 words listed in a pocket dictionary, to provide a comparison of fre-quency of occurrence in child and adult vocabularies. Five aspects of the fig-ures merit discussion.

First, the phoneme /b/ accounts for 22% of initial phonemes in words ac-quired between ages 11 and 19 months, again highlighting the extensive use of this phoneme in the early vocabularies of children learning to speak English. When contrasted with the vocabulary acquired from ages 20 to 30 months, pro-portional occurrence of word-initial /b/ declines dramatically, from 22% to 8.4%. The reverse pattern occurs with the voiceless bilabial cognate /p/. In ini-tial position, /p/ accounts for 4% of words from the early vocabulary but al-most 10% of the later vocabulary; in the adult set, initial /p/ accounts for 8.4% of the 20,000-word corpus.

Second, words beginning with /s/ were rare in the early vocabulary (only 3 of 100 words); but /s/ was the most frequent initial segment in the late vo-cabulary, occurring in 58 of the 498 words (11.6%). In the majority of target words, /s/ occurred as part of a consonant cluster. In the adult set, /s/ was the most frequently occurring initial consonant (9.5%).

Table 2. Developmental comparison of sound classes by position

	Ages 11–19 months (%)	Ages 20–30 months (%)		Ages 11–19 months (%)	Ages 20–30 months (%)
Manner of articulation			Manner of articulation		
	Initial position			Final position	
Stop	57	40	Stop	29	30
Fricative	8	21	Fricative	14	15
Affricate	4	3	Affricate	1	2
Nasal	8	7	Nasal	11	15
Liquid	2	7	Liquid	12	10
Glide	9	12	Vowel	33	27
Vowel	12	9			
Place of articulation			Place of articulation		
	Initial position			Final position	
Bilabial	33	27	Bilabial	2	9
Labiodental	3	5	Labiodental	1	2
Interdental	1	2	Interdental	3	0
Alveolar	26	33	Alveolar	48	46
Palatal	6	7	Palatal	3	4
Velar	13	11	Velar	10	11
Glottal	6	6	Vowel	33	27
Vowel	12	9			

Third, the proportion of vowel-initial words changes substantially from the children's vocabularies to the adult set. Across the three data sets, vowel-initial words account for 12% of early child vocabulary, 8.8% of later child vocabulary, and 23.1% of adult words.

Fourth, marked positional differences in frequency of occurrence are evident for /b/. In the first 100 words, /b/ occurs word initially in 22 words but never in final position. In the next 498 words acquired, initial /b/ occurs in 42 words (8.4%) and final /b/ occurs in 3 words (0.6%). For the adult set, initial /b/ accounts for 4.9% of the words and final /b/ for 0.6%.

Fifth, positional differences are also present for liquids, particularly in the early vocabulary, in which /l/ and /r/ each occur at the beginning of only one word (1% each); in final position, the proportional frequencies are 5% for /l/ (including syllabic /l/) and 7% for /r/ (the vocalic r [ɚ] of words like *cracker* and *diaper* was categorized as a vowel and thus was not considered in determining frequency of occurrence).

A final perspective on the relationship between frequency of occurrence and phonological acquisition compares the frequency of occurrence data based on the CDI with acquisition data from Templin's (1957) large-scale study. In Figure 6, the absolute frequency of occurrence of each initial consonant in

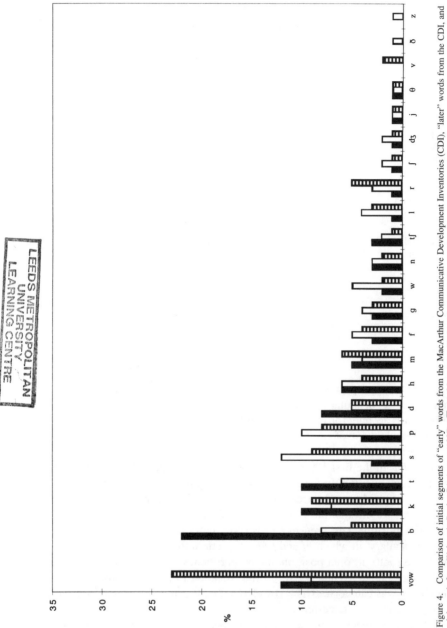

Figure 4. Comparison of initial segments of "early" words from the MacArthur Communicative Development Inventories (CDI), "later" words from the CDI, and adult words from *Webster's Pocket Dictionary* (1997). (■, 11–20 months; □, 21–30 months; ▦, adult.)

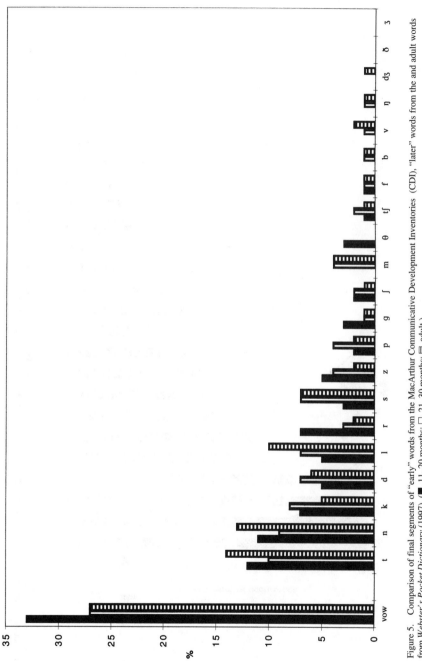

Figure 5. Comparison of final segments of "early" words from the MacArthur Communicative Development Inventories (CDI), "later" words from the and adult words from *Webster's Pocket Dictionary* (1997). (■, 11–20 months; □, 21–30 months; ▤, adult.)

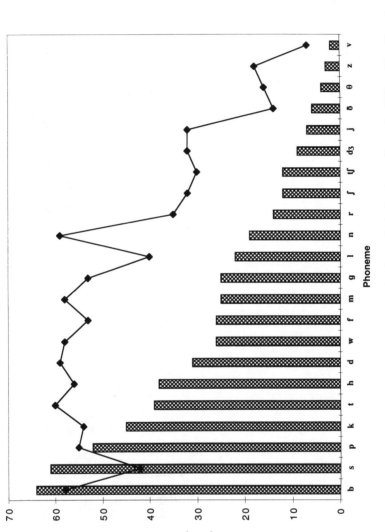

Figure 6.   Comparison of frequency of occurrence of initial consonants from the MacArthur Communicative Development Inventories (CDI) word list with number of 36-month-old individuals producing the consonant correctly. (■, frequency on CDI; ◆, correct production measured by number of subjects per 60-second interval.)

words from the CDI is indicated by the height of the bars, and the number of 36-month-old children producing that consonant correctly in word-initial position is shown by the continuous line. In general, phonemes that occur frequently are produced correctly by 3-year-old children, with a correlation of .71 between the two variables. Figure 7 presents the same type of analysis for consonants in final position. In this case, the correlation is not as strong ($r = .53$).

Despite the clear parallels between frequency of occurrence in early vocabulary and correct production at age 3 years, discrepancies are apparent. In initial position, for example, accuracy of production of /n/ and /j/ was greater than would be expected based on frequency of occurrence, whereas production of /s/ and /ɚ/ was less accurate than expected. In these cases, the variable of ease of articulation (however measured) seems to be a contributing factor. Phonemes that are easy to produce, such as stops, nasals, and glides, are produced correctly even though they may occur less frequently than phonemes that are lower on the ease of articulation variable—namely, fricatives, affricates, and liquids. The discrepancy between frequency of occurrence data and accuracy data for /s/ is compounded by the fact that although /s/ was the second most frequent consonant, occurring at the onset of 61 words, it was part of a consonant cluster in 40 of the 61 words, a factor that is likely to influence accuracy of production.

Summary

Comparisons of patterns of phonological acquisition and frequency of occurrence of phonological features reveal a strong relationship between the two (see Pye, Ingram, & List, 1987, for similar findings). At the level of individual phonemes, word and syllable shapes, and stress placement, those patterns that occur most often tend to be acquired early. This analysis, based on word types rather than tokens, suggests that the number of different forms stored in the mental lexicon is more important than the number of times the same form is used in output in terms of effects on phonological acquisition. In addition, it is clear that other factors must also be considered, in particular the relative ease of articulation of particular segments and syllable patterns.

INDIVIDUAL DIFFERENCES
IN PHONOLOGICAL AND LEXICAL DEVELOPMENT

Studies of individual differences in rate of lexical development also support the view of a strong relationship between lexical and phonological development. The basic finding in this domain is that children with large lexicons tend to have large inventories of speech sounds and syllable structures; conversely, children with smaller vocabularies have limited phonetic inventories. This section summarizes research on the two ends of the continuum: young children who exhibit exceptionally large vocabularies for their age and children with late onset of meaningful speech or unusually slow lexical development.

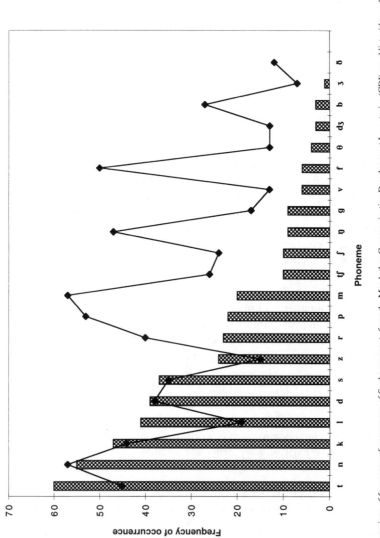

Figure 7. Comparison of frequency of occurrence of final consonants from the MacArthur Communicative Development Inventories (CDI) word list with number of 36-month-old individuals producing the consonant correctly. (■, frequency on CDI; ◆, correct production as measured by number of subjects per 60-second interval.)

Precocious Talkers

Stoel-Gammon and Dale (1988) examined the phonological patterns of a group of precocious talkers, that is, children who had productive vocabularies of 400–600 words at age 18 months, far exceeding the average vocabulary of 50–60 words. (The precocious children may also have been early talkers, but documentation regarding the age at which they acquired their first words was not available and thus the label of *early talker* is not appropriate.) Comparisons of the phonetic inventories of the 12 precocious talkers at age 20 months with a group of 32 typically developing children at ages 21 and 24 months revealed differences in both size and nature of the consonantal repertoire. (To be included in the child's inventory, a phone had to occur in a minimum of two different words in a 60-minute speech sample; accuracy of production was not considered.) At age 21 months, the inventories of the typically developing children contained, on average, 6.7 consonants in word-initial position and 3.6 consonants in final position. At age 24 months, the inventories had increased to 9.5 consonants in initial position and 5.7 consonants in final position. For the precocious talkers, the average phonetic inventory at age 20 months included 11.7 word-initial consonants and 7.4 word-final consonants. Thus, precocious talkers at age 20 months had larger phonetic inventories than the typically developing children at age 24 months.

Table 3 provides a summary of initial and final consonants present in the inventories of at least half the subjects of a given age group. As shown in the table, inventories of the typically developing subjects at age 21 months were limited in terms of place and manner of articulation, composed predominantly of stops and nasals. At age 24 months, these inventories had expanded to include glides, a few fricatives, and one liquid. By comparison, the precocious talkers at age 20 months produced a variety of place and manner classes, including several fricatives, an affricate, and final liquids, in addition to the stops, nasals, and glides that would be expected.

Late Talkers

Studies examining the relationship between lexical and phonological acquisition among late talkers suggest that a limited phonological system generally

Table 3.   Initial and final consonants used by typically developing children (*n* = 32) and precocious talkers (*n* = 12): Consonants appearing in 50% of subjects' inventories

Group (age)	Initial inventory	Final inventory
Typically developing (21 months)	b t d m n h	t n
Typically developing (24 months)	b* t d* k g m n w h f s	p t* k n s r
Precocious talkers (20 months)	p* b* t* d* k* g m* n w h* f* s ∫ t∫	p* t* k* n s z m n* r l

*Indicates consonants appearing in 90% of the inventories.

goes hand in hand with a small productive vocabulary (Stoel-Gammon, 1991a, 1991b). This finding holds true even when the corpus analyzed includes non-meaningful (i.e., uninterpretable) utterances as well as identifiable word productions. In one of the first studies, Paul and Jennings (1992) compared the phonologies of two groups of late talkers and controls matched for age, sex, and socioeconomic status. They reported that all of the late talkers were phonologically less advanced than their age-matched peers with regard to number of different consonants produced, complexity of syllable structures, and accuracy of consonants in word productions. In addition, the older late talkers, ages 24–34 months, were more advanced than the younger group, ages 18–23 months, on measures of size of consonantal inventory and accuracy of consonants in word productions. The two groups did not differ with respect to syllable structure. Because the sound classes and syllable structures used by the typically developing subjects and the late talkers were similar, the authors concluded that the late talkers were delayed but not deviant in their phonological development.

In a second study involving late talkers and typically developing age-matched peers, Rescorla and Ratner (1996) examined the speech patterns of 30 late talkers ages 24–31 months (mean age = 26 months) and compared them with 30 controls matched for age, sex, and socioeconomic status. The late talkers displayed significantly smaller inventories of consonants and vowels and greater proportional use of open syllables (vowel only or CV). In addition, the late talkers vocalized less frequently than the controls (a mean of 51.4 versus 118.2 vocalizations in the 10-minute spontaneous speech sample). The authors' conclusions are nearly identical to those of Paul and Jennings (1992): Phonological systems of the late talker group are characterized more accurately as delayed than as deviant, because they resemble the systems of younger, typically developing children. It was also hypothesized that, for the late talkers, the low rates of vocalization and phonological delay are interdependent.

Thal, Oroz, and McCaw (1995) also examined the phonological patterns of late talkers who scored below the 10th percentile on the CDI (Fenson et al., 1993) and compared the findings with two groups of controls, one matched for age and the other for language level. Late talkers in the premeaningful speech group (seven children, ages 18–33 months, who produced fewer than 10 different words in a 30-minute speech sample) performed like their language-matched controls on various phonological measures of syllable structure and consonant use in babble and speech but were significantly lower than their age-matched controls on all measures except two: number of different consonants in babbled utterances and proportion of true consonants in babble. For this group of children with substantial delays in the acquisition of a productive vocabulary, performance on phonological measures was similar to children with the same-size productive vocabulary who were, on average, 8 months younger.

For late talkers in the meaningful speech group (10 children, ages 19–28 months, who produced more than 10 words in the speech sample), the relationships between phonology and lexicon were somewhat more complex. The performance of late talkers in this group did not differ statistically from their language-matched controls on any of the phonological measures. At the same time, these late talkers differed from their age-matched controls on only one of the seven measures: number of different consonants produced in word-final position. These findings suggest that the phonological abilities of subjects in the meaningful speech group fell between the two control groups.

Summary

If lexicon size is used as the criterion for defining subject groups, investigations of children with exceptionally large (i.e., precocious talkers) or exceptionally small (i.e., late talkers) vocabularies yield the same findings. For both populations, lexicon size and phonological skills are commensurate: Precocious talkers are advanced in both domains, and late talkers are delayed in both. Although the correlation between the two factors is apparent, it is difficult to determine which of the two is the causal factor. The influence is undoubtedly bidirectional to some extent. Yet it seems reasonable to propose that phonological development may be a limiting factor that inhibits lexical growth among late talkers, whereas among precocious talkers the large vocabulary with a greater variety of phonetic targets may create a demand for a more advanced phonological system. This proposal awaits further research.

CONCLUSIONS

This chapter has summarized research on early speech and language development and documented the presence of ties across three domains: 1) the phonetics of babble, 2) a child's acquisition of a productive vocabulary, and 3) early phonological development. It was argued that, at the onset of meaningful speech, a child's phonological system plays a critical role in determining which words will be included in the productive vocabulary. The role of phonology declines as the vocabulary increases and the influences of the lexicon and phonology become bidirectional. It was shown that frequency of occurrence of target features (i.e., segments, sound classes, syllable shapes) is closely correlated to general patterns of phonological acquisition. In particular, accuracy of production of word-initial consonants at the age of 3 years is strongly associated with their frequency of occurrence in children's vocabularies.

One limitation of the research cited in this chapter is that it is based exclusively on studies of children acquiring English. Questions regarding influences of frequency of occurrence are best answered by examining developmental patterns of children acquiring languages with different phonological systems. A second limitation is that, although there are data on frequency of occurrence in terms of word tokens, relatively little is known about the role of frequency of occurrence of the input. One goal of future investigations should be documentation of lexical and phonological characteristics of speech directed to infants and toddlers. Findings regarding lexical and phonological development should be interpreted within a larger perspective of the general context in which language is acquired. These studies will help to determine the extent to which context is linked to common tendencies and individual differences observed in early language development.

REFERENCES

Coplan, J., & Gleason, J. (1988). Unclear speech: Recognition and significance of unintelligible speech in preschool children. *Pediatrics, 82,* 447–452.

Dale, P.S., & Fenson, L. (1993, July). *LEX: A Lexical Development Norms Database* [Computer program]. Seattle: University of Washington, Department of Psychology.

Dale, P.S., & Fenson, L. (1996). Lexical development norms for young children. *Behavior Research Methods, Instruments, & Computers, 28,* 125–127.

Fenson, L., Dale, P., Reznick, J.S., Thal, D., Bates, E., Hartung, J., Pethick, S., & Reilly, J. (1993). *MacArthur Communicative Development Inventories (CDI).* San Diego: Singular Publishing Group.

Ferguson, C.A., & Farwell, C. (1975). Words and sounds in early language acquisition: Initial consonants in the first fifty words. *Language, 51,* 419–439.

Jakobson, R. (1960). Why "Mama" and "Papa"? In B. Kaplan & S. Wapner (Eds.), *Perspectives in psychological theory: Essays in honor of Heinz Werner* (pp. 124–134). New York: International Universities Press.

Jensen, T.S., Boggild-Andersen, B., Schmidt, J., Ankerhus, J., & Hansen, E. (1988). Perinatal risk factors and first year vocalizations: Influence on preschool language and motor performance. *Developmental Medicine and Child Neurology, 30,* 153–161.

Kagan, J. (1971). *Change and continuity in infancy.* New York: John Wiley & Sons.

Leonard, L.B., & McGregor, K.K. (1991). Unusual phonological patterns and their underlying representations: A case study. *Journal of Child Language, 18,* 261–272.

Locke, J.L. (1985). The role of phonetic factors in parent reference. *Journal of Child Language, 12,* 215–220.

Macken, M.A. (1996). Prosodic constraints on features. In B. Bernhardt, J. Gilbert, & D. Ingram (Eds.), *Proceedings of the UBC International Conference on Phonological Acquisition* (pp. 159–172). Somerville, MA: Casadilla Press.

Menn, L. (1976). *Pattern, control and contrast in beginning speech: A case study in the development of word form and word function.* Unpublished doctoral dissertation, University of Illinois, Urbana-Champaign.

Menyuk, P., Liebergott, J., & Schultz, M. (1986). Predicting phonological development. In B. Lindstrom & R. Zetterstrom (Eds.), *Precursors of early speech* (pp. 70–93). New York: Stockton Press.

Messick, C. (1984). *Phonetic and contextual aspects of the transition to early words.* Unpublished doctoral dissertation, Purdue University, West Lafayette, IN.

Paynter, E., & Petty, N. (1974). Articulatory sound: Acquisition of two-year-old children. *Perceptual and Motor Skills, 39,* 1079–1085.

Paul, R., & Jennings, P. (1992). Phonological behavior in toddlers with specific expressive language delay. *Journal of Speech and Hearing Research, 35,* 99–107.

Prather, E., Hedrick, D., & Kern, D. (1975). Articulation development in children aged two to four years. *Journal of Speech and Hearing Disorders, 53,* 179–191.

Pye, C., Ingram, D., & List, H. (1987). A comparison of initial consonant acquisition in English and Quiché. In K.E. Nelson & A. Van Kleeck (Eds.), *Children's language* (Vol. 6, pp. 175–190). Hillsdale, NJ: Lawrence Erlbaum Associates.

Rescorla, L., & Ratner, N.B. (1996). Phonetic profiles of toddlers with specific expressive language impairment. *Journal of Speech and Hearing Research, 39,* 153–165.

Robb, M., Bauer, H., & Tyler, A. (1994). A quantitative analysis of the single-word stage. *First Language, 14,* 37–48.

Robb, M., & Bleile, K. (1994). Consonant inventories of young children from 8 to 25 months. *Clinical Linguistics and Phonetics, 8,* 295–320.

Schwartz, R., & Leonard, L. (1982). Do children pick and choose? An examination of phonological selection and avoidance in early lexical acquisition. *Journal of Child Language, 9,* 319–336.

Stoel-Gammon, C. (1985). Phonetic inventories, 15–24 months: A longitudinal study. *Journal of Speech and Hearing Research, 28,* 505–512.

Stoel-Gammon, C. (1987). The phonological skills of two-year-old children. *Language, Speech, and Hearing Services in Schools, 18,* 323–329.

Stoel-Gammon, C. (1989). Prespeech and early speech development of two late talkers. *First Language, 9,* 207–224.

Stoel-Gammon, C. (1991a). Issues in phonological development and disorders. In J.F. Miller (Ed.), *Research on child language disorders: A decade of progress* (pp. 255–265). Austin, TX: PRO-ED.

Stoel-Gammon, C. (1991b). Normal and disordered phonology in two-year-olds. *Topics in Language Disorders, 11,* 21–32.

Stoel-Gammon, C. (1992). Prelinguistic vocal development: Measurement and predictions. In C.A. Ferguson, L. Menn, & C. Stoel-Gammon (Eds.), *Phonological development: Models, research, implications* (pp. 439–456). Timonium, MD: York Press.

Stoel-Gammon, C. (1995). *What children say: A phonological analysis of the target words acquired by young American children.* Paper presented at Child Language Seminar, Bristol University, England.

Stoel-Gammon, C. (1998). Role of babbling and phonology in early linguistic development. In A.M. Wetherby, S.F. Warren, & J. Reichle (Eds.), *Communication and language intervention series: Vol. 7. Transitions in prelinguistic communication* (pp. 87–110). Baltimore: Paul H. Brookes Publishing Co.

Stoel-Gammon, C., & Cooper, J. (1984). Patterns of early lexical and phonological development. *Journal of Child Language, 11,* 247–271.

Stoel-Gammon, C., & Dale, P. (1988, May). *Aspects of phonological development of linguistically precocious children.* Paper presented at Child Phonology Conference, University of Illinois, Champaign-Urbana.

Stoel-Gammon, C., & Stone, J. (1991). Assessing phonology in young children. *Clinics in Communication Disorders, 1,* 25–39.

Templin, M. (1957). *Certain language skills in children.* Minneapolis: University of Minnesota Press.

Thal, D., Oroz, M., & McCaw, V. (1995). Phonological and lexical development in normal and late-talking toddlers. *Applied Psycholinguistics, 16,* 407–424.

Velleman, S.L. (1996). Metathesis highlights feature-by-position constraints. In B. Bernhardt, J. Gilbert, & D. Ingram (Eds.), *Proceedings of the UBC International Conference on Phonological Acquisition* (pp. 173–186). Somerville, MA: Casadilla Press.

Vihman, M. (1992). Early syllables and the construction of phonology. In C.A. Ferguson, L. Menn, & C. Stoel-Gammon (Eds.), *Phonological development: Models, research, implications* (pp. 393–422). Timonium, MD: York Press.

Vihman, M. (1996). *Phonological development: The origins of language in the child.* Cambridge, MA: Blackwell Publishers.

Vihman, M., Ferguson, C.A., & Elbert, M. (1987). Phonological development from babbling to speech: Common tendencies and individual differences. *Applied Psycholinguistics, 7,* 3–40.

Vihman, M.M., & Greenlee, M. (1987). Individual differences in phonological development: Ages one and three years. *Journal of Speech and Hearing Research, 30,* 503–521.

Waterson, N. (1971). Child phonology: A prosodic view. *Journal of Linguistics, 7,* 179–211.

Webster's Pocket Dictionary. (1997). Springfield, MA: Merriam-Webster.

Whitehurst, G., Smith, M., Fischel, J., Arnold, D., & Lonigan, C. (1991). The continuity of babble and speech in children with specific expressive language delay. *Journal of Speech and Hearing Research, 34,* 1121–1129.

3

Are Developmental Language Disorders Primarily Grammatical?
Speculations from an Evolutionary Model

John L. Locke

FOR ALL THAT HAS BEEN written about children with developmental language disorders, there is one thing that is known indisputably. On the day they enter the clinic for their initial evaluation, they are doing better than ever. The reason for this has far-reaching implications for the understanding of language and the conditions that impede its development.

Many researchers have come to associate full linguistic capacity with grammar, but the initial symptom of hard-core linguistic problems is not, paradoxically, grammatical failure. Rather, affected children appear on the clinic doorstep, usually at pregrammatical ages, because they are not talking often or saying many different words. Whether they have normal comprehension (Paul & Alforde, 1993) or are delayed in this area, too (Thal, Tobias, & Morrison, 1991), at least half these children will still have problems 1 year later.

Many of language delay's "first offenders" come to light at about 18–20 months of age. Infants of this age should be talking and, if typical, should be doing so with as many as 50 different words. Most of their individual utterances will usually comprise a single word or rote reproduction of a preassembled phrase that they have heard. Less frequently, they will personally assemble two-word phrases such as "Mommy go." With no more to talk with than this, it is not clear how listeners could detect an underlying grammatical problem even if a child had one.

The grammars of language do not usually emerge until later. I time the onset of grammar with the first creative exercise of regularizing operations based on learned linguistic principles. Marcus and his colleagues (Marcus,

---

The author is indebted to Thomas Dickins and Michael Studdert-Kennedy for helpful discussions of the subject matter in this chapter.

The term *normal* and non–person-first language are used throughout this chapter at the author's request.

1995; Marcus et al., 1992) traced the onset of verb tense and noun plural regularizations to an 18-month period that begins at about age 20 months. During that period, a previously correct irregular verb such as *went* may also be expressed as *goed*, and an irregular noun plural such as *feet* may continue to be said correctly but also as *foots*. Morphological operations such as these presuppose the phonological analyses that make /d/ and /s/ available for suffixing and the phrase processing that allows recognition of tense and plurality relations. It is therefore unsurprising that the age of creative morphology is consistent with most other forms of grammatical evidence, whether phonological, morphological, or syntactic (cf. Locke, 1997).

The cause of these problems must be understood, but our explanatory efforts may actually benefit from consideration of a hypothetical child, one who may never be seen in a clinic and may never need to be treated. Breaking from the usual "Why this?" motif, I ask below "Why not that?" Only after gleaning insights from the hypothetical child will we return to the question that is uppermost in most of our minds: Why do typical children with language delays have their typical problems?

A HYPOTHETICAL CHILD

Consider a child who acquires new utterances at the normal rate and then, as he or she approaches the age of grammaticality, fails to evince regularizing operations, ultimately slowing down in the rate of lexical acquisition. It makes perfect biolinguistic sense that such children should exist, should exist in fairly large numbers, and should even be typical. But they are neither typical nor abundant, and it is entirely likely that there are no such children.

To be sure, children with such a profile are occasionally reported. But when an otherwise normally advancing child suddenly slows down, one usually wonders if something outside the normal range of developmental events has just happened—perhaps a sudden change in hearing, health, emotional adjustment, or neurological status—and often the feared event has actually happened (e.g., Landau & Kleffner, 1957). The few cases that have come to my own attention later turned out to be red herrings. In every instance, the child did not merely slow down, as would presumably be the result of an underpowered grammatical system, but actually *lost* communicative and lexical behaviors that had developed earlier (e.g., "Tony" in Greenspan, 1992). These cases are even more difficult to interpret in developmental terms because the most that would be predicted under any extant ontogenetic model is a reduction in the rate of future lexical acquisitions.

Why is it rare for a child to uneventfully acquire vocabulary and then, as frankly grammatical behavior ought to commence, slow down? One possibility is that humans have a single language-learning system that, if improperly constituted, leaves the individual with less than the full amount of functional linguistic capacity. Limited to utterance data, this would seem to be a logical conclusion, and some have drawn it (Bates, Bretherton, & Snyder, 1988; Marchman & Bates, 1994). But there are other kinds of evidence that suggest that the logical conclusion may be incorrect. When these other types of evidence are considered, it becomes apparent that language presupposes the effective action of two functionally interrelated systems.

DUAL SYSTEMS

The acquisition of utterance material and the use of linguistic grammars to create and interpret language appear to be performed by different, disparately situated neural mechanisms (Locke, 1992, 1993). The system that acquires utterances supplies children with the words that they will need to talk to and to understand others and the material needed to learn the structure of language. It does this by interpreting vocal and facial emotion; observing, storing, and reproducing the superficial vocal and gestural behaviors of talking people; correlating eye movements with concurrent vocal behavior; and carrying out other operations that provide the child with utterances and helpful hints as to their deployment. Given its numerable functions, it is not surprising that this system constitutes a plurality of socially cognitive mechanisms (Karmiloff-Smith, Klima, Bellugi, Grant, & Baron-Cohen, 1995).

Although this acquisitive system is critical to the development of language, its functions have contemporaneous consequences that are not linguistic. These include person identification, affect monitoring, and affiliation. Fortunately, when language develops, it apparently does nothing to crowd out these functions. In fact, as far as we know, children who acquire language easily are no better or worse than their delayed peers at recognizing caregivers and other members of their social group, taking protective and affiliative action in response to vocal-emotional displays, and a range of other activities that require effective processing and storage of vocal behavior (Locke, 1996, in press b). It fits, then, that many of these behaviors are more likely to be performed in the "nonlinguistic" right hemisphere than in the left (cf. Locke, 1997).

That the human mind should house mechanisms that simultaneously serve both linguistic and nonlinguistic functions is not particularly surprising. Inasmuch as evolution acts on existing variation (Jacob, 1982), the brain systems that initially contributed to language must have had other reasons for existing. The advent of language would have had difficulty turning off these original functions, which other pressures would preserve to benefit the modern individual. These evolved cognitive mechanisms would thus resemble the inelegant "kludge" of the engineer or computer scientist, solutions that were "dictated by available materials and short-term expediency" (Clark, 1987, p. 283).

The grammatical system is less transparent and less easily reducible to a series of identifiable operations than the socially cognitive network, but there are four actions that can be identified:

1. Analysis of utterance material into smaller pieces that correspond to phonemes, syllables, and words
2. Detection of sequences and patterns of these pieces
3. In development, construction of a mental system that characterizes these patterns
4. Expressive use of that system to generate novel forms at and above the level of the word

This asocial specialization has no known use apart from linguistic communication and possibly the representation of experience, and it has no means of acquiring the data on which it operates. The overwhelming evidence, whether neuropathological or electrophysiological, is that these functions typically are performed by mechanisms that are housed primarily in the left cerebral hemisphere.

It is thus apparent that our species' capacity for linguistic communication represents the conjunction of disparate specializations, served by different brain systems, the first specialization chronologically preceding, as well as enabling and requiring, the second specialization. Because the typically delayed child displays less than the normal amount of word knowledge, socially cognitive behaviors will usually get the blame. It is imperative that we look more carefully at the precursive role of these behaviors.

SOCIALLY COGNITIVE PRECURSORS

Strictly defined, *precursors to language* are behaviors that precede the development of language and are not instances of language itself. It is assumed that in the evolution of language in the species, there were nonlinguistic behaviors—some of which may be witnessed today in similar though probably reduced form in nonhuman primates—that enhanced fitness and were therefore reinforced in the species. It is also assumed, with empirical support, that in the human infant's development of language there are prelinguistic behaviors that lay the groundwork for later developments that are more straightforwardly linguistic.

Several of the behaviors that precede later developments, of whatever type, are thought to facilitate those developments. The reasons are various (cf. Dunst, 1990). One is chronological: The precursors come first. Infants, it is believed, must be able to do some things before they can do other things. Another reason is linked to the first but is more mechanistic: Specific sensory, motoric, and conceptual developments must occur if the child is to progress to higher levels of behavior that specifically subsume functioning at the lower, earlier levels. A better reason for believing that precursive behaviors facilitate later developments is statistical, usually in the form of correlations.

There is hard evidence that infants who engage in high levels of some facilitative behaviors do actually score higher on language measures later. These demonstrated facilitators include joint attention, vocal development, and lexical imitation (Masur, 1995; Oller, 1995; Snow, 1989; Tomasello & Farrar, 1986). The interpretive danger here, of course, is that these behaviors could be epiphenomenally linked to anything that normally comes later, but these particular precursors at least enjoy a logical connection to language insofar as they relate to utterance storage and reproduction.

My own view is that the ontogenetic force of precursors resides less in the fact that they are laid down early in the developmental game than in their contemporaneous power to actively channel the infant toward behaviors that are linguistic. Thus, I assume here, after Mayr (1974), that joint attention, vocal imitation, and kindred behaviors comprise a feedback or guidance system that keeps infants on one or more growth paths that lead, more or less anticlimactically, to spoken language (Locke, 1993, in press b).

THE REAL CHILD

Language-delayed children display reduced socially cognitive activity; however, there is still little evidence for reduced joint attention, vocal imitation, and other precursors before the actual diagnosis of delayed language. The reason is that researchers do not know in advance who is going to be delayed and thus have not known at which infants they should be looking for evidence of precursors. The data from infants with danger signs like Down syndrome or very low birth weight may be interesting but are not really the most appropriate kind of evidence.

There are some other socially cognitive behaviors that relate to language-learning mechanisms less plausibly than joint attention and vocal imitation but are nonetheless reduced in language-delayed children.[1] Although the research is incomplete, it is beginning to appear that children who fall behind in the acquisition of vocabulary are less voluble than typically developing children. D'Odorico (1996) reported that Italian infants who are extremely voluble at 12 months of age have a higher word-to-nonword ratio 4 months later than their less voluble peers. Lexically delayed 2-year-olds evince fewer vocally communicative intentions per minute than typically developing children while displaying more gesturally communicative intentions (Paul & Shiffer, 1991), and

---

[1]In some studies, late-onset or atypical babbling has been found in infants who were later determined to have begun talking late (e.g., Oller, 1995; Stoel-Gammon, 1989), and of course we know that lexically delayed children appear to be incapable of a range of phonetic and phonological behaviors (cf. Mirak & Rescorla, 1997; Rescorla & Ratner, 1996). However, as similar as babbling and talking may be at the motor-phonetic level, the two activities are not obviously guided by similar socially cognitive mechanisms.

they produce far fewer utterances than normals, independent of their quality (Paul & Jennings, 1992). Thal, Oroz, and McCaw (1995) studied late-talking 18- to 33-month-olds who were still in the single-word stage of language development. The mean number of utterances produced by late talkers, especially those who produced few words in a play session, fell below that produced by age-matched controls and language-matched controls. Similar findings have been reported by Rescorla and Ratner (1996).

It is also apparent that lexically delayed children use the words they know less effectively in social situations than their more advanced peers. Craig and colleagues (Craig & Evans, 1989, 1993; Craig & Washington, 1993) found that receptively delayed children tend to be less adept at entering ongoing conversations and at assuming and yielding the floor than children with similarly small working vocabularies but good lexical comprehension. In a study of late-talking 2-year-olds, Paul, Looney, and Dahm (1991) found that of six children who also had receptive delays, five were socially retarded on a standardized measure that includes a range of nonverbal social behaviors (e.g., smiling). Moreover, they found that four of seven children with expressive (but no social or receptive) delays at 2 years of age had measurable social delays 1 year later. Because of the relative youth of the children, these findings suggest that language-delayed children may already have social delays before self-recognition of their problem and formal diagnosis.

What delays the early phases of language learning that are rooted in social cognition? Even other primates reveal some ability to do precursive behaviors that relate to utterance learning and, if reared appropriately (Tomasello, Savage-Rumbaugh, & Kruger, 1993), may even be capable of learning utterances (cf. Savage-Rumbaugh et al., 1993). Our evolutionary ancestors would have had this ability as well. However, nonhuman primates have no demonstrated grammatical ability. Why, then, is language delay initially manifested in the developmentally earlier socially cognitive operations and not in the later-emerging grammatical system? The former system would seem to be more robust, its individual operations having other proximal consequences or "causes" aside from their role in language (Locke, 1996). Even nonverbal children need to understand the motives and actions of other people, and a great deal of information about these is transmitted vocally.

The problem becomes even more puzzling when one considers comparative data showing that chimpanzees and humans, including those with Down syndrome, pass through the same stages of concept development in the same order and at approximately the same chronological ages (Antinucci, 1990; Dunst, 1990). When humans finally diverge from the other primates, they do so on late-developing concepts. The analogy in language would be grammar. The bonobo Kanzi has a larger receptive vocabulary than many children with fairly specific language delays (Savage-Raumbaugh et al., 1993). One assumes that he has not "gone grammatical," because he lacks the mechanism to make that possible. Why is this so for the late-developing child?

One possibility is that most lexically delayed children seem to develop language at the same rate as their typically developing peers but, for reasons unknown, get off to a late start. It is difficult to say why the starts are delayed, but vocabulary development is not the only area that is behind schedule. Indeed, it is difficult to find any behaviors that are not delayed in these children, from manual motor to visual perception tasks (cf. Locke, 1994, 1997).

As noted previously, it appears that about half of the language delays at 2 years of age eventually resolve. The other half turn into highly specific grammatical disorders (Paul & Riback, 1993; Paul & Shiffer, 1991; Paul & Smith, 1993; Rice, Wexler, & Cleave, 1995), with morphology frequently more impaired than syntax (Clahsen, 1989; Smith-Lock, 1993). Smith-Lock (1993) found that children who were 2 years behind their age-matched peers in language but equivalent on nonverbal measures were selectively delayed in the acquisition of inflectional morphology and displayed selective deficits in morphological analysis.

Under the first hypothesis, the proximal cause of utterance acquisition problems is the distal cause of grammatical problems. I have suggested elsewhere that grammatical mechanisms will not fully activate if there is less than the usual amount of work for them to do, just as the visual cortex fails to develop if there is less than the usual amount of patterned light (Locke, 1997). In the typical case, regularizing operations begin when children have about 400 words in their expressive vocabulary (Bates, Dale, & Thal, 1994; Marchman & Bates, 1994), an achievement that usually occurs in the third year of life. Expressed words are observable and measurable, but it appears to be the number of words in storage that counts. The size of a child's receptive lexicon is harder to estimate but could easily run to several thousand words at age 3. It is hypothesized that this burgeoning store of comprehended words triggers or reinforces the activation of analytical mechanisms. In the case of the persistently delayed child, this quantity of words is not attained until a far older age, presumably during a later stage of neural maturation.

Now, if there were no outer limit on how long a child could continue to acquire linguistic material and rules, late-developing children would eventually catch their faster peers and would not carry residual deficits into adulthood. However, residual deficits are characteristic of those who are late to develop vocabulary, even though children with lexical delays actually learn language at the same rate as typically developing children (Bishop & Edmundson, 1987a, 1987b). As of 1998, the most recent evidence (cf. Locke, 1998) suggested that if severely delayed children have not caught up by the age of 4 or 5 years, many of them never will. Thus, one assumes that the opportunity for activation of analytical and computational mechanisms can indeed come and go without optimal result, leaving lexically delayed children with an underpowered capacity to learn and use linguistic rules.

The second possible cause of specific grammatical deficits is also presumed to be genetic; but, instead of acting indirectly by first affecting socially cognitive behaviors, the hypothetical effect is direct. The most celebrated attempt to document a specifically grammatical genetic effect (Gopnik & Crago, 1991) was later convincingly challenged (Vargha-Khadem, Watkins, Alcock, Fletcher, & Passingham, 1995). Thus, at this writing, the collected evidence points to a tandem operation whereby socially cognitive deficits delimit lexical development, which causes grammatical deficits, but without any evidence of a primary grammatical deficiency.

WHY IS THE REAL CHILD POSSIBLE? AN EVOLUTIONARY PERSPECTIVE

Miller (1990) said that we know more about language than we understand, and it may be possible to solve the paradox if we think in new ways about research findings that already exist. For reasons that become clear later in this chapter, I believe the optimal framework may be an evolutionary one. This assertion is at least ironic because linguistic evolution is not at all understood and is purely a speculative affair as of 1998 and because one of the sources of evidence on evolution is ontogeny (Studdert-Kennedy, 1991). Nevertheless, consideration of how language-learning systems were assembled in evolutionary history seems to inspire a different type of thinking as to their functional interrelationships in the human infant of today. Conceptions of the probable course of linguistic evolution may help us to see which of various precursive behaviors are facilitative and which are nascent forms of the linguistic beast itself.

The capacity to learn and use language is buried deep in the biological makeup of our species. Once assumed to be a cultural invention, language is now claimed to be a property of all normally constituted humans, perhaps even an "instinct" (Pinker, 1994, 1995). Yet, a significant minority of children— seemingly about 7% of the otherwise normally developing 2-year-olds in middle-class American families—are identified each year with language ability that falls well below their measurable level of intellectual function (Rescorla, 1989; Tomblin, 1996). Because most of these children are free of obviously interfering conditions, including hearing loss, brain damage, and primary emotional disorder, a question arises immediately: If language is an "instinct," why do so many otherwise typical children fall below the biological norm for language? After all, there are no proportionate delays in walking, localization of sound, and recognition that objects removed from view continue to exist.

Are the linguistic criteria more cultural than functional, or is Pinker just plain wrong? It must be admitted that by the time language-delayed children mature, most speak well enough to be assimilated by their community, and the majority usually acquire the basic literacy and computational skills needed to survive in a competitive, industrialized society. But as typical as they may seem, many continue to display residual deficits in adulthood, whether in speaking behaviors (Tomblin, Freese, & Records, 1992) or in a range of reading, writing, and spelling difficulties (Aram, Ekelman, & Nation, 1984; Felsenfeld, Broen, & McGue, 1992; Klackenberg, 1980; Lewis & Freebairn, 1992; Tallal, Ross, & Curtiss, 1989). Perhaps, Pinker might say, these deficits are "flushed out" today by performance demands associated with literacy and would never have been noticed when language was evolving in our species, or even a few centuries ago in agrarian societies. The level of linguistic function that survives developmental language disorders, on this account, meets some species minimum that stretches across cultures.

Although it is possible that our species' capacity for grammatical behavior arose de novo, as some have claimed, I suggest that our hominid ancestors' disposition to engage in vocal behavior with other familiars led to such a proliferation of unparticulated utterances that an organizing mechanism became critical. I also suggest that those who were able to detect recurrent gestural patterns in their vocal behaviors were more likely to develop or commandeer such a mechanism, and, when they did, their ability to learn and manipulate large vocabularies of vocal material took a significant step forward. This, for reasons unknown, increased their reproductive fitness.[2]

Did the precursors of today also precede language in our prelinguistic ancestors? We cannot know for sure, but extrapolations from nonhuman primates suggest that our hominid ancestors would have possessed some level of ability in the socially cognitive behaviors that now precede and facilitate language development in the infant. But the level of word-learning ability of our hominid ancestors would have fallen below our own, just as nonhuman primates' ability to carry out most socially cognitive operations is surpassed by that of modern humans (cf. Brothers, 1990). Supporting evidence reviewed elsewhere (Locke, 1995) is summarized here. For example, indicating behaviors such as pointing and joint visual reference are correlated with lexical development in humans. In primates, however, some species appear to use eye movements indexically, whereas others seem not to engage in referential pointing. Whereas human infants recognize their mothers by their mother's voices—and in the process apparently develop a preference for some properties of her language—the evidence for kin recognition in nonhuman primates involves the mother recognizing the infant. In our own young, there are correlations between early vocal imitation and later lexical development; but in monkeys, who match vocal frequency during dyadic exchanges, there is little or no uncontested evidence of expressive vocal learning. Although maternal–infant vocal behavior has a conversation-like temporal structure in humans, the evidence for turn taking in monkeys is limited to mature animals.

---

[2]This discussion concerns phonetic and social aspects of the evolutionary process and excludes consideration of other aspects, such as the origins of representational capacity and vocal-motor control.

In human children, the effective use of language seems to require an "other minds" concept (cf. Hobson, 1993; Premack & Woodruff, 1978); but in nonhuman primates, there is still little evidence of other minds. With appropriate experience, certain of the apes may spontaneously display an ability to comprehend utterances and some disposition to use symbols creatively; but these talents fall short of what is done even by younger children. Nonhuman primates thus enjoy some level of ability in areas of social cognition that relate to language in the developing human infant, but, for the most part, it is a reduced level.

How did grammatical capacity emerge in our evolutionary ancestors? There is no accepted answer to this question. Some have ventured that grammatical capacity arose by genetic accident (Piatelli-Palmarini, 1989). Others assume that grammar could have evolved only through natural selection (cf. Pinker & Bloom, 1990), although the raw mental material may have been appropriated from some extracommunicative source (Bickerton, 1995; Wilkins & Wakefield, 1995). The central tenet of evolutionary psychology is that highly specialized cognitive systems are available to modern humans because the systems solved problems experienced by our evolutionary ancestors (cf. Cosmides & Tooby, 1987, 1994). For example, our ancestors needed to tell one individual from another; thus, there are cognitive (and neural) mechanisms that activate at the appearance of faces and the sound of voices. Lacking a reason to suppose that the evolution of grammatical capacity was somehow exempted from this general principle, it can be assumed that it, too, arose as an adaptation. But if grammar solved ancestral problems, what were these problems? Perhaps better, how did grammar increase the fitness of hominids?

If there were intermediate stages in the evolution of language, our ancestors did not become grammatical overnight. In evolution, as in ontogeny, it is assumed that social sound making preceded grammar (Locke, in press a) and that such speechlike behaviors would have helped hominids to avoid and resolve conflict and to create and maintain social relationships (Dunbar, 1993; Morris, 1967). That they could have engaged in speechlike behavior seems obvious. First, girneys, peeps, and a variety of other vocal forms are heard when familiar nonhuman primates are gathered together under relaxed circumstances. Second, given that talking involves no more than a social sound-making frame and some minimal stock of learned forms, it is unlikely to have eluded the conceptual grasp of hominids. It may also have fallen within their motoric and perceptual capabilities; nonhuman primates naturally learn to recognize the vocal patterns that identify other conspecifics and to interpret vocalizations that signal emotional states and intentions of other animals, as well as various calls that signal food, copulation, and predators. Third, although the cortical or conceptual groundwork for a linguistic grammar could have become available in a variety of ways, it is illogical to assume that a dedicated and specialized utterance analytic and utterance computation system would have developed prior to its first obvious need and its first social applications in talking (Locke, in press a).

However, prosodically organized vocal patterns are not, by definition, particulated at levels corresponding to the units that are so freely recombined in linguistic phonologies (cf. Abler, 1989). Lacking analysis at the level of the segment, there would have been no way to store or to manipulate anything like the number of utterance units that characterize modern levels of language. Thus, the solution to the first problem gave rise to a second problem: As the capacity for reference expanded, stereotyped utterances would have proliferated to an unmanageable level without some implicit recognition of phonetic regularities—the organizational basis of their burgeoning store of vocal utterances. When this need arose, it is less than daring to suppose that our hominid ancestors, like modern primates, already enjoyed some ability to identify patterns and detect the organization in hierarchically organized material (cf. Greenfield, 1991). Because primates are adaptive, it is likely that hominids had some level of a domain-general ability to organize their own behavior (cf. Thelen, 1991; Thelen & Fogel, 1989).

How do we bridge this general ability to detect patterns and organization with the speech domain? How would our evolutionary ancestors have discovered and hence created a segmental organization for their stereotyped vocalizations? The answer may be linked to the process of social sound making. To achieve surface discriminability for more than a handful of vocal patterns, hominids would have needed to modify phonated signals with movements of the tongue, lips, and other movable parts of the vocal tract. However, our species can chop up the sound stream in only so many ways, as archives of phonological and sound-making behavior reveal (cf. Locke, 1983). Thus, ancestral talkers would have quickly discovered, from feeling and sound, the regular recycling of particular gestures. Utterances in need of formal organization would already have enjoyed some intrinsic organization at the level of the gesture, a level that corresponds to linguistic segments (Browman & Goldstein, 1989). Implicit recognition of this level of utterance organization would have created the basis for an elementary phonetic and, later, a phonological system.

One assumes that those who discovered the segment and its recombinability excelled in vocal behavior, and the ability to proliferate diverse utterances would thus have been enhanced through attested processes of natural selection.[3] The ability to learn the form and social significance of vocal patterns would also have been further elevated by selection after grammatical analysis began and speech became even more ornate.

---

[3]The specific processes supporting such changes have been understood at least since Waddington's (1953) studies revealed that when environmental pressures force usually dormant properties to the surface, their perceptible expression causes them to fall within the reach of natural selection. Thus, I assume, first, that minor degrees of variability in the hominid's vocal-support systems were brought out under increased pressures to communicate and, second, that small increments enhanced social fitness.

When linguistic behavior was enhanced by selection, there were two sets of beneficial consequences of vocal learning in the infant: 1) the earlier, prelinguistic ones relating to indexical and affective communication (Locke, 1996) and 2) the newer, linguistic ones relating to whatever factors favored the knowledge or use of language. The evolution of language would thus have raised abilities in all areas that contributed to linguistic proficiency, however elementary or "primitive" these areas might seem. This would have produced increases in vocal learning beyond that which existed prelinguistically because, other things being equal, the better vocal learners would have been advantaged vis-á-vis development of large vocabularies of stereotyped vocal patterns. In effect, the species-typical level of precursive behaviors would have risen.

What I am claiming is that the utterance acquisition systems of hominids would have worked well enough to produce a store of holistic forms sufficiently large to require the action of a weak utterance analytic mechanism. Adaptively, this mechanism would have grown more powerful as selection increasingly acted on the utterance acquisition system, in turn adding to the acquisitive efficiency of socially cognitive mechanisms, and so forth. High levels of precursive abilities in modern infants may thus represent the incipient action of a gradually maturing grammatical mechanism.

Figure 1 is a schematic proposal of the evolutionary process. The solid bars on the extreme left refer to various evolutionary precursors to language (e.g., vocal learning, joint attention). With some systemic (pattern detection and utterance analytic) ability, these precursive capabilities continued to develop and reciprocally reinforced systemic mechanisms. As these socially cog-

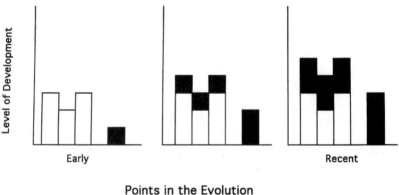

**Points in the Evolution
of Language**

Figure 1. Levels of various evolutionary precursors to language (e.g., vocal learning, joint attention) developing in response to and contributing to systemic (pattern detection and utterance analytic) mechanisms that ultimately evolved to undertake grammatical operations. (□, precursors; ■, grammar.)

nitive and systematizing operations continued to rise, utterances proliferated to the point where a full-fledged grammatical system was needed.

Those of our hominid ancestors who trafficked heavily in vocal behavior developed a store of useful forms. The more voluble hominids would have had larger stores. They would have benefited from an analytical mechanism, even a very weak one, that could chop prosodies into their segmental constituents. Such a mechanism would have taken the pressure off a prosodic type of storage system, enabling increases in the size of their vocal repertoire. As vocabularies grew, the benefits to those having better analytical and computational systems would also have increased. With segments and syllables emancipated from prosodies, our hominid ancestors would also have achieved a basic property of human language (Humboldt, 1836/1972): the ability to obtain infinitely variegated vocal displays, and hence messages, from finite means.

Because utterance complexity enhanced reproductive fitness, and because complexity was jointly a function of utterance acquisition and grammar, both systems were enhanced in tandem. Those who were high in the precursors—call them A, B, and C—typically benefited from and thus passed on the genes for a grammatical system—call it D. A, B, and C are still individual systems; but where language is concerned, they have been stitched together with D by 100,000 years of acquisition. The factors that "cause" language acquisition are thus conjoined with language itself. Precursive behaviors like joint attention retain their nonlinguistic status but ontogenetically have become prolinguistic. A consequence is that modern infants with advanced precursive skills are likely to be intrinsically prepared for high levels of grammaticality.

REAL CHILD REDUX

If grammar was an evolutionarily late-developing capacity, then it makes sense that children who sail through the socially cognitive phases of vocabulary learning can still slow down when they reach that phase in which grammatical mechanisms ordinarily activate. However, this is not what happens in the typical case. Rather, children who do not behave in a fully fledged grammatical way experience what is only the last in a long series of setbacks. The paradox is resolved if we find that language-disordered children's deficits are limited to the "topped-up" level of social cognition that was created by the advent of grammatical capacity.

Higher levels of utterance acquisition may be a form of systemic learning that is made possible by a gradually maturing, moderately empowered grammatical capacity. It would be unusual if a brain system did not develop gradually, and, if the grammatical machinery did so, there could be subtle effects that precede full-blown grammatical generativity. This would contribute to a seamlessness that could disguise the operation of multiple systems. Systemic learning would naturally include a native language bias that has been observed just before the end of the first year of life, in both structured listening tasks (Jusczyk, Friederici, Wessels, Svenkerud, & Jusczyk, 1993) and spontaneous vocalization (Boysson-Bardies et al., 1992), as well as in speech perception tasks (Werker & Polka, 1993). The familiar increase in the rate of lexical learning that occurs at about 18 months of age may reflect this sort of systemic functioning, for example, by making it easier to parse words as well as discover their segmental constituents. If grammatical mechanisms develop late in children with developmental language disorders, this delay could be revealed initially in a previously unsuspected place: the ineffective operation of receptive and expressive word-learning mechanisms.

CONCLUSIONS

In ways not yet understood, nonlinguistic behaviors such as volubility seem to be statistically related to language. The reasons for this are unknown. It is possible that those with an "appetite" for vocal behavior are more likely to enjoy, pay attention to, play with, and learn about the vocalizations of others, thereby storing and reproducing more speech than less voluble infants. If participation in social sound making caused our hominid ancestors to recognize oral gestures that correspond to articulatory segments, it is reasonable to suppose that talking in the second year of life contributes to the developing infant's discovery of phonetic regularities that function in the ambient language. According to this conception, first receptive and then expressive vocabulary systems work together adaptively to activate and reinforce mechanisms needed for grammatical language. A rapidly enlarging stock of segmentally underanalyzed utterances causes storage problems for the infant, pressuring him to identify regularities that underlie the organization of the system. As the infant plunges more deeply into talk, the natural patterning of vocal tract activity provides input to analytic mechanisms that perform the solution.

I suggested earlier in the chapter that there may be two causes of grammatical deficiency. The first is revealed by children with genetic deficiencies in the brain mechanisms that usually handle grammatical operations. The existence of such problems has never been proved; but if this group of children did exist, their grammatical deficit might be revealed as a systemic effect late in the first year of life. Because systemic effects have not yet been linked directly to grammatical problems, there is currently no real evidence that this possible group actually exists. The second hypothesized cause of grammatical deficiency is revealed by children who fall so far behind in socially cognitive operations that a critical moment for activation of linguistic mechanisms comes and goes before activation is complete, leaving them with residual deficits (cf. Tomblin et al., 1992). This proposed tandem action also needs to be confirmed, but there is no lack of research strategies for doing so (Locke, 1997).

Some children may have a conflation of these theoretically separable disorders. Poor word learning in the second year of life could reflect an intrinsically deficient grammatical mechanism that fails to parse utterances, learn patterns, and point the infant in the direction of lexical candidates. To turn fully on, this mechanism would require typical if not elevated levels of pressure from accumulating utterances in need of segmental analysis. Because these children are behind in lexical acquisition, however, they would be hit by a one–two punch: an inherently weak grammatical mechanism paired with too little of the material that precipitates the development of such a mechanism. If children with intrinsically impaired grammatical mechanisms do exist, we might conclude that language is a unitary system, as Bates et al. (1994) did.

How will these theoretical-diagnostic questions eventually be answered? One way is to sort infants according to their level of precursive behaviors and then look at their development of vocabulary. This is becoming increasingly possible as research methods are developed that steadily lower the estimated onset of lexical comprehension (cf. Mandel, Jusczyk, & Pisoni, 1995). It will be interesting to see whether any observed deficiencies occur in the first 8 or 9 months of life—for example, in vocal turn taking, perceptual learning, gestural and indexical gaze behavior—or 1 or 2 months later in the infant's processing and display of vocal behaviors during the systemic phase.

As functional neuroimaging becomes increasingly available as a research tool, it will be possible to ask whether language-listening experience activates the same neural sites in children suspected of primary grammatical deficits and equally delayed children who are thought to have primary deficits of social cognition. The neural and cognitive implications of the stimulus material and processing requirement will be critical in such tests, as will the developmental phase at the time of observation. But even if images of the brain are consulted, the challenges to the developmental psycholinguist will be the same: Find the behaviors that produce the groups, and find the stimuli that produce the behaviors.

REFERENCES

Abler, W.L. (1989). On the particulate principle of self-diversifying systems. *Journal of Social and Biological Structure, 12,* 1–13.

Antinucci, F. (1990). The comparative study of cognitive ontogeny in four primate species. In S.T. Parker & K.R. Gibson (Eds.), *"Language" and intelligence in monkeys and apes: Comparative developmental perspectives* (pp. 157–171). New York: Cambridge University Press.

Aram, D.M., Ekelman, B.L., & Nation, J.E. (1984). Preschoolers with language disorders: 10 years later. *Journal of Speech and Hearing Research, 27,* 232–244.

Bates, E., Bretherton, I., & Snyder, L. (1988). *From first words to grammar: Individual differences and dissociable mechanisms.* Cambridge, England: Cambridge University Press.

Bates, E., Dale, P.S., & Thal, D. (1994). Individual differences and their implications for theories of language development. In P. Fletcher & B. MacWhinney (Eds.), *Handbook of child language* (pp. 96–151). Oxford, England: Basil Blackwell.

Bickerton, D. (1995). *Language and human behaviour.* London: UCL Press.

Bishop, D.V.M., & Edmundson, A. (1987a). Language-impaired 4-year-olds: Distinguishing transient from persistent impairment. *Journal of Speech and Hearing Disorders, 52,* 156–173.

Bishop, D.V.M., & Edmundson, A. (1987b). Specific language impairment as a maturational lag: Evidence from longitudinal data on language and motor development. *Developmental Medicine and Child Neurology, 29,* 442–459.

Boysson-Bardies, B., Vihman, M.M., Rough-Hellichius, L., Durand, C., Landberg, I., & Arao, F. (1992). Material evidence of infant selection from the target language: A cross-linguistic phonetic study. In C. Ferguson, L. Menn, & C. Stoel-Gammon (Eds.), *Phonological development: Models, research, implications* (pp. 369–392). Timonium, MD: York Press.

Brothers, L. (1990). The social brain: A project for integrating primate behavior and neurophysiology in a new domain. *Concepts in Neuroscience, 1,* 27–51.

Browman, C.P., & Goldstein, L. (1989). Articulatory gestures as phonological units. *Phonology, 6,* 201–251.

Clahsen, H. (1989). The grammatical characterization of developmental dysphasia. *Linguistics, 27,* 897–920.

Clark, A. (1987). The kludge in the machine. *Mind and Language, 2,* 277–300.

Cosmides, L., & Tooby, J. (1987). From evolution to behavior: Evolutionary psychology as the missing link. In J. Dupré (Ed.), *The latest on the best: Essays on evolution and optimality* (pp. 277–306). Cambridge, MA: MIT Press.

Cosmides, L., & Tooby, J. (1994). Origins of domain specificity: The evolution of functional organization. In L.A. Hirschfeld, & S.A. Gelman (Eds.), *Mapping the mind: Domain specificity in cognition and culture* (pp. 85–116). Cambridge, England: Cambridge University Press.

Craig, H.K., & Evans, J.L. (1989). Turn exchange characteristics of SLI children's simultaneous and nonsimultaneous speech. *Journal of Speech and Hearing Disorders, 54,* 334–347.

Craig, H.K., & Evans, J.L. (1993). Pragmatics and SLI: Within-group variations in discourse behaviors. *Journal of Speech and Hearing Research, 36,* 777–789.

Craig, H.K., & Washington, J.A. (1993). Access behaviors of children with specific language impairment. *Journal of Speech and Hearing Research, 36,* 322–337.

D'Odorico, L. (1996, April). *Continuity and discontinuity in the transition between prelinguistic communication and language.* Paper presented at the Second European Research Conference on the Development of Sensory, Motor and Cognitive Abilities in Early Infancy: Antecedents of Language and the Symbolic Function, San Feliu de Guixois, Spain.

Dunbar, R.I.M. (1993). Coevolution of neocortical size, group size and language in humans. *Behavioral and Brain Sciences, 16,* 681–694.

Dunst, C.J. (1990). Sensorimotor development of infants with Down syndrome. In D. Cicchetti & M. Beeghly (Eds.), *Children with Down syndrome: A developmental perspective* (pp. 180–230). Cambridge, England: Cambridge University Press.

Felsenfeld, S., Broen, P.A., & McGue, M. (1992). A 28-year follow-up of adults with a history of moderate phonological disorder: Linguistic and personality results. *Journal of Speech and Hearing Research, 35,* 1114–1125.

Gopnik, M., & Crago, M. (1991). Familial aggregation of a developmental language disorder. *Cognition, 39,* 1–50.

Greenfield, P.M. (1991). Language, tools and brain: The ontogeny and phylogeny of hierarchically organized sequential behavior. *Behavioral and Brain Sciences, 14,* 531–595.

Greenspan, S.I. (1992). *Infancy and early childhood: The practice of clinical assessment and intervention with emotional and developmental challenges.* Madison, CT: International Universities Press.

Hobson, R.P. (1993). *Autism and the development of mind.* East Sussex, England: Lawrence Erlbaum Associates.

Humboldt, W. von. (1972). *Linguistic variability and intellectual development* (G.C. Buck & F.A. Raven, trans.). Philadelphia: University of Pennsylvania Press. (Original work published 1836)

Jacob, F. (1982). *The possible and the actual.* New York: Pantheon.

Jusczyk, P.W., Friederici, A.D., Wessels, J.M.I., Svenkerud, V.Y., & Jusczyk, A.M. (1993). Infants' sensitivity to the sound patterns of native language words. *Journal of Memory and Language, 32,* 402–420.

Karmiloff-Smith, A., Klima, E., Bellugi, U., Grant, J., & Baron-Cohen, S. (1995). Is there a social module? Language, face processing, and theory of mind in individuals with Williams syndrome. *Journal of Cognitive Neuroscience, 7,* 196–208.

Klackenberg, G. (1980). What happens to children with retarded speech at 3? *Acta Paediatrica Scandinavica, 69,* 681–685.

Landau, W.U., & Kleffner, F.R. (1957). Syndrome of acquired aphasia with convulsive disorder in children. *Neurology, 7,* 523–530.

Lewis, B.A., & Freebairn, L. (1992). Residual effects of preschool phonology disorders in grade school, adolescence, and adulthood. *Journal of Speech and Hearing Research, 35,* 819–831.

Locke, J.L. (1983). *Phonological acquisition and change.* New York: Academic Press.

Locke, J.L. (1992). Neural specializations for language: A developmental perspective. *Seminars in the Neurosciences, 4,* 425–431.

Locke, J.L. (1993). *The child's path to spoken language.* Cambridge, MA: Harvard University Press.

Locke, J.L. (1994). Gradual emergence of developmental language disorders. *Journal of Speech and Hearing Research, 37,* 608–616.

Locke, J.L. (1995). Linguistic capacity: An ontogenetic theory with evolutionary implications. In E. Zimmerman, J. Newman, & U. Jurgens (Eds.), *Current topics in primate vocal communication* (pp. 253–272). New York: Plenum.

Locke, J.L. (1996). Why do infants begin to talk? Language as an unintended consequence. *Journal of Child Language, 23,* 251–268.

Locke, J.L. (1997). A theory of neurolinguistic development. *Brain and Language, 58,* 265–326.

Locke, J.L. (1998). *The de-voicing of society: Why we don't talk to each other anymore.* New York: Simon & Schuster.

Locke, J.L. (in press a). Social sound-making as a precursor to spoken language. In J.R. Hurford, M. Studdert-Kennedy, & C. Knight (Eds.), *Approaches to the evolution of language: Social and cognitive bases.* Cambridge, England: Cambridge University Press.

Locke, J.L. (in press b). Towards a biological science of language development. In M. Barrett (Ed.), *The development of language.* Hove, England: Psychology Press.

Mandel, D.R., Jusczyk, P.W., & Pisoni, D.B. (1995). Infants' recognition of the sound patterns of their own names. *Psychological Science, 6,* 314–317.

Marchman, V.A., & Bates, E. (1994). Continuity in lexical and morphological development: A test of the critical mass hypothesis. *Journal of Child Language, 21,* 339–366.

Marcus, G.F. (1995). Children's overregularization of English plurals: A quantitative analysis. *Journal of Child Language, 22*, 447–459.

Marcus, G.F., Pinker, S., Ullman, M., Hollander, M., Rosen, T.J., & Xu, F. (1992). Overregularization in language acquisition. *Monograph of the Society for Research in Child Development, 57*(Serial No. 228).

Masur, E.F. (1995). Infants' early verbal imitation and their later lexical development. *Merrill-Palmer Quarterly, 41*, 286–306.

Mayr, E. (1974). Teleological and teleonomic: A new analysis. *Boston Studies in the Philosophy of Science, 14*, 91–117.

Miller, G.A. (1990). The place of language in a scientific psychology. *Psychological Science, 1*, 7–14.

Mirak, J., & Rescorla, L. (1997). *Phonetic skills and vocabulary size in late talkers: Concurrent and predictive relationships.* Manuscript submitted for publication.

Morris, D. (1967). *The naked ape: A zoologist's study of the human animal.* New York: McGraw-Hill.

Oller, D.K. (1995, December). *Emerging theories of etiology in specific language disorders.* Paper presented at American Speech-Language-Hearing Association, Orlando, FL.

Paul, R., & Alforde, S. (1993). Grammatical morpheme acquisition in 4-year-olds with normal, impaired and late-developing language. *Journal of Speech and Hearing Research, 36*, 1271–1275.

Paul, R., & Jennings, P. (1992). Phonological behavior in toddlers with slow expressive language development. *Journal of Speech and Hearing Research, 35*, 99–107.

Paul, R., Looney, S.S., & Dahm, P.S. (1991). Communication and socialization skills at ages 2 and 3 in "late-talking" young children. *Journal of Speech and Hearing Research, 34*, 858–865.

Paul, R., & Riback, M. (1993, June). *Sentence structure development in late talkers.* Poster presentation at the Symposium for Research in Child Language Disorders, Madison, WI.

Paul, R., & Shiffer, M.E. (1991). Communicative initiations in normal and late-talking toddlers. *Applied Psycholinguistics, 12*, 419–431.

Paul, R., & Smith, R.L. (1993). Narrative skills in 4-year-olds with normal, impaired, and late-developing language. *Journal of Speech and Hearing Research, 36*, 592–598.

Piatelli-Palmarini, M. (1989). Evolution, selection and cognition: From "learning" to parameter setting in biology and the study of language. *Cognition, 31*, 1–44.

Pinker, S. (1994). *The language instinct: The new science of language and mind.* London: Penguin Press.

Pinker, S. (1995). Facts about human language relevant to its evolution. In J.-P. Changeux & J. Chavaillon (Eds.), *Origins of the human brain* (pp. 262–283). Oxford, England: Clarendon Press.

Pinker, S., & Bloom, P. (1990). Natural language and natural selection. *Behavioral and Brain Sciences, 13*, 707–784.

Premack, D., & Woodruff, G. (1978). Does the chimpanzee have a theory of mind? *Behavioral and Brain Sciences, 4*, 515–526.

Rescorla, L. (1989). The language development survey: A screening tool for delayed language in toddlers. *Journal of Speech and Hearing Disorders, 54*, 587–599.

Rescorla, L., & Ratner, N.B. (1996). Phonetic profiles of toddlers with specific expressive language impairment (SLI-E). *Journal of Speech and Hearing Research, 39*, 153–165.

Rice, M.L., Wexler, K., & Cleave, P.L. (1995). Specific language impairment as a period of extended optional infinitive. *Journal of Speech and Hearing Research, 38*, 850–863.

Savage-Rumbaugh, E.S., Murphy, J., Sevcik, R.A., Brakke, K.E., Williams, S.L., & Rumbaugh, D.M. (1993). Language comprehension in ape and child. *Monographs of the Society for Research on Child Development, 58*(Serial No. 233).

Smith-Lock, K.M. (1993). Morphological analysis and the acquisition of morphology and syntax in specifically-language-impaired children. *Haskins Laboratories Status Report on Speech Research, SR-144,* 113–138.

Snow, C.E. (1989). Imitativeness: A trait or a skill? In G.E. Speidel & K.E. Nelson (Eds.), *The many faces of imitation in language learning.* New York: Springer-Verlag.

Stoel-Gammon, C. (1989). Prespeech and early speech development of two late talkers. *First Language, 9,* 207–224.

Studdert-Kennedy, M. (1991). Language development from an evolutionary perspective. In N.A. Krasnegor, D.M. Rumbaugh, R.L. Schiefelbusch, & M. Studdert-Kennedy (Eds.), *Language acquisition: Biological and behavioral determinants* (pp. 5–24). Hillsdale, NJ: Lawrence Erlbaum Associates.

Tallal, P., Ross, R., & Curtiss, S. (1989). Familial aggregation in specific language impairment. *Journal of Speech and Hearing Disorders, 54,* 167–173.

Thal, D., Oroz, M., & McCaw, V. (1995). Phonological and lexical development in normal and late talking toddlers. *Applied Psycholinguistics, 16,* 407–424.

Thal, D., Tobias, S., & Morrison, D. (1991). Language and gesture in late talkers: A one-year follow-up. *Journal of Speech and Hearing Research, 34,* 604–612.

Thelen, E. (1991). Motor aspects of emergent speech: A dynamic approach. In N.A. Krasnegor, D.M. Rumbaugh, R.L. Schiefelbusch, & M. Studdert-Kennedy (Eds.), *Language acquisition: Biological and behavioral determinants* (pp. 339–362). Hillsdale, NJ: Lawrence Erlbaum Associates.

Thelen, E., & Fogel, A. (1989). Toward an action-based theory of infant development. In J. Lockman & N. Hazen (Eds.), *Action in a social context: Perspectives on early development.* New York: Plenum.

Tomasello, M., & Farrar, M.J. (1986). Joint attention and early language. *Child Development, 57,* 1454–1463.

Tomasello, M., Savage-Rumbaugh, S., & Kruger, A.C. (1993). Imitative learning of actions on objects by children, chimpanzees, and enculturated chimpanzees. *Child Development, 64,* 1688–1705.

Tomblin, B. (1996, June). *The big picture of SLI: Results of an epidemiologic study of SLI among kindergarten children.* Paper presented at the 17th Annual Symposium on Research in Child Language Disorders, Madison, WI.

Tomblin, J.B., Freese, P.R., & Records, N.L. (1992). Diagnosing specific language impairment in adults for the purpose of pedigree analysis. *Journal of Speech and Hearing Research, 35,* 832–843.

Vargha-Khadem, F., Watkins, K., Alcock, K., Fletcher, P., & Passingham, R. (1995). Praxic and nonverbal cognitive deficits in a large family with a genetically transmitted speech and language disorder. *Proceedings of the National Academy of Sciences of the United States of America, 92,* 930–933.

Waddington, C.H. (1953). Genetic assimilation of an acquired character. *Evolution, 7,* 118–126.

Werker, J.F., & Polka, L. (1993). Developmental changes in speech perception: New challenges and new directions. *Journal of Phonetics, 21,* 83–101.

Wilkins, W.K., & Wakefield, J. (1995). Brain evolution and neurolinguistic preconditions. *Behavioral and Brain Sciences, 18,* 161–226.

4

Comorbidity of
Speech-Language Disorder
Implications for a
Phenotype Marker for Speech Delay

Lawrence D. Shriberg and Diane Austin

COMORBIDITY, AS DEFINED IN AN epidemiological context, refers to "disease(s) that coexist in a study participant in addition to the index condition that is the subject of the study" (Last, 1988, p. 28). Information on the comorbidity of diseases within individuals is used by public health researchers and health care providers. For research purposes, comorbidity data can provide unique, descriptive, explanatory perspectives on the nature and origins of diseases, possibly leading to hypotheses about etiologic processes and alternative forms of treatment. For example, insights about the nature of a newly identified disease might be gained if comorbidity data indicated that it frequently co-occurred in individuals with a related and well-described disease. For applied concerns, comorbidity data guide health care providers in allocating the resources needed to identify and serve people with the co-occurring disorders in question. Thus, as a special type of epidemiological data, comorbidity information has the potential to significantly contribute to the study, treatment, and prevention of disease.

This chapter examines data on the comorbidity of two relatively prevalent public health concerns: child speech disorders and child language disorders. The focus is on measurement issues in child speech disorders, specifically on the potential contributions of comorbidity data to the goal of identifying a phe-

This chapter was supported by Grants DC00496, DC00528, and DC02746 from the National Institute on Deafness and Other Communication Disorders, National Institutes of Health.

The authors express sincere thanks to the following colleagues and collaborators, who provided subject data, research assistance, and research guidance at different stages of this project: Phil Connell, Karen Cruickshanks, Rebecca Hinke, Joan Kwiatkowski, Barbara Lewis, Jane McSweeny, Carmen Rasmussen, Dennis Ruscello, Bruce Tomblin, Catherine Trost-Steffen, Dee Vetter, Carol Widder, and Xuyang Zhang.

notype marker for a genetically transmitted form of child speech disorders. Do comorbidity data suggest strong speech–language associations, supporting the likelihood of a common phenotype marker at a processing level that does not involve productive speech? Alternatively, do they suggest significant independence of the two disorders, which would support the need for a phenotype involving speech production? These issues relate to the general focus of this volume, that is, ways in which speech and language converge or diverge in development and disorders.

To appreciate historical, theoretical, and methodological perspectives on this issue, this chapter begins with a brief overview of research in child speech disorders and some background in contemporary speech-genetics research. A sample of available comorbidity data on speech-language disorders is then examined. The third section reviews a classification system for child speech disorders developed specifically for etiology studies, including genetics research. The fourth section is a presentation of results from four comorbidity studies using the new classification system. Findings suggest that the comorbidity of speech-language disorders is lower than previously reported, supporting a perspective that an autonomous phenotype for speech disorders is a valid need in speech-genetics research. As is discussed, findings also support a greater divergence of at least the productive aspects of phonological development and disorder relative to language development and disorder.

DEVELOPMENTAL PHONOLOGICAL DISORDERS

This section provides an overview of nosology and research trends in child speech disorders. Also discussed are relevant issues in speech-genetics research.

Nosology

Child speech disorders is the suggested cover term for all speech-sound disorders occurring during the developmental period for speech acquisition, nominally from birth to 9 years. The most prevalent form of child speech disorders is referenced by a number of labels, including functional articulation disorder; developmental phonological disorder; hybrids such as articulation/phonological disorder; and less theoretically committed terms such as multiple phoneme disorder, speech delay, or intelligibility impairments. The discipline of communicative disorders continues to accommodate this multiplicity of terms at least in part because of the lack of theoretical clarity on the role of cognitive-linguistic, sensorimotor, and psychosocial substrates as original and/or maintaining causes of speech disorder. Whichever is the preferred term, this form of child speech disorder is distinguished from those forms for which causal origins have been identified (e.g., speech disorders associated with craniofacial dysmorphologies, sensorimotor impairments, pervasive developmental disabilities). As described in this chapter, the term *special populations* subsumes all developmental phonological disorders associated with known etiologies. The authors of this chapter use the term *developmental phonological disorder* (DPD) for the form of child speech disorder characterized by mild to severe speech involvement of unknown origin.

The terminological situation described is familiar to those involved in the study and treatment of language disorders in children, where a parallel literature on classification systems and alternative clinical-research labels includes equally lively dialogue (e.g., Aram, Morris, & Hall, 1993). It would be efficient to use *child language disorders* as the companion cover term to child speech disorders and, in turn, the term *developmental language disorder* (DLD) for children with language disorders of unknown origin. However, to avoid adding another term to the mix, we use the well-entrenched, albeit contentious, term *specific language impairment* (SLI) for children with DLD of unknown origin. In cases where researchers may not adhere to or provide information on inclusionary and exclusionary criteria associated with SLI, DLD is a useful cover and companion term to DPD.

Research Trends

A brief review of research in developmental phonological disorders suggests why there are few reliable data on the comorbidity of DPD and SLI (viz., DLD). For this purpose, the 60 years of research in developmental phonological disorders between 1930 and 1990 can be divided into two 30-year periods.

1930–1960 From approximately the 1930s through the 1950s, there was considerable research activity attempting to associate the origins of all forms of child speech disorders to clinical or subclinical (i.e., suspect) differences in children's speech-hearing mechanisms, cognitive-linguistic functions, or psychosocial processes. Although impressive gains were made in understanding why and how children in special populations had difficulties producing intelligible speech, syntheses of the classic studies of this period conclude that no single cause for DPD was identified (Bernthal & Bankson, 1993; Creaghead, Newman, & Secord, 1989; Shriberg, 1980; Stoel-Gammon & Dunn, 1985; Weiss, Gordon, & Lillywhite, 1987; Winitz, 1969; Winitz & Darley, 1980). A crucial methodological observation is that studies undertaken during this period treated DPD as a unitary disorder that varied in severity of involvement. That is, compared with theoretical perspectives and measurement approaches to phonological comprehension, phonological organization, and speech production in the 1990s, the measurement of both speech and language status in the studies of 1930–1960 reflected a limited sector of the relevant variables.

1960–1990 A second period of research, from approximately the 1960s to the late 1980s, was characterized by the absence of widespread programmatic explanatory studies of child speech disorders, both within special populations and in DPD. This period included paradigmatic research shifts to alternative methods for linguistic description of the speech of children with all forms of child speech disorders, regardless of etiology, and acquisition and treatment strategies stressing associationist psychology. Some theoretical evolutions from these linguistic and behaviorist lineages, respectively, are emerging nonlinear phonological theories that describe developmental phonological disorders (e.g., Bernhardt & Stemberger, 1997; Goldsmith, 1995; Schwartz, 1992) and emerging neural network models of speech-sound acquisition and performance (e.g., Menn, Markey, Mozer, & Lewis, 1993; Stemberger, 1992). Consistent with the explanatory levels in such frameworks, individual differences in distal causes (i.e., etiology) are not represented as relevant independent variables.

1990s The 1990s mark the onset of a third period of research in child speech disorders in which there is a notable return to studies directed at pathogenesis, including both distal and proximal causes, and to clinical subtyping. Among other putative etiologic origins of speech-language disorders, perhaps most promising is the possibility that there may be a familial form expressed as a genetically transmitted trait. As introduced previously, a crucial need in pursuit of this hypothesis is the development of one or more phenotype markers for use in behavioral and molecular genetics designs. The following discussion is an overview of the relevant issues.

Speech-Genetics Research

The hypothesis that genetic transmission is the distal origin of the most common form of a speech-language disorder has gained a significant base of support in classic and emerging findings using twin and familial aggregation designs (e.g., Arnold, 1961; Beitchman, Hood, & Inglis, 1992; Bishop, 1992; Bishop, North, & Donlan, 1995; Borges-Orsorio & Salzano, 1985; Felsenfeld, Broen, & McGue, 1992; Gopnik & Crago, 1991; Hurst, Baraitser, Auger, Grahm, & Norell, 1990; Ingram, 1959; Lahey & Edwards, 1995; Lewis, Cox, & Byard, 1993; Lewis, Ekelman, & Aram, 1989; Lewis & Thompson, 1992; Locke & Mather, 1989; Matheny & Bruggeman, 1973; Neils & Aram, 1986; Samples & Lane, 1985; Schuele & Rice, 1996; Shriberg & Kwiatkowski, 1994; Stromswold & Rifkin, 1996; Tallal, Ross, & Curtiss, 1989; Tallal, Townsend, Curtiss, & Wulfeck, 1991; Tomblin, 1989). The data on familial aggregation, for example, indicate that more than half of the children with SLI have at least one other family member with a history of speech-language and/or learning disorders (usefully termed SLLD in Lahey & Edwards, 1995), including the widely cited highest proportion of .77 reported by Tallal et al.

(1989). Whitehurst et al. (1991) did not find higher proportions of family members with SLLD in the families of the children they studied; but, as these authors pointed out, the probands were young children whose language involvements were limited to expressive language disorder. Perhaps the most significant finding in behavioral genetic studies was reported by Felsenfeld and Plomin (1997), who tested children followed in the Colorado Adoption Project. These authors examined speech outcomes in 156 adopted and non-adopted children at varying risk for speech disorder based on self-reported parental speech history. Children with an affected biological parent were significantly more likely to have a speech disorder (approximately three times the risk) compared with children raised by an affected parent and children with no parental history. Rice (1996) provides excellent coverage of the scope of genetic research in SLI, and Gilger (1995) provides an informative tutorial on genetic methods applied to communicative disorders.

As emphasized in all other areas of human genetics, the major methodological problem in speech-genetics research is the development of an appropriate phenotype (cf. Brzustowicz, 1996). The techniques for behavioral analysis of family and twin data and molecular analysis of tissue samples are increasingly accessible, including procedures to assess how the disorder is genetically transmitted and eventually the genetic coding for the disorder. It is the identification of a phenotype marker for speech-genetics research that presents the formidable challenge. Candidate markers are likely to arise from one of three sources:

1. Clinical diagnostic marker
2. Research diagnostic marker
3. Autonomous speech marker

Clinical Diagnostic Marker   It might turn out that one of the common diagnostic markers used to classify a child as having a speech disorder in educational or clinical environments, for example, a score on a standardized articulation test, will have the sensitivity and specificity required for a phenotype marker in genetics studies. Most behavioral genetics studies have used articulation test scores to identify affected children. When classification of probands or relatives is based on presence or absence of a disorder, the diagnostic marker provides only a qualitative index. Several of the diagnostic classifications in the Speech Disorders Classification System (SDCS) (Shriberg, 1993), described later in this chapter, could also serve as a qualitative phenotype marker. When a score or standardized score is used, a common practice in twin concordance studies, the diagnostic marker is a quantitative index (cf. Pennington, 1986). If the history of research in medical and psychiatric genetics is instructive for speech-language genetics, diagnostic markers taken directly from the clinic are not likely to have the sensitivity and specificity needed for genetics research (cf. Smith, Pennington, & DeFries, 1996; Tomblin, Freese, & Records, 1992).

Research Diagnostic Marker A second possibility is that speech and language measures will need to be developed or modified to identify a phenotype marker that meets behavioral and molecular genetics research needs. Some specific linguistic and psychometric needs for speech testing in multigenerational, multidialectal, and multicultural populations have been considered elsewhere (Shriberg, 1993). Potential phenotype markers may come from levels of speech processing other than natural speech production, especially processing levels that might claim closer association with developmental neurobiological processes (cf. Pennington, 1986). Thus, in addition to phenotypes based on productive speech errors on traditional citation form tasks (e.g., Felsenfeld et al., 1992) and conversational speech samples (e.g., Shriberg, 1993; Shriberg, Austin, Lewis, McSweeny, & Wilson, 1997a, 1997b), the speech-genetics and related literature includes potential phenotype markers based on auditory-processing tasks (cf. Farmer & Klein, 1995), speech perception (e.g., Boada et al., 1998), multisyllabic and nonsense word repetition tasks (e.g., Bishop, 1994; Lewis & Freebairn, 1992), and phonological awareness tasks (e.g., Bird, Bishop, & Freeman, 1995).

Autonomous Speech Marker A third possibility is that whichever the level of assessment, the phenotype for developmental phonological disorders might need to differ from markers associated with other verbal trait disorders. Such a marker might be called an autonomous speech phenotype to differentiate it from all processing markers that do not directly assess the speech signal. There are many places to look for such markers in relation to the developmental neurobiology of central and peripheral speech systems (Christman, 1995). Although academic and clinical disciplines treat developmental speech disorders and developmental language disorders as distinct entities for the purposes of diagnostic classification (cf. American Psychiatric Association, 1994), the distinction between speech processing and language processing is often blurred in genetics research.

Our own research focuses on the utility of identifying a phenotype marker of DPD in conversational speech. The primary constraint on such a marker is that it may no longer be available in people (i.e., relatives of probands) whose speech has normalized, that is, those who no longer have speech production errors. We are currently using acoustic analysis techniques to determine if markers for prior or continuing disorder might be retrievable at the level of subphonemic description. The magnitude of comorbidity estimates for co-occurring speech-language disorders should inform research among the three possibilities previously described. At least for a first approximation, the higher the comorbidity rates, the less likely the need for an autonomous speech phenotype.

Summary

The 1990s mark the onset of an exciting period in speech-language disorders in which there is a real possibility to learn why some children have significant difficulty acquiring speech and language. Toward that end, data on the co-morbidity of child speech and language disorders might provide important insights. Useful comorbidity research requires classification systems for the disorders under study and consensus on diagnostic criteria for each of the disorders. In a widely cited review and study of the prevalence of speech and language disorders, Beitchman, Nair, Clegg, and Patel stated, "The lack of a comprehensive classification system for speech and language disorders is . . . a serious barrier to developing useful and accurate prevalence estimates" (1986, p. 98). The following section describes a classification system for speech-sound disorders that is used in four new comorbidity studies described later in this chapter.

THE SPEECH DISORDERS CLASSIFICATION SYSTEM

The SDCS shown in Figure 1 was designed to classify speech disorders throughout the life span. It includes primary classification categories that account for number and type of speech errors, suspected etiological subtypes, and course of the disorder. The latter is particularly important in genetics research, as gene regulation issues affecting the onset of disorder may also underlie the relative time course of normalization and topographic changes within different time periods. The SDCS was first described in Shriberg (1993), updated in Shriberg (1994), and finalized in Shriberg et al. (1997b). Formally, the system is structured to reflect both descriptive classification (solid lines) and etiologic explanatory classification (dashed lines; cf. Shriberg, 1982). The eight boxes in the top two rows of Figure 1 indicate the major typological classifications in the SDCS system. Developmental phonological disorders subsumes two forms of child speech disorders: speech delay and residual errors. Speech delay subsumes four etiological subtypes, shown in dashed lines, as well as speech delays of known origin in special populations. Residual errors, the other form of a developmental phonological disorder, subsumes six descriptive subtypes.

The discussion in this section, which closely follows another description of the SDCS (Shriberg, 1997), highlights emerging research findings for the 20 classification categories that compose the SDCS portrayed in Figure 1. Preliminary prevalence estimates are included for each disorder classification, data that bear on comorbidity and phenotype issues. Especially for the reader less familiar with the speech side of the speech–language connection, this review provides a perspective on what was described prior to the 1990s as a monolithic functional articulation problem.

Normal and Normalized Speech

The upper-left-most box in Figure 1 includes two descriptive classifications, which accounts for the 20 SDCS classifications in 19 boxes. Speakers with normal speech for their age at assessment and no history of nonnormal speech are classified as having normal speech acquisition (NSA). The SDCS program uses tables of reference data and a set of inclusionary and exclusionary criteria to determine if a conversational speech sample from a speaker meets criteria for NSA (Shriberg, 1993; Shriberg et al., 1997b). People with documented histories of earlier speech delay are classified as having normalized speech acquisition. Longitudinal studies estimate 9 years as the approximate end point of the typical developmental period, with additional productive speech development at allophonic and prosodic levels occurring up to 12 years of age (cf. Shriberg, Gruber, & Kwiatkowski, 1994; Shriberg, Kwiatkowski, & Gruber, 1994). Another important point in time for biobehavioral development observed in our longitudinal studies appears to be 6 years of age, when 75% of children with speech delay normalize their speech disorders (i.e., are classified as NSA by the SDCS program) (Shriberg, Gruber, et al., 1994).

Nondevelopmental Speech Disorders and Speech Differences

The two right-most boxes in Figure 1 represent two categories of speech patterns in children or adults that either are not developmental in origin or are not appropriately classified as a speech disorder. Nondevelopmental speech disorders is an appropriate classification for all speech disorders that occur after the developmental period for speech, nominally 9 years of age. This classification includes the full scope of adult disorders, including those due to trauma, disease, and various physical and emotional illnesses. The study and treatment of adult-onset speech disorders is a complex topic, but differential diagnosis is not complicated by those speech-hearing mechanism, cognitive-linguistic, and psychosocial processes that are associated with children's growth and development.

The right-most classification in the first row of Figure 1 is a category for child and adult speakers with speech differences. This category includes all speech and prosody-voice differences that speakers might elect to modify, such as those associated with mastery of English as a second language or the speech and prosody-voice patterns of children or adults speaking an English vernacular. As indicated by the dashed line connecting this box to the others, the discipline of speech-language pathology clearly differentiates speech differences from speech disorders. However, because of the similarity in assessment and instructional techniques for differences and disorders, it is useful to tie this classification category to the categories of speech disorder in the SDCS. Service providers increasingly need information on the comorbidity of

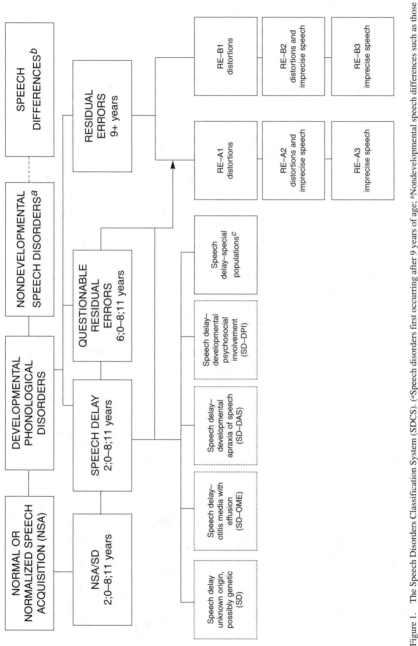

Figure 1. The Speech Disorders Classification System (SDCS). ([a]Speech disorders first occurring after 9 years of age; [b]Nondevelopmental speech differences such as those associated with cultural diversity and accent reduction; [c]Speech delay in special populations such as those associated with craniofacial and sensorimotor involvements.)

speech-language disorders in children from diverse linguistic and multicultural backgrounds.

Normal Speech Acquisition/Speech Delay

The need for a hybrid classification termed *normal* (or *normalized*) *speech acquisition/speech delay* (NSA/SD) is a familiar issue in epidemiologic research. Although accounting needs in service delivery systems typically require dichotomous classifications of people as either normal or affected, few diseases or disorders divide in this fashion. Especially if the underlying trait or disorder is continuously distributed in a population, arbitrary cutoff points yield children whose status is actually intermediate between normal and affected. An example is the procedure used to classify children in the Collaborative Perinatal Project of the National Institute of Neurological and Communicative Disorders and Stroke (NINCDS) (Lassman, Fisch, Vetter, & La Benz, 1980), discussed later in this chapter. Using statistical criteria not relevant here, researchers classified all speech, language, and hearing scores into three categories: normal, suspect, and abnormal. An intermediate category was needed for both initial identification of disorder and for classification preceding complete normalization of many disorders. Similarly, in addition to NSA and SD, the SDCS classification NSA/SD indicates status between normal or normalized speech acquisition and speech delay. As shown in Figure 1, children classified as NSA/SD may meet criteria for questionable residual errors (QREs) at 6 years of age, may normalize completely at any age up to 8 years, or may meet criteria for residual errors (REs) at 9 years of age if they continue to have speech errors.

The data in Figure 2 support the validity of NSA/SD as a classification category. These data are the SDCS classifications of 586 children whose conversational speech was sampled in several different studies (Shriberg, 1997). The metric used to assess speech in conversation, the Percentage of Consonants Correct–Revised (PCC–R), scores all correct sounds and distortion er-

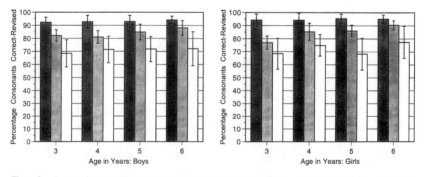

Figure 2. Age trends (means, standard deviations) for 3- to 6-year-old boys and girls classified by the SDCS as having normal or normalized speech acquisition (NSA), intermediate status (NSA/SD), or speech delay (SD). (■, normal speech acquisition; ▨, normal speech acquisition/speech delay; □, speech delay.)

rors as phonemically correct (Shriberg, Austin, et al., 1997a), with incorrect sounds including all phoneme deletions and substitutions. The means and standard deviation bars in Figure 2 indicate that the PCC–R scores differ for 3- to 6-year-old children classified as NSA, NSA/SD, and SD. The mean PCC–R scores for children classified as NSA/SD fall generally between the trends for NSA and SD at each age. The standard deviation bars also indicate good separation among the distributions for each classification group, suggesting that the scores of most children in this group fall in between the scores of most children in the other two groups. As described in the next section, we use the term *subclinical* as the diagnostic label for children classified as NSA/SD by the SDCS program. This classification is important in the comorbidity studies reported later in this chapter.

Speech Delay

Speech delay, or *SD*, has been proposed as the appropriate nosological term for the estimated 2%–3% of preschool children with a developmental phonological disorder of unknown origin (Leske, 1981). The SDCS classifies a child as having SD when age-inappropriate speech-sound deletions and/or substitutions occur in a conversational speech sample. As described, some children normalize SD by 6 years of age, some completely normalize between 6 and 8 years of age, some retain QRE from 6 to 8 years, and some retain residual errors after 9 years of age. Such different normalization histories might be important to the development of a behavioral phenotype for speech disorders, with gene-to-behavior pathways being a possible governing source for mechanisms underlying different normalization histories. In a study of language acquisition in which trends for heritability coefficients were higher in older monozygotic twin pairs, Stromswold and Rifkin (1996) suggested that the role of genetic factors in language acquisition may increase as children get older. From a methodological perspective, as considered in the studies reported later in this chapter, normalization rates play an important role in the interpretation of prevalence and comorbidity estimates.

The boxes subsumed under speech delay in Figure 1 comprise four proposed etiological subtypes of developmental phonological disorders and a classification for children in special populations with known causes. Information on the biolinguistic and sociolinguistic correlates of each disorder will inform research in the others, toward an eventual account of the origin and course of all child speech disorders. This section continues with brief comments on each of the proposed etiological subtypes; rationale and preliminary estimates of epidemiological and other nonspeech data (e.g., prevalence, gender ratio, language status, speech-sound normalization history, residual error status, familial aggregation) are provided in Shriberg (1994).

Speech Delay The most prevalent type of SD is simply termed *speech delay*. Based solely on a clinical database of approximately 350 children referred to a university phonology clinic for assessment or treatment of a phonological problem of unknown origin, a preliminary estimate is that this form of SD occurs in perhaps 60% of preschool children identified by speech-language pathologists as having a developmental phonological disorder (Shriberg, 1994). These are essentially the children whose case data and assessment results suggest no significant involvement in speech-mechanism, cognitive-linguistic, or psychosocial processes. That is, there is no one area of involvement or information in the case data that could be posited as a sufficient explanation for the presenting speech problem.

Emerging support for the possibility of a genetic origin for this form of a child speech disorder was cited previously. The primary source of evidence for genetic transmission of SD is the high prevalence of verbal trait impairments in nuclear and extended families of children with speech-language disorders. Studies have reported familial aggregation in 20% to nearly 60% of children (i.e., probands) ascertained on the basis of a speech-language disorder (cf. Felsenfeld, McGue, & Broen, 1995; Lahey & Edwards, 1995). The authors' data indicate that 56% of a sample of 84 children with SD had one or more family members with (or who previously had) the same speech problem (Shriberg & Kwiatkowski, 1994). For this proposed subtype of speech delay, the research challenges are to explicate the underlying neurolinguistic processing deficits and eventually the sociobiological origins of those deficits. In the context of this chapter, the focus is on the crucial importance for genetics studies of identifying the correct phenotype markers for SD.

Speech Delay–Otitis Media with Effusion   A second possible more proximal origin of speech delay is linguistic processing deficits associated with fluctuant conductive hearing loss due to early recurrent otitis media with effusion (i.e., speech delay–otitis media with effusion [SD–OME]). Many children referred to our speech clinic for suspected speech delay have had nearly continuous OME during some period of the first 3 years of life and beyond. The case histories of such children typically include ample evidence of fluctuant hearing loss in one or both ears. Analysis of two cohorts of children, one group followed in a university pediatrics clinic and another group followed in a Native American tribal health clinic, indicated that early recurrent OME is a significant risk factor for speech disorder (Shriberg, Flipsen, et al., 1997). Based on the percentage of children with SD in a university phonology clinic who have suspected SD–OME, a preliminary prevalence estimate is that this form of SD constitutes approximately 30% of preschool children with speech delay of unknown origin.

The language characteristics of children with SD–OME have yet to be compared with the language profiles of children with other forms of SD as well as with profiles for children with other forms of SLI. The auditory-perceptual consequences of fluctuant conductive hearing loss can be used to generate hypotheses about effects of OME and the acquisition of certain lexical and morphosyntactic forms. The primary finding is that SD–OME appears to be associated with reduced intelligibility, lower than expected for a child's speech status (Shriberg, Flipsen, et al., 1997). The intelligibility deficit is likely to reflect an interaction with language variables. Neither the prevalence nor the potentially unique speech-language consequences of this proposed subtype of SD (which, like the other suspected forms of SD, could also have unique distal genetic origins) can be estimated until one or more diagnostic markers for SD–OME are identified.

Speech Delay–Developmental Apraxia of Speech   A third possible subtype of SD shown in Figure 1 is a form suspected to resemble acquired apraxia of speech in adults. The acquired form of apraxia (adult apraxia of speech) meets criteria for one of the SDCS classifications aggregated within the category termed nondevelopmental speech disorder (see Figure 1). To be consistent with the most widely used term for this form of speech delay, the SDCS classification for this subtype is *speech delay–developmental apraxia of speech* (SD–DAS).

In a study series, we reported that approximately half of a total of 53 children with suspected DAS have inappropriate sentential stress (Shriberg, Aram, & Kwiatkowski, 1997). The specific pattern observed in this work and assessed in subsequent linguistic analyses (e.g., Velleman & Shriberg, 1997) is one of excessive-equal stress. This prosodic difference is proposed as a diagnostic marker for at least a subgroup of children with suspected SD–DAS. Inappropriate stress of the type coded in these studies is seldom observed in children acquiring speech typically or with any of the other suspected forms of SD shown in Figure 1. The reported high familial aggregation in suspected SD–DAS (Hall, Jordan, & Robin, 1993) suggests that this prosodic diagnostic marker might also serve as a phenotype marker. Using the same clinical population as previously cited, we estimate that children with this suspected subtype of SD compose 3%–5% of all children referred for a developmental speech disorder of unknown origin.

Speech Delay–Developmental Psychosocial Involvement   The fourth type of speech delay shown in Figure 1, speech delay–developmental psychosocial involvement (SD–DPI), is the most speculative of the SD subtypes in the SDCS. The proposal that psychosocial issues can be causally sufficient for speech delay is predicated on the observations of pioneer speech pathologists such as Charles Van Riper, Wendall Johnson, and Muriel Morley. Each of these perceptive clinical researchers has reported psychosocial needs in some children with speech delay. These observations are supported in several surveys (e.g., Baker & Cantwell, 1982; Beitchman, Nair, Clegg, & Patel, 1986) and follow-up studies (e.g., Shriberg & Kwiatkowski, 1988) documenting psychosocial needs in some children with suspected SD–DPI. Based solely on the authors' local clinical referral estimates, children with SD–DPI and/or some other form of SD compose approximately 7% of the remaining children referred for speech delay of unknown origin (i.e., SD: 60%; SD–OME: 30%; SD–DAS: 3%; SD–DPI and others: 7%).

There are only preliminary proposals for diagnostic markers for children with SD–DPI. A leading candidate is in the prosody-voice domain during discourse, the feature of speech that reflects affective states and traits. Children with suspected SD-DPI exhibit moment-to-moment variability in prosody-voice domains as well as retest variability on indices of segmental competence. Relative to language characteristics, some children with suspected SD–DPI seem to have considerable difficulty with the types of dyadic activities that most children like and from which they learn. As with each of the other proposed etiological subtypes, eventual validation of a subtype of speech delay associated with psychosocial issues would be presumed to have useful implications for the form and content of treatment.

Speech Delay–Special Populations The many special populations within the current scope of practice in speech pathology demand ever-increasing clinical competencies. Inclusion of this cover term for children with exceptional needs in addition to their speech needs emphasizes two considerations: 1) These children have developmentally related speech needs in addition to their unique speech involvements, and 2) clinical decision making for these children is informed by findings in other proposed subtypes of speech delay. This perspective also emphasizes the need for integrated speech-language research, as discussed in several chapters in this volume. However, much of the large-scale research in special populations since the 1970s has focused on either the speech domain or the language domain but seldom on both using well-developed methods in the same project. Thus, the inclusion of special populations in the SDCS encourages clinical–research rapprochement among all types of speech disorders and among speech-language domains in the same individual that too often are studied and treated as independent systems.

Questionable Residual Errors

During the period from ages 6 to 8 years, there is one other type of developmental speech disorder that a child can have in addition to SD or NSA/SD. The classification QRE is used for children who have one or more speech-sound distortions or common substitutions (e.g., distortions of fricatives or liquids, substitutions of /θ/ for /s/ or /w/ for /r/ and others), errors that do not meet SDCS criteria for SD or NSA/SD (which would require significant age-inappropriate deletions and substitutions). Some children with QRE could be children who normalized from SD or NSA/SD status, or, as shown in Figure 1, they could have no such history. The importance of this distinction in the time course of the disorder is discussed in the following section.

Residual Errors

As noted previously, speech errors may continue as the residuals of a speech delay, or they may occur without such histories. Residual errors is the classification for children and adults with speech-sound errors that are developmental in onset and persistent beyond 9 years of age, whereas QRE is the appropriate classification for children with articulatory errors occurring from the 6- to 8-year-old period when they may still normalize.

The SDCS has six subtypes of RE based on a speaker's history and error pattern. Speakers ages 9 years and older with histories of SD are classified as RE-A. Children or adults with speech errors but no history of speech delay are classified as RE-B. The three numbered RE subtypes in Figure 1 can be used to further classify error patterns first occurring during the developmental period. Those following a history of some form of SD are included in the A alternatives; those not associated with SD are included in the B alternatives. RE-A1 or RE-B1 is for residual common distortion errors (see Shriberg, 1993; Appendix). RE-A2 and RE-B2 are for residual common distortions and imprecise speech (omissions and substitutions). RE-A3 and RE-B3 are for imprecise speech. Although there are no reliable prevalence data, preliminary findings indicate that each of these error types occurs in adult speech (Shriberg et al., 1997b). In one study of 112 adult relatives of children identified as having speech errors, there were some notable gender trends for distortion errors (e.g., dentalized fricatives versus derhotacized /r/, /ɝ/, and /ɚ/) that persisted in all age groups, including speakers older than 50 years of age (Lewis & Shriberg, 1994). As observed elsewhere in our database studies, fricative distortions may be more prevalent in females and derhotacized /r/ and rhotic vowels more prevalent in males. For phenotype issues as well as more general questions about the origin of speech-sound distortions, large-scale studies of RE could be productive. Decreased articulatory precision, as it may first occur in some adult populations, would be classified in the first row in Figure 1 as a nondevelopmental speech disorder if associated with a disorder or specific event (e.g., stroke, traumatic brain injury); it would be classified as a speech difference if associated with typical aging.

What is important about children with RE and QRE is whether they should be included in a tabulation of people with speech disorders in prevalence or comorbidity studies. If they do not have an earlier history of SD, are such behavioral differences consistent with the genotype posited to underlie speech delay? Specifically, does RE reflect simply a less severe expression of the genes that code for SD, or do common distortions and substitutions arise from sources different than those posited to underlie SD? If considered the same disorder, are children who persist from QRE to RE more severely involved than children who normalize QRE, or do they differ in some qualitative way from children who normalize QRE during the developmental period?

These questions and the extended review of the SDCS were provided to highlight both the complexity and the importance of such detail for the speech side of the speech-language comorbidity research reviewed in the next section of this chapter.

COMORBIDITY OF SPEECH AND LANGUAGE DISORDERS

It is useful to begin a discussion of comorbidity (also termed *concomitant* [Paul, 1995] or *coexisting* [St. Louis, Ruscello, & Lundeen, 1992] disorders) with a brief review of some alternative ways to express the prevalence and comorbidity of diseases or disorders.

Prevalence Estimates

In genetics research, prevalence estimates for a disorder provide the unconditional probabilities or liabilities against which the prevalence of a disorder in a specific target group (e.g., an extended family) is compared. The prevalence percentage of a disorder or disease is computed by dividing the number of people positive for the disorder (i.e., affected) by the number of people in the population or population sample at that period of time, multiplying the result by 100 (e.g., 6 affected, 1,000 people: prevalence $=$ .6%). A prevalence rate expresses a similar concept, but it is referenced to a standard unit (e.g., 60 affected people per 10,000 people: prevalence rate $=$ .60). Prevalence percentages are typically used to describe a given sample or population, whereas prevalence rates are useful to estimate or compare health service needs in relation to population size. Burd, Hammes, Bornhoeft, and Fisher (1988) provided an example of an epidemiological study in communicative disorders that uses prevalence rates to estimate the number of people expected to be affected in a population of interest.

Comorbidity Estimates

Estimates of the comorbidity of speech disorders and language disorders are obtained in two ways, a possible source of confusion to the casual reader. One type of comorbidity percentage or comorbidity rate reflects the same information as a prevalence estimate obtained for a single disorder. The difference is that the statistic reflects people in the sample who are positive for two or more disorders. Thus, in addition to prevalence percentages for each disorder, an epidemiological study may provide a separate percentage or rate for the joint occurrence of disorders in the sample. Comorbidity percentages estimated in this way typically are relatively small in absolute magnitude and not too discrepant from the individual prevalence of each disorder.

The second and more frequently reported type of comorbidity estimate reflects the percentage of children identified as positive for one disorder who are also identified as positive for one or more other disorders. This is the definition of *comorbidity* given at the outset of this chapter and is likely to be of greater relevance for the issues raised in this chapter. The denominator for this second type of comorbidity estimate is the number of individuals affected with the first or index disorder, and the numerator is the number of those people positive for the second or other disorders. Continuing the previous examples, if 15 of 60 people positive for the index disorder or condition were also positive for another disorder, the comorbidity percentage would be 25%. For the reader interested in epidemiological method, Kahn and Sempos (1989), Khoury, Beaty, and Cohen (1993), and Last (1988) are useful references; for a brief explanation, see Streiner, Norman, and Munroe Blum (1989).

The generalizability and utility of both types of comorbidity estimates depend on the validity and reliability of the methods used to obtain the sample. Comorbidity estimates of the first type typically are undertaken on large samples, which requires testing protocols that are time and cost efficient. Comorbidity estimates of the second type are generally based on considerably smaller samples, typically convenience samples ascertained from available clinical sources or databases. Thus, they do not have the external validity associated with epidemiologic data. However, smaller sample sizes typically permit more detailed assessment data on either or both the index disorder and the other disorder, depending on the focus of the study. Even when based on a relatively small number of cases, well-developed comorbidity data of the second type can be quite useful to generate and test hypotheses.

A set of comorbidity estimates for speech and language disorders ideally should include both types of comorbidity estimates, with estimates of the second type being based on both language and speech as the index group. Although there are many available prevalence estimates individually for speech disorders and language disorders (see reviews in Beitchman, et al., 1986; Silva, 1987; Tomblin et al., in press; Tomblin, Records, & Zhang, 1996), there are few reported comorbidity data of either type.

Epidemiology Studies in the United States

It is important for future research planning to understand why detailed comorbidity data of the first type have not been obtained in each of the three large-scale epidemiologic projects on communicative disorders conducted in the United States.

The National Speech and Hearing Survey   The National Speech and Hearing Survey (NSHS; Hull, Mielke, Timmons, & Welleford, 1971) conducted in the 1960s randomly selected and assessed 38,884 children in first through twelfth grades in 100 school districts in nine U.S. census regions. Although spontaneous and imitative language samples were obtained on audiotape, there was no standardized measure of language considered appropriate for inclusion in the protocol at that time. St. Louis et al. (1992) provided a thorough historical and methodological description of the NSHS. Moreover, based on retranscription of a small sample of the original audiotapes, St. Louis and colleagues have completed comorbidity studies in several target disorders, including speech and language (see Table 1). The files and audiotapes have been archived, and interested researchers are invited to make arrangements to gain access to this substantial resource.

The NINCDS Collaborative Perinatal Project The massive nationwide NINCDS Collaborative Perinatal Project conducted in the 1970s (Lassman et al., 1980) assessed approximately 20,000 children at 3 years of age and again at age 8 years. Although the published volume of findings provides percentages for children classified as normal, suspect, and abnormal on many speech and language variables, the tables and figures do not provide or allow the reader to derive per-subject data on the comorbidity of speech-language in-

Table 1. Estimates of the comorbidity of speech and language disorders

Study	n	Mean age[a]	Comorbidity estimates by index disorder	
			Speech index	Language index
Paul (1993)	37	3[b]		37%
Whitehurst et al. (1991)	22	3		35
Connell, Elbert, and Dinnsen (1991)	23	4	43%	
Shriberg, Kwiatkowski, Best, Hengst, and Terselic-Weber (1986)	33	4	60	
Shriberg and Kwiatkowski (1994)	64	4	66	
Bishop and Edmundson (1987)	66	4[c]		74
Paul (1993)	37	4[b]		16
Tallal, Ross, and Curtiss (1989)	76	4		60
Bishop and Edmundson (1987)	67	4.5[c]		55
Shriberg et al. (1986)	38	5	50	
Bishop and Edmundson (1987)	68	5[c]		34
Tomblin (1996a)	862	5		25
Paul and Shriberg (1982)	30	6	66	
Shriberg and Kwiatkowski (1982)	43	6	77	
Schery (1985)	718	7	75[d]	75[d]
St. Louis, Ruscello, Grafton, and Hershman (1994)	20	7[e]	45	
St. Louis et al. (1994)	20	7[e]		65
Ruscello, St. Louis, and Mason (1991)	24	12.5	54[f]	
Ruscello et al. (1991)	24	12.5	21[g]	

[a] Ages rounded up at .5, unless mean age was provided within narrow age range
[b,c] Same children followed longitudinally
[d] No index disorder in this survey
[e] Estimated
[f] Classified as having delayed articulation
[g] Classified as having residual errors

volvement. D. Vetter (personal communication, February 1997) suggested that cross-tabulation output allowing for these comorbidity comparisons may still be accessible to the interested researcher.

Epidemiology of Specific Language Impairment Project   The Epidemiology of Specific Language Impairment (EpiSLI) study conducted in the 1990s (Tomblin, 1996a; Tomblin et al., in press) used stratified cluster sampling procedures to assess more than 7,000 kindergartners living in three midwestern areas. Estimates of the prevalence of speech disorder and comorbidity of speech and language disorders were not goals of this project. However, because the diagnostic protocol in the Iowa studies did include the Word Articulation subtest of the Test of Language Development–2: Primary (TOLD–P; Newcomer & Hammill, 1988), a 20-item single-word articulation test administered by imitation, it was possible for Tomblin and colleagues to provide a preliminary estimate of the comorbidity of language and speech disorders using a subsample of children in the EpiSLI study (comorbidity of the second type; see Table 1). Additional data from this project are presented in the final section of this chapter, including a description of the criteria used to define SLI.

Comorbidity Data: Studies and Findings

Table 1 is a sample of estimates of the comorbidity of speech and language disorders arranged by increasing age and the index disorder. Not all studies used the inclusionary and exclusionary criteria typically associated with SLI. Each of the studies in Table 1 used diagnostic markers based on natural or evoked speech production to classify children's speech status, rather than phonological processing tasks or challenging speech production tasks. The studies in Table 1 undoubtedly only sample the available estimates, but they do include those located in a reasonably wide literature search. Several are discussed in the monograph by St. Louis et al. (1992). Evaluative review of the studies generating the entries in Table 1 would extend beyond the scope of this chapter. The focus here is only on the implications of trends in Table 1 for phenotype issues in speech disorders. Three observations are of interest.

First, in comparison with studies that ascertained children by language disorder, studies in which the index disorder is speech appear to report somewhat higher comorbidity estimates. The average comorbidity of the 10 estimates in which children were ascertained by speech was 55.7%, whereas the average comorbidity of the 10 estimates based on language as the index disorder was 47.6%. Second, our own previous estimate of the percentage of preschool children with speech delays who also have a language disorder was 50%–75% (Shriberg & Kwiatkowski, 1994). Based on the studies in Table 1, using just the six studies of children ages 3–6 years with speech as the index disorder, the average is approximately 60%. The third and most important observation about the entries in Table 1 underscores the variability in estimates, even for children of the same age ascertained by the same index disorder and obtained in studies conducted by the same research group. Given the similarities in the subjects and speech-testing procedures in the five independent estimates from our own studies, ranging from 50% to 77%, it is likely that the sources for these differences are in the language domain, including differences in the language measures used in each study and in the criteria used to classify children as having language disorders.

Comorbidity Data: Some Preliminary Observations

It is challenging to speculate on what the comorbidity estimates in Table 1 might suggest about associations between speech and language disorders and their implications for a phenotype marker for speech disorders. After a presentation of findings from four comorbidity estimates in the next section of the chapter, we provide some summary observations. This section comments on three possible methodological explanations for the previous observations and makes one preliminary observation on implications for the phenotype issue.

First, on the issue of differences in comorbidity estimates based on index disorder, one explanation could invoke the concept of ascertainment bias. Shaywitz, Shaywitz, Fletcher, and Escobar (1990) provided a signal call for the possibility that the social-behavioral characteristics of children with dyslexia might bias prevalence rates and gender ratios when ascertainment was by clinical referral as opposed to population surveys. On similar grounds, comorbidity data obtained by clinical referral could also be biased by a number of social factors affecting sampling.

A second related possibility concerns possible differences in the impact of speech versus language disorders on the likelihood of clinical referral, an issue discussed by Tomblin (1996a). Tomblin noted that in comparison to the 7.4% prevalence of SLI found for kindergarten children in the EpiSLI Project, the generally lower SLI prevalence estimates from clinical referral studies could be due to the social salience of speech versus language disorders. The premise is that if a speech disorder is more noticeable than a language disorder, milder forms of language disorder might go unidentified unless co-occurring with a speech disorder. This hypothesis might be invoked to directly explain differences in prevalence estimates based on clinical referral, but it predicts the opposite of the present findings, that is, that comorbidity estimates were higher for those indexed by speech disorder. If severity of language disorder is at least moderately associated with severity of speech disorder, co-morbidity estimates for children ascertained by language disorder should be higher than when ascertained by speech disorder. That is, if language disorder is less salient than speech disorder, children who are identified as having a language disorder should be more severely involved and hence more likely to have a speech disorder.

A third possible explanation for the differences in estimates associated with index disorder could relate to differences in the normalization (i.e., recovery) rates of speech versus language disorders. This explanation is conditional on the validity of two assumptions. The first assumption is the same as for the second possibility—that the more severely involved a child is in one disorder, speech or language, the more likely the child is to be clinically involved at least to some degree in the other. The second assumption, based on data on typical speech and language acquisition, is that speech disorders normalize sooner than language disorders. If these two assumptions are valid, it would follow that the comorbidity rates for children with persistent speech disorder should be higher than for children with persisting language disorder, the trends observed in Table 1. That is, comorbidity is higher in children ascertained by speech disorder because only those who have not normalized are eligible for inclusion; such children have more severe speech involvement and hence are more likely also to retain language involvement.

Finally, measurement issues and possible biases notwithstanding, the data in Table 1 appear to support more independence between speech and language disorder than is generally reported, including discussions elsewhere in this volume. Comorbidity for speech-language disorders was less than 50% in 8 of the 20 comorbidity estimates in Table 1. Thus, a substantial number of children appear to have one disorder but not the other, at least at some time during the developmental period. As suggested at the outset of this chapter, if these findings are cross-validated in well-developed epidemiological studies, comorbidity data can generate useful hypotheses about shared and nonshared substrates of developmental speech disorder and developmental language disorder.

COMORBIDITY OF DPD AND SLI IN FOUR STUDY SAMPLES

The following is a preliminary report of four studies that address some of the methodological differences among studies noted in Table 1. First, the SDCS system is used in all four studies; therefore, speech status across studies is determined by the same criteria. Second, although language measures vary across studies, we provide detailed rationale for the definition of subclinical and clinical involvement for each measure, based primarily on the work of Lahey and Edwards (1995) and Tomblin et al. (1996). Third, we calculated comorbidity at the level of both clinical and subclinical involvement for both language and speech to allow a look at possible differences associated with severity of involvement. Fourth, we address possible contributions of gender to the magnitude of comorbidity estimates. Finally, to provide more detail on language variables, findings are arranged by language modality (i.e., receptive, expressive) and language domain (i.e., vocabulary, grammar, vocabulary/grammar).

Participants and Ascertainment Procedures

Table 2 is a summary of the gender, age, and speech status of 219 children in four study samples drawn from several projects. The number of children in each study ranged from 40 to 79, percentage of boys from approximately 62% to 68%, and mean age from approximately 4 to 6 years. In Studies 1, 2, and 3, children were ascertained by referral from speech-language pathologists asked to identify children with developmental speech disorders or intelligibility problems, regardless of language status. Children in Study 4 were identified as SLI in an epidemiological study of language disorders in kindergarten children. In each of the four studies, associated measures and case history data ensured that children were free of significant involvements of the speech and hearing mechanism, cognitive-linguistic function, or psychosocial processes. In keeping with the previous discussion on the importance of method in prevalence and comorbidity research, the following sections provide detailed information on subject ascertainment and measurement procedures.

Study 1 Study 1 included 58 of 64 children obtained by referral from speech-language pathologists in the Madison, Wisconsin, Metropolitan School District (cf. Shriberg & Kwiatkowski, 1994) for a descriptive study conducted in the mid-1980s. The six children not included in Study 1 did not meet criteria for NSA/SD or SD in the revised SDCS system.

Study 2 Study 2 included two cohorts of children (25 children in Cohort 1, 20 in Cohort 2) whose speech was assessed at 6-month intervals in the early 1990s until normalization (cf. Kwiatkowski & Shriberg, 1997; Shriberg, Gruber, & Kwiatkowski, 1994). Data are reported from the initial assessment of these children, who were also recruited by referral from clinicians in the Madison, Wisconsin, area. All 25 of the children in Cohort 1 and 17 of the children in Cohort 2 met revised SDCS criteria for NSA/SD or SD.

Study 3 Study 3 included 40 children from a collaborative study of familial aggregation of speech disorders initiated in the early 1990s (cf. Lewis & Shriberg, 1994). Children with speech delay were recruited through referrals from speech-language pathologists in the Cleveland, Ohio, area. Probands and nuclear family members received a speech and language assessment appropriate for their age. Of the original 53 probands whose speech was transcribed in our laboratory, 16 had speech errors that did not meet criteria for NSA/SD or SD at the time of conversational speech sampling. Five probands were excluded from this report because they did not meet age criteria for the TOLD–P (two were younger than age 4 years, one was older than age 7 years) or did not have subscores available. The 40 children reported here include 32 of the original 53 probands and eight 4- to 7-year-old siblings of probands meeting criteria for NSA/SD or SD in the revised SDCS system.

Study 4 Study 4 included 79 children classified as SLI in an epidemiological study of language disorders in kindergarten children conducted in Iowa and western Illinois (Tomblin et al., 1996). Conversational speech samples

Table 2. Descriptive statistics for children in four study samples, including age (in months), gender, and speech characteristics (subclinical, clinical)

	Speech Status																							Total														
	Subclinical												Clinical																									
	Male				Female				Both				Male				Female				Both				Male				Female				Both			
			Age				Age			Age				Age				Age			Age				Age				Age			Age	
Study	n	%	M	SD	n	%	M	SD	n	M	SD	n	%	M	SD	n	%	M	SD	n	M	SD	n	%	M	SD	n	%	M	SD	n	M	SD
1	9	64.3	53.0	8.7	5	35.7	54.0	4.5	14	53.4	7.3	28	63.6	50.8	9.2	16	36.4	49.0	7.8	44	50.1	8.7	37	63.8	51.3	9.0	21	36.2	50.2	7.4	58	50.9	8.4
2[a]	5	71.4	47.8	4.5	2	28.6	45.0	2.8	7	47.0	4.1	23	65.7	48.3	7.6	12	34.3	48.9	5.9	35	48.5	7.0	28	66.7	48.2	7.1	14	33.3	48.4	5.6	42	48.3	6.6
3	10	58.8	65.3	16.7	7	41.2	74.3	15.8	17	69.0	16.5	17	73.9	60.5	11.2	6	26.1	59.0	9.0	23	60.1	10.5	27	67.5	62.3	13.4	13	32.5	67.2	14.9	40	63.9	13.9
4[b]	—				—				—			—				—				—			49	62.0	71.8	3.6	30	38.0	70.8	4.3	79	71.4	3.9
All	24	64.8	55.4		14	35.2	57.8		38	56.5		68	67.7	53.2		34	32.3	52.3		102	52.9		141	65.0	58.4		78	35.0	59.2		219	58.6	

M, mean; SD, standard deviation.

[a] Study 2 includes two cohorts of children followed prospectively (see text).

[b] Study 4 subjects were selected on the basis of language disorder rather than speech (see text). The numbers of children with speech involvement are reported in Figure 4.

were obtained from a randomly selected subsample of children from the epidemiology project: 6 speech samples from the pilot phase of this study and 73 speech samples from two study cohorts collected in successive years of the project. Five additional speech samples were excluded because transcripts could not be classified reliably (too few usable words) by the SDCS program.

Conversational Speech Sampling and Classification of Speech Status

Conversational speech samples were obtained from each child in each study using a standard protocol followed by all research collaborators to maximize technical quality and linguistic productivity (Shriberg, 1993). High-quality monaural audiocassette recorders, matching external microphones, and high-quality audiocassette tapes were used, with microphone-to-lip distance monitored at 15 centimeters. Children were asked to discuss favorite home and school activities and recent events. For some children, pictures were used to suggest topics. Examiners verbally glossed speech that was likely to be unintelligible to transcribers, following a protocol that was minimally intrusive to the child. The average number of utterances per sample was 68 (Study 1, 78; Study 2, 147; Study 3, 77; Study 4, 46).

All speech samples were transcribed by one of three research transcriptionists trained in systems for narrow phonetic transcription (Shriberg & Kent, 1995), consensus transcription (Shriberg, Kwiatkowski, & Hoffmann, 1984), and formatting transcripts for computer analysis (Shriberg, 1986). Research assistants entered transcripts in the PEPPER program (Shriberg, 1986) running in a VAX environment. The SDCS program, which was included in the suite of PEPPER analyses, classified the sample as a variant of NSA, QRE, NSA/SD, or SD. For our purposes, additional information from the SDCS system (i.e., subclassifications not described in the previous review) was collapsed to yield two clinical classification groups: subclinical speech disorder and clinical speech disorder. The subclinical group included children classified as NSA/SD, and the clinical group included children classified as SD. Children classified as NSA or QRE were included only in Study 4.

Classification of Language Status

As previously discussed, definitions of language involvement have included varying measures of language domains and modalities and varying cutoff scores to index disorder. Commonly used cutoff criteria for clinical involvement on standardized language tests include a range of scores from 1 to 1.3 standard deviation units below the mean. For example, Lahey and Edwards (1995) used a score 1.3 standard deviation units below the mean to define clinical involvement, whereas Lewis et al. (1993) used 1 standard deviation below the mean to define clinical involvement. In Tomblin et al. (1996), z scores below -1.25 in two of five areas of language performance were found to yield the greatest sensitivity and specificity based on concurrent validity assessment using the Iowa Severity Rating Scales (Jeffrey & Freilinger, 1986).

Children in these four study samples were given tests of both receptive and expressive language modalities, with vocabulary and grammar domains evaluated in separate subtests or combined in a single test or score. The children in Study 4 also were given a measure of narrative comprehension and production. Table 3 includes a list of the measures used in the four studies and the criteria used to code language status. Each study used a different set of language measures, including standardized measures and analysis of the conversational speech sample to assign structural stage. Standardized measures differed in the way scores were calculated and reported, with most measures using normal curve equivalents (i.e., z scores, standard scores, percentile scores), others using age-equivalent scores, and structural stage expressed as a difference between the expected and emerging stage.

For each of the language measures in Table 3, a score of 1.25 standard deviation units below the mean (whether expressed as a z score, standard score, or percentile score) was adopted as the scoring criteria for clinical involvement for all measures that provided a score of that type, which was consistent with the scoring criteria for Study 4. For measures whose reference data provide only age-level scores, a 1-year or greater delay was considered clinical involvement, with a two-stage gap between the emerging and expected structural stage also considered clinical involvement. To retain maximum sensitivity to language problems, scores that were greater than 1 and less than 1.25 standard deviation units below the mean were classified as reflecting subclinical involvement for a measure. For measures providing age-level scores, greater than 6-month and less than 1-year delays were considered subclinical involvement, with a one-stage gap between emerging and expected structural stage also considered subclinical involvement. To present information consistently across studies, an ordinal coding system was developed to index normal language, subclinical involvement, or clinical involvement on each language measure. (See the Appendix to this chapter for additional subject and language classification information for each of the four studies.)

Subtypes of Language Disorders

Subtypes of language disorders (i.e., receptive only versus expressive only versus both receptive and expressive) are of interest in most studies of developmental language disorders. A variety of criteria have been used to define subtypes. For example, Lahey and Edwards (1995) defined an *expressive only disorder* by requiring all scores from receptive measures to be within 1 standard deviation of the mean, two measures of expressive language to be −1.3 standard deviation units or more below the mean, and the difference between the expressive and receptive language scores to be greater than 2 standard errors of measurement of the difference. Although the rationale for this model is

Table 3. Language measures reported for the four study samples and criteria used to code language status

Measure	Study 1	Study 2	Study 3	Study 4	Modality Receptive	Modality Expressive	Domain Vocabulary	Domain Grammar	Coding criteria[a] A	Coding criteria[a] B	Coding criteria[a] C	Coding criteria[a] D
Peabody Picture Vocabulary Test–Revised (PPVT–R) (Dunn & Dunn, 1981)	X	X			X		X		X			
Preschool Language Scale (PLS) (Zimmerman, Steiner, & Pond, 1979)	X				X		X	X		X		
Structural Stage (StruSt)[b] (Miller, 1981; Miller & Chapman, 1986; Paul & Shriberg, 1982)	X	X				X		X			X	
Test for Auditory Comprehension of Language–Revised (TACL–R)[c] (Carrow-Woolfolk, 1985)												
Elaborated Sentences (TALC–ES)		X			X			X	X			
Grammatical Morphemes (TACL–GM)		X			X			X	X			
Word Classes and Relations (TACL–WC)		X			X		X		X			
Sequenced Inventory of Communication Development (SICD)[d] (Hedrick, Prather, & Tobin, 1975)		X			X		X	X			X	
Test of Language Development–2: Primary (TOLD–2) (Newcomer & Hammill, 1988)												

Subtest[e]				
Grammatic Completion (TOLD–GC)	X		X	X	X
Grammatic Understanding (TOLD–GU)	X		X	X	X
Picture Vocabulary (TOLD–PV)	X		X	X	
Sentence Imitation (TOLD–SI)	X		X		
Quotients					
Listening Quotient (TOLD–LiQ)	X	X	X	X	X
Speaking Quotient (TOLD–SpQ)	X	X		X	X
Spoken Language Quotient (TOLD–SLQ)	X		X	X	X

[a] Coding criteria:

A   *Normal:*   z score −1.0 or higher, standard score 85 or higher, or 16th percentile or higher

     Subclinical: z score between −1.25 and −1.0 (exclusive), standard score of 82–84, or 11th–15th percentile

     Clinical: z score −1.25 and lower, standard score 81 and lower, or 10th percentile or lower

B   *Normal:*   Scored 6 months below age level or higher

     Subclinical: Scored more than 6 months but less than 1 year below age level

     Clinical: Scored 1 year or more below age level

C   *Normal:*   Emerging stage at or above expected stage

     Subclinical: Emerging stage one stage below expected stage

     Clinical: Emerging stage two or more stages below expected stage

[b] Structural stage was evaluated for all children in Cohort 1 and all 3-year-old children in Cohort 2 (N = 33).

[c] TACL–R subtests were given to subjects ages 3 and older in Cohort 1 (N = 23).

[d] SICD was given to subjects younger than age 3 years in Cohort 1 (N = 2).

[e] TOLD was given to subjects ages 4 years and older in Cohort 2 (N = 10). The TOLD Oral Vocabulary subtest was also given but is not reported here, because it was the only independent measure of expressive vocabulary in the four studies.

attractive, the variety of measures used in Studies 1–3 did not allow us to use differences between receptive and expressive scores. Instead of focusing on subtypes, we have focused on Modality × Domain performance on individual measures. In Table 3, each measure is classified by modality (i.e., receptive, expressive, both) and domain (i.e., vocabulary, grammar, both). In the following discussion of findings, subclinical or clinical involvement in a Modality × Domain category is defined by the most severe involvement (i.e., normal, subclinical, clinical) on any measure in that category. For example, some children in Study 2 received both the Peabody Picture Vocabulary Test–Revised (PPVT–R) (Dunn & Dunn, 1981) and the Word Classes and Relations subtest of the Test for Auditory Comprehension of Language–Revised (TACL–WC) (Carrow-Woolfolk, 1985), which are both measures of receptive vocabulary. A child coded normal language for the PPVT–R and subclinical language for the TACL–WC would be coded subclinical language for receptive vocabulary.

Results: Comorbidity of Language Disorder in Children with Speech Disorder

Figures 3 and 4 are summaries of the comorbidity findings for children in Studies 1–3. The children in these three studies were ascertained by clinical referral on the basis of their speech problems of unknown origin and by their classification as NSA/SD or SD on the SDCS. Figure 3 includes percentages for children with co-occuring impairments on receptive language measures, and Figure 4 includes percentages for children with co-occurring impairments on expressive language measures. Comorbidity estimates are provided by gender, language modality, and level of involvement (i.e., clinical, subclinical) in each domain. The number of children contributing to each percentage calculation is provided below each bar. The information in Figures 3 and 4, which bears on three questions, is now examined.

What Is the Comorbidity of Receptive and Expressive Language Disorder in Children with Speech Disorder? The right-most percentage in each panel containing data reflects the comorbidity percentage collapsed by gender and level of clinical involvement. There are five such estimates available in Figure 3 and three in Figure 4, totaling eight estimates of the comorbidity of speech and language disorder. For receptive involvement (Figure 3), the estimated comorbidity of speech-language disorder, in increasing order, is 6% (Study 1, vocabulary and grammar), 15% (Study 1, vocabulary), 17% (Study 2, vocabulary), 20% (Study 3, vocabulary and grammar), and 21% (Study 2, grammar). Thus, the range of comorbidity estimates is 6%–21%, with most (5/6) between 15% and 21%. For expressive involvement (Figure 4), the three summary comorbidity statistics in increasing order are 38% (Study 3, vocabulary and grammar), 43% (Study 2, grammar), and 62% (Study 1, grammar). Thus, estimates range from 38% to 62%, with two of the three estimates being less than 45%.

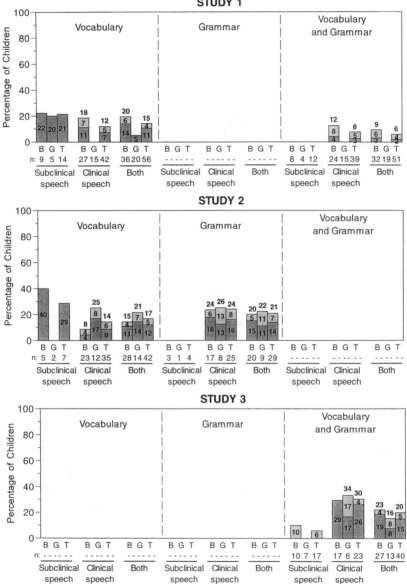

Figure 3. Estimates of the comorbidity of speech disorder and receptive language disorder in Studies 1, 2, and 3. The index disorder is speech disorder. (B, boys; G, girls; T, total; ■, subclinical language; ■, clinical language.)

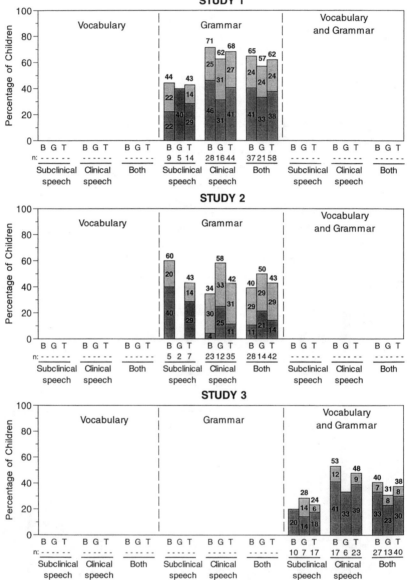

Figure 4. Estimates of the comorbidity of speech disorder and expressive language disorder in Studies 1, 2, and 3. The index disorder is speech disorder. (B, boys; G, girls; T, total; ■, subclinical language; ■, clinical language.)

These findings indicate that for children with speech involvement as ascertained from clinicians, the risk for co-occurring expressive language involvement is approximately two to three times greater than the risk for co-occurring receptive language involvement. The range of estimates within each modality underscores the variability across estimates observed previously in Table 1. The two estimates of receptive vocabulary are close in agreement (Study 1, 15%; Study 2, 17%), but the two estimates of receptive vocabulary and grammar (Study 1, 6%; Study 3, 20%) and expressive grammar (Study 1, 62%; Study 2, 43%) are not close in agreement. These differences are not likely to be due to differences in subjects, because children in Study 1 and Study 2 were ascertained similarly from the same population. Moreover, differences are not likely to be due to speech measurement issues, because speech status was determined in exactly the same way in each study. Other than possible differences associated with severity of involvement, the likely source of variance in comorbidity estimates within the same language domain is differences inherent in the variety of language measures, measure composites, and/or cutoff criteria used to classify language involvement (see Table 3).

Compared with previous estimates of 10%–40% comorbidity of speech disorder and language comprehension disorder (Shriberg & Kwiatkowski, 1994), the present findings (Figure 3) estimate comorbidity at 6%–20%. Furthermore, compared with previous estimates of 50%–75% comorbidity of speech disorder and expressive language disorder (Shriberg & Kwiatkowski, 1994), the present findings (Figure 4) estimate comorbidity at 38%–62%. Additional comment is deferred to summary discussion.

Does the Comorbidity of Speech and Receptive or Expressive Speech Language Disorder Vary by Gender? Of the eight summary estimates of speech-language disorder comorbidity in Figures 3 and 4 (i.e., gender estimates collapsed over severity of speech involvement), five have higher values for boys than girls. For the five panels assessing the comorbidity of speech and receptive language disorder in Figure 3, comorbidity percentages were higher for boys in Study 1, vocabulary (boys, 20%; girls, 5%); Study 1, vocabulary and grammar (boys, 9%; girls: 0%); and Study 3, vocabulary and grammar (boys, 23%; girls, 16%). Comorbidity percentages were higher for girls in Study 2, vocabulary (girls, 21%; boys, 15%); and Study 2, grammar (girls, 22%; boys, 20%). For the three estimates of the comorbidity of speech and expressive language disorder in Figure 4, estimates were higher for boys in Study 1, grammar (boys, 65%; girls, 57%); and Study 3, vocabulary and grammar (boys, 40%; girls; 31%); and higher for girls in Study 2, grammar (girls, 50%; boys, 40%).

These data suggest that there are no reliable gender trends for the comorbidity of speech and receptive or expressive language involvement. Gender differences range from only 2% to 15% across the eight estimates, and two of the three estimates of the same language domain disagree in directional trend.

For this question, the diversity of measures might be viewed as support for an interim conclusion of no differences in comorbidity associated with gender. To further assess gender and language, we completed Fisher exact tests on the proportions of boys and girls with normal versus clinical and/or subclinical language involvement in the three studies. None of the comparisons were statistically significant at .05 alpha levels.

Does the Comorbidity of Receptive or Expressive Language Disorder Increase with the Severity of the Speech Disorder? As noted previously, a number of theoretical perspectives would predict that the comorbidity of speech and language disorders would increase with increasing severity of the index disorder. In these data, support for this prediction can be assessed by comparing comorbidity questions for children with subclinical speech involvement with estimates for children with clinical speech involvement. Although the histograms in these figures provide separate percentages for subclinical and clinical language disorders (see Table 3 for per-measure criteria), only the totals (subclinical plus clinical language disorder) are used in these and all other comparisons. The reader may want to break out language severity findings for each of the three questions posed here, using the percentages provided in Figures 3 and 4. Differences in the ages and procedures for classifying language disorders in children in the first three studies compared with Study 4 prohibit a look at the other severity-related issue noted previously concerning its possible effects on ascertainment.

For the comorbidity of speech and receptive language disorder in Figure 3, there is modest support for a speech-language association based on severity of speech involvement, but only for language measures involving grammar. In comparison with children with subclinical speech disorders, children with clinical speech disorders had higher comorbidity estimates in the three comparisons involving receptive grammar: 1) Study 1, vocabulary and grammar (subclinical: 0%; clinical: 8%); 2) Study 2, grammar (subclinical, 0%; clinical, 24%); and 3) Study 3, vocabulary and grammar (subclinical, 6%; clinical, 30%). For the two measures involving receptive vocabulary, however, children with subclinical involvement had higher comorbidity rates in Study 1, vocabulary (subclinical, 21%; clinical, 12%), and Study 2, vocabulary (subclinical, 29%; clinical, 14%).

The data for expressive language disorders also support higher comorbidity rates for children with clinical compared with subclinical levels of speech involvement, including findings for both grammar and grammar and vocabulary (as shown in Figure 4, no data are reported for expressive vocabulary alone; see Table 3). Children with clinical speech involvements had higher comorbidity rates for grammar in Study 1 (subclinical, 43%; clinical, 68%), essentially equal rates for grammar in Study 2 (subclinical, 43%; clinical, 42%), and higher comorbidity rates for vocabulary and grammar in Study 3 (subclinical, 24%; clinical, 48%). Thus, although not attested in all comparisons, increased severity of speech disorder appears to be related to increased probability of receptive and expressive language disorder in the domain of grammar.

Results: Comorbidity of Speech
Disorder in Children with Language Disorder

The data from Study 4 provide information on the comorbidity of speech disorder in children ascertained by language disorder. The data of Study 4 are constrained by the age of these children, which at the time of speech testing averaged 71.4 months, or nearly 6 years, of age (Table 2). Thus, for each of the questions asked in this section, the answers are limited to comorbidity estimates for speech-language disorder at an age when, as noted previously, an estimated 75% of children with earlier clinical or subclinical speech disorder have normalized. Although the sampling and measurement operations for both speech and language are well developed in Study 4, this age constraint limits the point prevalence estimate of comorbidity to this relatively late period in speech acquisition. Figure 5 includes findings for performance on measures of receptive and expressive language disorders, with separate comorbidity percentages shown by gender, level of language involvement, and level of speech involvement. The same three questions as those for comorbidity of language disorder are posed of these comorbidity estimates.

What Is the Comorbidity of Speech Disorder in Children with Receptive and Expressive Language Disorder? The data in the top panel, reflecting SLI as defined in Tomblin et al. (in press), indicate that 9% of 6-year-old children with SLI have clinical speech disorder, and an additional 29% have subclinical speech disorder, for an overall comorbidity estimate of 38%. This estimate is within 13 percentage points of the 25% estimate found by Tomblin using a larger sample of children from this study but using different procedures to classify children's speech status (see Table 1). When SLI is defined by involvement in a particular domain, as shown in the two other panels in Figure 5, the overall comorbidity estimates are fairly similar for children meeting criteria for receptive language disorder (28% subclinical speech disorder and 6% clinical speech disorder, totaling 34%) and expressive language disorder (31% subclinical and 9% clinical, totaling 40%). Unlike the differences in receptive and expressive comorbidity data observed in Figures 3 and 4, children ascertained by receptive and/or expressive language involvements in Study 4 are at approximately similar risk for continuing speech involvement, 34% and 40%, respectively. Tomblin (1996b) commented on the lack of utility of observing traditional distinctions between receptive and language domains for SLI classifications in children at this age.

Does the Comorbidity of Language and Speech Disorder Vary by Gender? Of the three summary gender comparisons in Figure 5, each indicates that boys with language disorder have slightly higher comorbidity of speech disorder than girls: for the EpiSLI system: boys, 43%; girls, 30%; for recep-

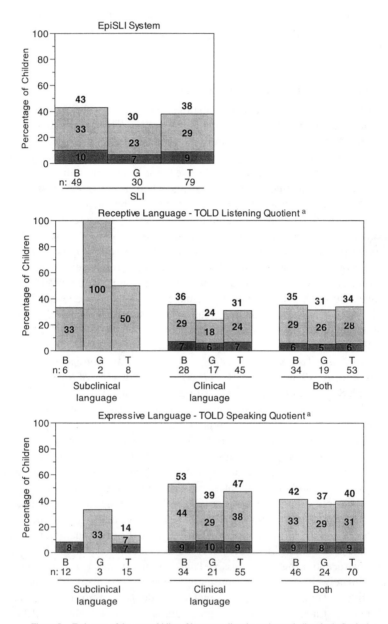

Figure 5. Estimates of the comorbidity of language disorder and speech disorder in Study 4. The index disorder is language disorder. (*a*Only children with subclinical or clinical performance on this measure are reported in this panel.) (B, boys; G, girls; T, total; ■, subclinical speech; ■, clinical speech.)

tive language involvement: boys, 35%; girls, 31%; and for expressive language involvement: boys, 42%; girls, 37%. As with the gender findings for the co-occurrence of language disorders in younger speech-involved children, the small absolute differences in percentages (4%–13%) provide only the most modest support for a theoretically significant gender difference in persisting speech disorder in children with language disorder. Most of the differences were associated with subclinical speech involvement, with gender differences of only 1%–3% separating comorbidity rates for children with clinical speech involvement.

Does the Comorbidity of Speech Disorder Increase with the Severity of the Receptive or Expressive Language Disorder? There are few data in Figure 5 to assess severity issues because the EpiSLI definition of *language disorder* does not include a subclinical classification and does not classify involvement by modality. Only 8 children and 15 children, respectively, were classified as subclinical language on the composite receptive and expressive measures. The receptive data for the eight children with subclinical language involvement appear unruly (each of the two girls with subclinical language had subclinical speech disorder, yielding 100% comorbidity) but, taken together with data for boys, suggest no differences in comorbidity associated with severity of language involvement. For children with expressive language involvement, the data seem to point more clearly to higher comorbidity rates associated with clinical language involvement, with differences primarily involving the percentages for subclinical speech involvement. In sum, the few data available to assess severity as a moderating variable in comorbidity rates are inconclusive for receptive language involvement and supportive of a positive association for expressive language disorder, with the latter effects primarily associated with increased risk for the persistence of subclinical speech disorder.

CONCLUSIONS

This chapter has reviewed some information on the comorbidity of speech-language disorders from the perspective of emerging research in the genetics of speech and language disorders. Comorbidity findings from approximately two dozen studies indicate that developmental phonological and language disorders do not always co-occur, even when assessed in very young children. Some variables that appear to be associated with the magnitude of comorbidity estimates include the index disorder (speech disorder > language disorder), the language modality (expressive language disorder > receptive language disorder), the language domain (grammatical [i.e., syntactic, morphologic] disorder > vocabulary [i.e., semantic] disorder), and perhaps gender (boys > girls). However, although each of these variables may contribute to the magnitude of the comorbidity estimate, none of the observed combinations of influential variables were associated with estimates greater than approximately 70% in the four study samples examined. The largest comorbidity estimates in these four studies typically averaged considerably lower.

Are these findings readily explainable by measurement error, which, if removed from these estimates, would yield 100% comorbidity, especially at the earliest ages? As we concluded in response to the estimates in Table 1, the substantial gap between 100% comorbidity and the percentages obtained in these four studies suggests that measurement error is not a sufficient explanation for the lower-than-expected magnitude of the estimates. Certainly, different ways to measure SLI and different statistical criteria to define SLI have a large influence on comorbidity estimates, with the more stringent criteria for SLI associated with lower comorbidity estimates. However, comorbidity estimates were not higher in the four study samples when subclinical forms of both speech and language disorders were included in the estimates, nor were they higher when the classification of speech disorder ensured that children had what are considered phonological rather than only articulatory involvements (i.e., SD and NSA/SD rather than QRE or RE), with the latter presumably not being associated with language disorder.

Rather than attributing lower comorbidity estimates to measurement issues, our strongest suspicion is that some phonological disorders occurring without concomitant language disorder represent one of the other forms of SD described in review of the SDCS. In our preliminary estimates, only approximately 60% of children with SD may have the suspected inherited form, with the other approximately 40% being associated with one of the other three proposed etiologic origins of childhood speech disorders (i.e., SD–OME, SD–DAS, SD–DPI). As summarized previously, the comorbidity estimates in Table 1 and Figures 3–5 reflecting speech and expressive language disorder in children of preschool age are consistent with this 50%–60% prevalence estimate. We are especially interested in the estimated approximately 30% of children referred for speech delay whose disorder is suspected to be due to the fluctuant conductive hearing loss associated with early recurrent otitis media with effusion (SD–OME). Although evidence for significant language disorder as a sequela of OME remains equivocal, there is good reason to suspect earlier and more salient effects on speech (cf. Shriberg et al., 1998).

These comorbidity data illustrate the complex issues that must be addressed in the development of a phenotype for developmental phonological disorders. It may be that an inherited phonological disorder arises as a variant of an inherited language or verbal trait disorder. If so, it would not require an autonomous phenotype as proposed at the outset of this chapter, and children reflecting the diverse forms of the inherited verbal or language deficit could be treated as one undifferentiated group in molecular genetics studies to identify the genotype. However, if the relatively low reported comorbidity estimates are not explained by measurement error or by appeal to other etiologic subtypes, we are left with a sizable proportion of children—converging on 50% in the estimates in Table 1 and even higher percentages in the estimates in Figures 3–5—with only a speech disorder or only a language disorder.

A key element needed to resolve issues associated with the comorbidity findings reviewed is a set of diagnostic markers for each of the four suspected subtypes of SD. Once children with other subtypes of SD can be reliably excluded from study samples of children suspected to have the inherited form, researchers can assess whether there are differences in the speech profiles or normalization histories of children with only speech disorder compared with children with speech-language disorder. Also, performance on all proposed phenotype markers (e.g., phenotypes based on natural speech production, challenging speech production tasks, phonological awareness tasks, nonsense word repetition tasks) can be compared to determine if there are some children whose only linguistic problem is a mild to significant delay in the correct production of speech sounds. We think the existence of such children will eventually be documented, with consequent implications for effective and efficient treatment.

The data presented also highlight the questions raised in other chapters in this volume regarding relations between speech and language in development and disorders. If specific speech disorders turn out to be a distinct phenotype, separable by both behavioral and genetic markers from more pervasive disorders involving both speech and language, this finding would have important implications for understanding the mechanisms of the development of both speech-sound production and language formulation. If distinct genetic mechanisms for specific speech disorders can be identified, this would imply that discrete biochemical pathways subserve the speech acquisition system, more or less independent of the processes that enable language development. This would suggest that some aspects of speech development do not rely, or do not rely entirely, on a substrate of language, contrary to the view that a phonological orientation to speech-sound development would imply.

Finally, our views on treatment of childhood speech disorders might also be affected by the implications of these comorbidity findings. There has been a trend to see developmental speech-sound disorders as one manifestation of language disorder (cf. Bishop & Edmundson, 1987). That is, the phonological perspective, with its emphasis on underlying representations and simplification processes, has viewed child speech disorders as arising from faulty rule learning and treatable by approaches used to remediate language problems. If, however, certain child speech disorders arise from pathways distinct from those of language disorders, such an approach for these types would be called into question. Additional research to elaborate the phenotype of specific speech disorders and link it to identifiable biological markers is needed to illuminate the complex associations between child speech and child language disorders.

REFERENCES

American Psychiatric Association. (1994). *Diagnostic and statistical manual of mental disorders* (4th ed.). Washington, DC: Author.

Aram, D.M., Morris, R., & Hall, N.E. (1993). Clinical and research congruence in identifying children with specific language impairment. *Journal of Speech and Hearing Research, 36,* 580–591.

Arnold, G.E. (1961). The genetic background of developmental language disorders. *Folia Phoniatrica, 13,* 246–254.

Baker, L., & Cantwell, D.P. (1982). Developmental, social, and behavioral characteristics of speech and language disordered children. *Child Psychiatry and Human Development, 12,* 195–206.

Beitchman, J.H., Hood, J., & Inglis, A. (1992). Familial transmission of speech and language impairment: A preliminary investigation. *Canadian Journal of Psychiatry, 37,* 151–156.

Beitchman, J.H., Nair, R., Clegg, M., & Patel, P.G. (1986). Prevalence of speech and language disorders in 5-year-old kindergarten children in the Ottawa-Carleton region. *Journal of Speech and Hearing Disorders, 51,* 98–110.

Bernhardt, B.H., & Stemberger, J.P. (1997). *Handbook of phonological development.* New York: Academic Press.

Bernthal, J.E., & Bankson, N.W. (1993). *Articulation and phonological disorders* (3rd ed.). Englewood Cliffs, NJ: Prentice-Hall.

Bird, J., Bishop, D.V.M., & Freeman, N.H. (1995). Phonological awareness and literacy development in children with expressive phonological impairments. *Journal of Speech and Hearing Research, 38,* 446–462.

Bishop, D.V.M. (1992). Biological basis of developmental language disorders. In P. Fletcher & D. Hall (Eds.), *Specific speech and language disorders in children* (pp. 2–17). San Diego: Singular Publishing Group.

Bishop, D.V.M. (1994). Is specific language impairment a valid diagnostic category? Genetic and psycholinguistic evidence. *Philosophical Transactions of the Royal Society, 346,* 105–111.

Bishop, D.V.M., & Edmundson, A. (1987). Language-impaired 4-year-olds: Distinguishing transient from persistent impairment. *Journal of Speech and Hearing Disorders, 52,* 156–173.

Bishop, D.V.M., North, T., & Donlan, C. (1995). Genetic basis of specific language impairment: Evidence from a twin study. *Developmental Medicine and Child Neurology, 37,* 56–71.

Boada, R., Shriberg, L.D., Nittrouer, S., Markey, K., Lefly, D., & Pennington, B. (1998). *Speech perception and production in young familial dyslexics.* Manuscript in preparation.

Borges-Orsorio, M.R., & Salzano, F.M. (1985). Language disabilities in 3 twin pairs and their relatives. *Acta Geneticae Medicae et Gemellologiae (Roma), 34,* 95–100.

Brzustowicz, L. (1996). Looking for language genes: Lessons from complex disorder studies. In M.L. Rice (Ed.), *Toward a genetics of language* (pp. 3–25). Mahwah, NJ: Lawrence Erlbaum Associates.

Burd, L., Hammes, K., Bornhoeft, D.M., & Fisher, W. (1988). A North Dakota prevalence study of nonverbal school-age children. *Language, Speech, and Hearing Services in Schools, 19,* 371–383.

Carrow-Woolfolk, E. (1985). *Test for Auditory Comprehension of Language–Revised (TACL–R).* Allen, TX: DLM Teaching Resources.

Christman, S.S. (1995, May). *Neurological aspects of phonological development: The first year.* Paper presented at the Child Phonology Meeting, Memphis, TN.

Connell, P., Elbert, M., & Dinnsen, D. (1991, June). *A syntax-delayed subgroup of phonologically delayed children.* Paper presented at the Symposium on Research in Child Language Disorders, Madison, WI.

Creaghead, N.A., Newman, P.W., & Secord, W. (1989). *Assessment and remediation of articulatory and phonological disorders* (2nd ed.). Columbus, OH: Charles E. Merrill.

Culatta, B., Page, J.L., & Ellis, J. (1983). Story retelling as a communicative performance screening tool. *Language, Speech, and Hearing Services in Schools, 14,* 66–74.

Dunn, L.M., & Dunn, L.M. (1981). *Peabody Picture Vocabulary Test–Revised.* Circle Pines, MN: American Guidance Service.

Farmer, M.E., & Klein, R.M. (1995). The evidence for a temporal processing deficit linked to dyslexia: A review. *Psychonomic Bulletin and Review, 2,* 460–493.

Felsenfeld, S., Broen, P., & McGue, M. (1992). A 28-year-follow-up of adults with a history of phonological disorder: Linguistic and personality results. *Journal of Speech and Hearing Disorders, 38,* 1114–1125.

Felsenfeld, S., McGue, M., & Broen, P.A. (1995). Familial aggregation of phonological disorders: Results from a 28-year follow-up. *Journal of Speech and Hearing Research, 38,* 1091–1107.

Felsenfeld, S., & Plomin, R. (1997). Epidemiological and offspring analyses of developmental speech disorders using data from the Colorado Adoption Project. *Journal of Speech and Hearing Research, 40,* 778–791.

Gilger, J.W. (1995). Behavioral genetics: Concepts for research and practice in language development and disorders. *Journal of Speech and Hearing Research, 38,* 1126–1142.

Goldsmith, J.A. (Ed.). (1995). *The handbook of phonological theory.* Cambridge, MA: Blackwell Publishers.

Gopnik, M., & Crago, M. (1991). Familial aggregation of a developmental language disorder. *Cognition, 39,* 1–50.

Hall, P.K., Jordan, L.S., & Robin, D.A. (1993). *Developmental apraxia of speech: Theory and clinical practice.* Austin, TX: PRO-ED.

Hedrick, D.L., Prather, E.M., & Tobin, A.R. (1975). *Sequenced Inventory of Communication Development* (SICD) (Rev. ed.). Seattle: University of Washington Press.

Hull, F.M., Mielke, P.W., Timmons, R.J., & Welleford, J.A. (1971). The National Speech and Hearing Survey: Preliminary results. *Asha, 13,* 501–509.

Hurst, J.A., Baraitser, M., Auger, E., Grahm, F., & Norell, S. (1990). An extended family with a dominantly inherited speech disorder. *Developmental Medicine and Child Neurology, 32,* 352–355.

Ingram, T. (1959). Specific developmental disorders of speech in childhood. *Brain, 82,* 450–467.

Jeffrey, R., & Freilinger, J. (1986). *Iowa's Severity Rating Scales for Speech and Language Impairments.* Des Moines: Iowa Department of Education.

Kahn, H.A., & Sempos, C.T. (1989). *Statistical methods in epidemiology.* New York: Oxford University Press.

Khoury, M.J., Beaty, T.H., & Cohen, B.H. (1993). *Fundamentals in genetic epidemiology.* New York: Oxford University Press.

Kwiatkowski, J., & Shriberg, L.D. (1997). *The capability-focus framework for treatment of child speech disorders.* Manuscript submitted for publication.

Lahey, M., & Edwards, J. (1995). Specific language impairment: Preliminary investigation of factors associated with family history and with patterns of language performance. *Journal of Speech and Hearing Research, 38,* 643–657.

Lassman, F.M., Fisch, R.O., Vetter, D.K., & La Benz, E.S. (1980). *Early correlates of speech language, and hearing.* Littleton, MA: PSG Publishing.

Last, J.M. (Ed.). (1988). *A dictionary of epidemiology* (2nd ed.). New York: Oxford University Press.

Leske, M. (1981). Prevalence estimates of communicative disorders in the United States: Speech disorders. *Asha, 23,* 217–228.

Lewis, B.A., Cox, N.J., & Byard, P.J. (1993). Segregation analysis of speech and language disorders. *Behavior Genetics, 23,* 291–299.

Lewis, B.A., Ekelman, B.L., & Aram, D.M. (1989). A familial study of severe phonological disorders. *Journal of Speech and Hearing Research, 32,* 713–724.

Lewis, B.A., & Freebairn, L. (1992). Residual effects of preschool phonology disorders in grade school, adolescence, and adulthood. *Journal of Speech and Hearing Research, 35,* 819–831.

Lewis, B.A., & Shriberg, L.D. (1994, November). *Life span interrelationships among speech, prosody-voice, and nontraditional phonological measures.* Miniseminar presented at the Annual Convention of the American Speech-Language-Hearing Association, New Orleans, LA.

Lewis, B.A., & Thompson, L.A. (1992). A study of developmental speech and language disorders in twins. *Journal of Speech and Hearing Research, 35,* 1086–1094.

Locke, J.L., & Mather, P.L. (1989). Genetic factors in the ontogeny of spoken language: Evidence from monozygotic and dizygotic twins. *Journal of Child Language, 16,* 553–559.

Matheny, A.P., & Bruggeman, C.E. (1973). Children's speech: Heredity components and sex differences. *Folia Phoniatrica, 25,* 442–449.

Menn, L., Markey, K., Mozer, M., & Lewis, C. (1993). Connectionist modeling and the microstructure of phonological development: A progress report. In B. Boysson-Bardies, S. Schonen, P. Jusczyk, P.F. MacNeilage, & J. Morton (Eds.), *Developmental neurocognition: Models, research, implications* (pp. 421–434). Timonium, MD: York Press.

Miller, J.F. (1981). *Assessing language production in children.* Austin, TX: PRO-ED.

Miller, J.F., & Chapman, R. (1986). *Systematic Analysis of Language Transcripts (SALT).* Madison: University of Wisconsin.

Neils, J., & Aram, D.M. (1986). Family history of children with developmental language disorders. *Perceptual and Motor Skills: Part 1, 63*(2), 655–658.

Newcomer, P., & Hammill, D. (1988). *Test of Language Development–2: Primary* (TOLD–2). Austin, TX: PRO-ED.

Paul, R. (1993). Patterns of development in late talkers: Preschool years. *Journal of Childhood Communication Disorders, 15,* 7–14.

Paul, R. (1995). *Language disorders from infancy through adolescence: Assessment and intervention.* St. Louis: Mosby–Year Book.

Paul, R., & Shriberg, L.D. (1982). Associations between phonology and syntax in speech-delayed children. *Journal of Speech and Hearing Research, 25,* 536–547.

Pennington, B.F. (1986). Issues in the diagnosis and phenotype analysis of dyslexia: Implications for family studies. In S.D. Smith (Ed.), *Genetics and learning disabilities* (pp. 69–96). San Diego: College-Hill Press.

Rice, M.L. (Ed.). (1996). *Toward a genetics of language.* Mahwah, NJ: Lawrence Erlbaum Associates.

Ruscello, D.M., St. Louis, K.O., & Mason, N. (1991). School-aged children with phonological disorders: Coexistence with other speech/language disorders. *Journal of Speech and Hearing Research, 34,* 236–242.

Samples, J.M., & Lane, V.W. (1985). Genetic possibilities in six siblings with specific language learning disorders. *Asha, 27,* 167–173.

Schery, T.K. (1985). Correlates of language development in language-disordered children. *Journal of Speech and Hearing Disorders, 50,* 73–83.

Schuele, C.M., & Rice, M.L. (1996, June). *Specific language impairment: A family case study.* Paper presented at the Symposium on Research in Child Language Disorders, Madison, WI.

Schwartz, R.G. (1992). Nonlinear phonology as a framework for phonological acquisition. In R. Chapman (Ed.), *Processes in language acquisition and disorders* (pp. 108–124). St. Louis: Mosby–Year Book.

Shaywitz, S.E., Shaywitz, B.A., Fletcher, J.M., & Escobar, M.D. (1990). Prevalence of reading disability in boys and girls. *Journal of the American Medical Association, 264,* 998–1002.

Shriberg, L.D. (1980). Developmental phonological disorders. In T.J. Hixon, L.D. Shriberg, & J.S. Saxman (Eds.), *Introduction to communicative disorders* (pp. 262–309). Englewood Cliffs, NJ: Prentice-Hall.

Shriberg, L.D. (1982). Toward classification of developmental phonological disorders. In N.J. Lass (Ed.), *Speech and language: Advances in basic research and practice* (Vol. 8, pp. 2–18). New York: Academic Press.

Shriberg, L.D. (1986). *PEPPER: Programs to examine phonetic and phonologic evaluation records.* Hillsdale, NJ: Lawrence Erlbaum Associates.

Shriberg, L.D. (1993). Four new speech and prosody-voice measures for genetics research and other studies in developmental phonological disorders. *Journal of Speech and Hearing Research, 36,* 105–140.

Shriberg, L.D. (1994). Five subtypes of developmental phonological disorders. *Clinics in Communication Disorders, 4*(1), 38–53.

Shriberg, L.D. (1997). Developmental phonological disorder(s): One or many? In B.W. Hodson & M.L. Edwards (Eds.), *Applied phonology: Perspectives and clinical applications* (pp. 105–127). Gaithersburg, MD: Aspen Publishers.

Shriberg, L.D., Aram, D.M., & Kwiatkowski, J. (1997). Developmental apraxia of speech: III. A subtype marked by inappropriate stress. *Journal of Speech, Language, and Hearing Research, 40,* 313–337.

Shriberg, L.D., Austin, D., Lewis, B.A., McSweeny, J.L., & Wilson, D.L. (1997a). The Percentage of Consonants Correct (PCC) metric: Extensions and reliability data. *Journal of Speech, Language, and Hearing Research, 40,* 708–722.

Shriberg, L.D., Austin, D., Lewis, B.A., McSweeny, J.L., & Wilson, D.L. (1997b). The Speech Disorders Classification System (SDCS): Extensions and lifespan reference data. *Journal of Speech, Language, and Hearing Research, 40,* 723–740.

Shriberg, L.D., Flipsen, P., Jr., Thielke, H., Kwiatkowski, J., Kertoy, M., Katcher, M., Nellis, R., & Block, M. (1998). *Risk for speech delay associated with early recurrent otitis media with effusion.* Manuscript submitted for publication.

Shriberg, L.D., Gruber, F.A., & Kwiatkowski, J. (1994). Developmental phonological disorders. III: Long-term speech-sound normalization. *Journal of Speech and Hearing Research, 37,* 1151–1177.

Shriberg, L.D., & Kent, R.D. (1995). *Clinical phonetics* (2nd ed.). Needham Heights, MA: Allyn & Bacon.

Shriberg, L.D., & Kwiatkowski, J. (1982). Phonological disorders: I. A diagnostic classification system. *Journal of Speech and Hearing Disorders, 47,* 226–241.

Shriberg, L.D., & Kwiatkowski, J. (1988). A follow-up study of children with phonologic disorders of unknown origin. *Journal of Speech and Hearing Disorders, 53,* 144–155.

Shriberg, L.D., & Kwiatkowski, J. (1994). Developmental phonological disorders: I. A clinical profile. *Journal of Speech and Hearing Research, 37,* 1100–1126.

Shriberg, L.D., Kwiatkowski, J., Best, S., Hengst, J., & Terselic-Weber, B. (1986). Characteristics of children with phonologic disorders of unknown origin. *Journal of Speech and Hearing Disorders, 51,* 140–161.

Shriberg, L.D., Kwiatkowski, J., & Gruber, F.A. (1994). Developmental phonological disorders. II: Short-term speech-sound normalization. *Journal of Speech and Hearing Research, 37,* 1127–1150.

Shriberg, L.D., Kwiatkowski, J., & Hoffmann, K.A. (1984). A procedure for phonetic transcription by consensus. *Journal of Speech and Hearing Research, 27,* 456–465.

Silva, P.A. (1987). Epidemiology, longitudinal course, and some associated factors: An update. In W. Yule & M. Rutter (Eds.), *Language development and disorders* (pp. 1–15). Philadelphia: J.B. Lippincott.

Smith, S.D., Pennington, B.F., & DeFries, J.C. (1996). Linkage analysis with complex behavioral traits. In M.L. Rice (Ed.), *Toward a genetics of language* (pp. 29–44). Mahwah, NJ: Lawrence Erlbaum Associates.

Stemberger, J.P. (1992). A connectionist view of child phonology: Phonological processing without phonological processes. In C.A. Ferguson, L. Menn, & C. Stoel-Gammon (Eds.), *Phonological development: Models, research, implications* (pp. 65–90). Timonium, MD: York Press.

St. Louis, K.O., Ruscello, D.M., & Lundeen, C. (1992). *Coexistence of communication disorders in schoolchildren* (ASHA Monographs No. 27). Rockville, MD: American Speech-Language-Hearing Association.

St. Louis, K.O., Ruscello, D.M., Grafton, S.J., & Hershman, K.T. (1994, November). *Coexistence of communication disorders in clinical populations over four decades.* Poster presented at the Annual Convention of the Speech-Language-Hearing Association, New Orleans, LA.

Stoel-Gammon, C., & Dunn, C. (1985). *Normal and disordered phonology in children.* Baltimore: University Park Press.

Streiner, D.L., Norman, G.R., & Munroe Blum, H. (1989). *PDO epidemiology.* Toronto: B.C. Decker.

Stromswold, K., & Rifkin, J.I. (1996, June). *Language acquisition by identical versus fraternal twins.* Paper presented at the Symposium on Research in Child Language Disorders, Madison, WI.

Tallal, P., Ross, R., & Curtiss, S. (1989). Familial aggregation in specific language impairment. *Journal of Speech and Hearing Disorders, 54,* 167–173.

Tallal, P., Townsend, J., Curtiss, S., & Wulfeck, B. (1991). Phenotypic profiles of language-impaired children based on genetic/family history. *Brain and Language, 41,* 81–95.

Tomblin, J.B. (1989). Familial concentration of developmental language impairment. *Journal of Speech and Hearing Disorders, 54,* 287–295.

Tomblin, J.B. (1996a, April). *Epidemiology of SLI: The association of speech sound disorder with SLI.* Paper presented at the Child Phonology Conference, Iowa City, IA.

Tomblin, J.B. (1996b, June). *The big picture of SLI: Results of an epidemiologic study of SLI among kindergarten children.* Paper presented at the Symposium on Research in Child Language Disorders, Madison, WI.

Tomblin, J.B., Freese, P.R., & Records, N.L. (1992). Diagnosing specific language impairment in adults for the purpose of pedigree analysis. *Journal of Speech and Hearing Research, 35,* 832–843.

Tomblin, J.B., Records, N.L., Buckwalter, P., Zhang, X., Smith, E., & O'Brien, M. (in press). The prevalence of SLI in kindergarten children. *Journal of Speech, Language, and Hearing Research.*

Tomblin, J.B., Records, N.L., & Zhang, X. (1996). A system for the diagnosis of specific language impairment in kindergarten children. *Journal of Speech and Hearing Research, 39,* 1284–1294.

Velleman, S.L., & Shriberg, L.D. (1997). *Syllabic stress constraints as the proximal loci of a subtype of developmental apraxia of speech (DAS).* Manuscript in preparation.

Weiss, C.E., Gordon, M.E., & Lillywhite, H.S. (1987). *Clinical management of articulatory and phonological disorders* (2nd ed.). Baltimore: Williams & Wilkins.

Whitehurst, G.J., Arnold, D.S., Smith, M., Fischel, J.E., Lonigan, C.J., & Valdez-Menchaca, M.C. (1991). Family history in developmental expressive language delay. *Journal of Speech and Hearing Research, 34,* 1150–1157.

Winitz, H. (1969). *Articulatory acquisition and behavior.* Englewood Cliffs, NJ: Prentice-Hall.

Winitz, H., & Darley, F. (1980). Speech production. In P. LaBenz & A. LaBenz (Eds.), *Early correlates of speech, language, and hearing* (pp. 232–265). Littleton, MA: PSG Publishing.

Zimmerman, I.L., Steiner, V.G., & Pond, R.E. (1979). *Preschool Language Scale (PLS)* (Rev. ed.). Columbus, OH: Charles E. Merrill.

Appendix: Assessment Information for the Four Comorbidity Studies

STUDY 1

A total of 56 of the 58 children in Study 1 were given the Peabody Picture Vocabulary Test–Revised (PPVT–R; Dunn & Dunn, 1981) as a measure of receptive vocabulary and the Auditory Comprehension subtests of the Preschool Language Scale (Zimmerman, Steiner, & Pond, 1979) to measure receptive language skills (both vocabulary and grammar). Structural stage (StruSt), a measure of expressive grammar, was determined by analyzing conversational speech samples for syntactic performance using procedures and reference data described in Miller (1981), Miller and Chapman (1986), and Paul and Shriberg (1982). Results for other receptive and expressive language measures administered to the original group of 64 children are reported in Shriberg and Kwiatkowski (1994) and are not considered in this chapter.

STUDY 2

All 42 children in Study 2 were given the PPVT–R to assess receptive vocabulary. A total of 23 children in Cohort 1 received the Test for Auditory Comprehension of Language (TACL–R; Carrow-Woolfolk, 1985). The TACL–R includes three subtests: Word Classes and Relations (WC), a measure of receptive vocabulary; and Grammatical Morphemes (GM) and Elaborated Sentences (ES), two measures of receptive grammar. Percentile scores for all subtests and a total score were recorded. A total of 12 children achieved baseline performance on all subtests, 22 (15 M, 7 F) achieved baseline for WC, 15 (11 M, 4 F) for GM, and 16 (11 M, 5 F) for ES. Two children who were not yet 3 years of age at initial assessment received the receptive portion of the Sequenced Inventory of Communication Development (Hedrick, Prather, & Tobin, 1975) as an overall estimate of receptive language skills. Ten children in Cohort 2 who were at least 4 years old at initial assessment received five subtests of the Test of Language Development–2: Primary (TOLD–P; Newcomer & Hammill, 1988). Subtests administered were Picture Vocabulary (PV), a measure of receptive vocabulary; Grammatic Understanding (GU), a measure of receptive grammar; Oral Vocabulary (OV), a measure of expressive vocabulary; and Grammatic Completion (GC) and Sentence Imitation (SI), two measures of expressive grammar. Two subtests of phonology (Word Discrimination and Word Articulation) were not administered. Finally, as a measure of expressive grammar, structural stage was determined using the same procedures as used in Study 1 for all of the children in Cohort 1 and the seven 3-year-old children in Cohort 2.

STUDY 3

All children in Study 3 were given six subtests of the TOLD–P, including the five subtests listed for Study 2, and the Word Discrimination (WD) subtest, a measure of phonological awareness. We were provided with standard scores calculated from national norms in the TOLD–P manual for the Spoken Language Quotient (SLQ), which included all six subtests, and the Listening Quotient (LiQ), which included the PV, GU, and WD subtests for all 40 of the subjects reported here. We were also provided with the Speaking Quotient (SpQ), which included the OV, GC, and SI subtests, for 14 subjects. The LiQ was used as a measure of receptive language skills, and the SpQ was used as a measure of expressive skills, with both measures including subtests in the vocabulary and grammar domains. SpQ scores were not available for 26 of the children; therefore, the SLQ was used as an estimate of the child's expressive skills.

STUDY 4

All children in Study 4 were given the five subtests of the TOLD–P described for Study 2, and we were provided with LiQ and SpQ z scores as well as the child's status on the EpiSLI system (Tomblin et al., 1996). The z scores were calculated using local norms established by the Iowa project as described in Tomblin et al.

We also received each child's classification (normal language or SLI) on the EpiSLI system developed as part of the Iowa project. The EpiSLI system includes five subtests from the TOLD–P and results of a narrative comprehension and production measure based on the work of Culatta, Page, and Ellis (1983). The subtests were used to calculate composite scores in three domains (vocabulary, grammar, and narrative) and two modalities (comprehension and expression). Each domain composite included at least one receptive and one expressive measure, and the receptive and expressive composites included measures from each of the three domains: vocabulary, grammar, and narrative. As discussed previously, z scores of less than or equal to -1.25 based on local norms on two of these five composites yielded the greatest sensitivity and specificity when compared with a clinical rating system (Tomblin et al., 1996). As a result, children were classified as SLI in the EpiSLI system when they received z scores less than or equal to -1.25 for two of the five composite scores.

5

Where Words Come From
The Origins of Expressive Language

Ken M. Bleile

NEAR THE BEGINNING OF THEIR second year of life, most children begin using words to communicate. Some of the keenest interest and sharpest debate among those who study speech and language connections revolves around those first few words. Types of questions that investigators ask include the following: Why do words emerge when they do? What principles guide the organization of the child's early expressive vocabulary? How does the child learn to pronounce the sounds and syllables that compose these words?

The relationship between prespeech vocalizations and children's first words has been a major topic in the study of language acquisition since the early 1940s. An approach to the study of this topic involves the analysis of case studies of children who for medical reasons were not permitted to vocalize during infancy. One such child is identified as *E* (Bleile, Stark, & Silverman McGowan, 1993).

> *E* experienced a severe lung disability shortly after birth and had been tracheostomized for the first 2 years of her life. During that time, *E* had communicated entirely through pointing and signing because the tracheostomy that made her life possible also precluded any chance for her to vocalize. The tracheostomy was removed when *E* was slightly more than 24 months of age, and for the first time in her life *E* was able to speak. *E* remained silent for a few days after the surgery. Then, one day while sitting at a table, *E* opened her mouth and a little voiced sound emerged. Her eyes widened. It was the first voiced sound *E* had ever made with her mouth, and its occurrence appeared to surprise her as much as it appeared to delight her parents.

Children such as *E* test the degree of elasticity in the human capacity to acquire speech and language. The opportunity to study the development that such children provide is one that an ethical society can obtain by no other means. This chapter explores how the experiences of *E* and other children with tracheostomies illuminate the knowledge of the connection between prespeech vocalizations (henceforth called *babbling*) and the use of sounds and syllables in words (henceforth called *expressive language*). This chapter describes conceptual and methodological issues, the results of previous studies, and the developmental and clinical implications of tracheostomy research.

BABBLING AND EXPRESSIVE LANGUAGE

The study of babbling arguably began in 1941 with the publication of Jakobson's (1968) *Kindersprache, Aphasia, und allgemeine Lautgesetze* (henceforth abbreviated as *Kindersprache*). Ironically, *Kindersprache* contains little discussion of babbling, nor is the relationship between babbling and expressive language of central importance to the hypothesis Jakobson was exploring. A further irony is that Jakobson, the father of an academic field dedicated to exploring relationships between babbling and language, did not believe such a relationship existed.

The central hypothesis explored in *Kindersprache* pertains to the relationship among child language, aphasia, and language universals. To illustrate, in *Kindersprache*, Jakobson hypothesized that phonological distinctions made earliest in language acquisition are likely to be most widespread across languages and most likely to be lost latest by people with aphasia. For example, Jakobson claimed that the opposition between the distinctive feature of grave and acute (e.g., /p/ versus /t/) was acquired early by children and thus was likely to be a language universal and to be lost latest by people with neurological difficulties. More important, this hypothesis does not depend on whether a relationship exists between babbling and expressive language (Menn, 1980). Jakobson's well-known proposal was that babbling was unrelated to expressive language and that a period of silence sometimes occurred between babbling and the onset of meaningful language, indicating the separateness of the two activities.

Jakobson's conception of the relationship between babbling and expressive language arose from structuralism, a theory of phonology that Jakobson helped found and of which he was a chief advocate. An apocryphal though illuminating story is that Jakobson's inspiration for structuralism was a showing of cubist paintings in Paris in the 1920s. Like its artistic counterpart, Jakobson's linguistic theory hypothesized that a complex reality of opposites and contrasts underlay a seemingly ordinary surface appearance. For example, Jakobson hypothesized that the phonemes /p/ and /t/ were composed of distinctive features that opposed each other in the dimensions of grave and acute. Jakobson and many other structuralists were less concerned with the phonetic nature of sounds, which they considered a mere surface manifestation rather than the true nature of a phoneme.

Jakobson's views on babbling might be interpreted as both a natural outgrowth of structuralism and an attempt to demonstrate the reality of distinctive features. Jakobson's structuralist orientation tended to make him dismiss babbling as mere sound making; thus, it was outside the realm of phonological theory. Jakobson sought to demonstrate the reality of distinctive features in *Kindersprache* by emphasizing changes in children's language behavior with the onset of meaningful communication. Jakobson's contention that some children were actually silent between the end of babbling and the onset of expressive language further served to emphasize the difference between sound making and acquiring contrasts between distinctive features. Velten (1943) was perhaps the first to question the factual nature of Jakobson's view about the relationship between babbling and the development of expressive language. However, the debate ignited by *Kindersprache* waited to burst into full flame until 1968, when the book was translated into English.

Since the 1980s, babbling is typically conceived as a mechanism through which children learn to coordinate the activities of their vocal apparatus in speechlike ways (Locke, 1983; Stark, 1980; Vihman, 1996). One investigative team has likened babbling to serving the speech-motor system as a random noise generator that activates movements and feeds the results back to the sensory system (Braitenberg & Schüz, 1992). A particularly important milestone in the development of babbling is thought to occur at around 6 months of age, when children typically begin to combine consonant- and vowel-like sounds into syllables (Oller, 1986). By their first birthday, children are thought to begin recruiting the sounds and syllables used in babbling to make their first words.

There is evidence to support the existence of a relationship between babbling and expressive language. First, investigators have demonstrated that a developmental progression exists in vocalizations during the first year of life (see Chapters 2 and 3 for further discussion). For example, throughout the first year, the timing characteristics of vocalizations become increasingly more speechlike, providing a plausible series of steps through which the sounds and syllables used in words might gradually be acquired (Oller, 1980; Stark, 1980). Second, investigators have discovered continuity between the sounds and syllables occurring in late babbling and those found in children's early words (Boysson-Bardies & Vihman, 1991; Vihman, Ferguson, & Elbert, 1986). The continuity reflects both differences in language input as well as individual differences.

Although investigators have demonstrated continuity between the sounds and syllables of babbling and those found in early words, they have not demonstrated that babbling facilitates the development of expressive language. Behaviors that precede and follow each other need not be related. For example, although during the first weeks of life infants engage in walking-type motions of the legs, most investigators do not believe that these motions facilitate the later development of walking (Bleile et al., 1993). The occurrence of babbling before the onset of expressive language similarly does not necessarily indicate that the former facilitates the latter.

To demonstrate possible facilitating effects of babbling requires that investigators compare the expressive language outcomes of children who babble with those who do not. If babbling does not facilitate later development, the phonetic inventories of toddlers who babbled and those who were nonbabblers should be comparable. However, if babbling facilitates the development of expressive language, the phonetic inventories of toddlers who babbled should be developmentally advanced compared with children who did not babble.

Comparison of the expressive language outcomes of former babblers and nonbabblers is fraught with methodological and logical difficulties. A primary methodological concern is that children identified as nonbabblers may have babbled when other people were not present. Researchers have long known that during certain developmental periods infants seem to prefer to babble when adults are absent. An important logical concern is that a poorer outcome in children who did not babble may not be related to failure to babble. Failure to babble possibly may result from cognitive or environmental factors, and these other factors rather than the absence of babbling may lead to a poorer expressive language outcome.

Clarification of the relationship between babbling and expressive language would improve the knowledge of an important connection between speech and language. Furthermore, the issue has important clinical relevance to the growing population of children who have communication disorders during the first years of life. If babbling is unrelated to expressive language development, little reason exists to believe that stimulating vocal development in the prelinguistic period is a reasonable therapeutic activity. If babbling is actually practice for expressive language, however, then promoting vocal development in children in the prelinguistic stage becomes an important therapeutic goal.

LANGUAGE ACQUISITION IN EXTREME CIRCUMSTANCES

Language studies of children raised in extreme circumstances have a long history. Herodutus reported that the pharaoh Psammetichus (7th century B.C.E.) ordered two children to be raised by goats to determine the children's natural language. (Psammetichus claimed they spoke Phrygian.) During the Middle Ages and the Renaissance, such monarchs as the Emperor Frederick II, the Mogul Emperor Akbar, and King James IV of Scotland all subjected children to language deprivation experiments for reasons similar to those that motivated Psammetichus (Hewes, 1992). In the 19th century, scholars studied the language of the so-called wild boy of Aveyron (Humphrey & Humphrey, 1932), and the story of a child in India reportedly raised by wolves served as the inspiration for Kipling's *The Jungle Book* (1895). The case of Genie inspired a similar interest among both scholars and the popular press in the 1970s (Curtiss, 1977; Rymer, 1993).

Few circumstances in life are more extreme than being deprived of speech during the first years of life. Such a situation may arise when, for medical reasons, an infant receives a tracheostomy, which is an artificial airway made in the anterior neck below the vocal folds (Handler, 1993). When a tracheostomy is in place, air follows the course of least resistance and flows from the neck to the lungs, bypassing the mouth and nose. The tracheostomy remains patent through a tube (cannula) fitted into the opening. When the cannula is removed (decannulation), the child reverts to breathing through the mouth and nose.

In 1967, Lenneberg speculated that children with tracheostomies constituted a type of natural experiment that might be used to test hypotheses related to babbling and language development. The general research strategy proposed by Lenneberg was to study the expressive language outcome of children after decannulation. If babbling were unrelated to the development of expressive language, then the outcomes of these children would be comparable to those of their peers because failure to babble would not adversely affect expressive language. If, however, babbling facilitated expressive language, the expressive language of these children should be less developed than that of their peers because the failure to babble would represent the loss of an important developmental prerequisite. Lenneberg also speculated that children with tracheostomies may provide evidence of whether there exists a critical (or sensitive) period during which language must be acquired. If, similar to the visual system, acquisition of expressive language must be initiated within a certain time frame, children with tracheostomies who are decannulated outside this time frame should have less successful expressive language outcomes than those decannulated at earlier ages.

Children with Tracheostomies

Approximately 15 years elapsed between Lenneberg's observation and the first study that used children with tracheostomies to systematically explore the relationship between babbling and language development. This delay at first seems confusing because it occurred during a period in which studies of babbling flourished. One possible reason for the lack of research is that investigators were unable to obtain subjects because of the relative rarity of tracheostomy surgery in children. It is estimated that only 884–2,600 children undergo a tracheostomy annually in the United States (Office of Technology Assessment, 1987). Nonetheless, this cannot be the sole reason. Although not a large number, 2,000 children per year is more than enough for many studies.

An additional and more important reason for the lack of studies is that most children with tracheostomies fail to meet basic inclusion requirements for investigations of the relationship between babbling and expressive language. In addition to being cannulated during the babbling period, such requirements minimally include a relatively intact oral mechanism, at least typical cognitive abilities, and a lack of vocal experience while tracheostomized. Minimal inclusion requirements and factors that make it difficult to obtain children who meet these requirements are now described and are summarized in Tables 1 and 2.

An intact oral mechanism and typical cognition are needed to preclude the possibility that a delay in expressive language development after decannulation results from physical impairment or from general slowing in cognitive development. Common physical impairments affecting the oral mechanism among children with tracheostomies include tracheomalacia, tracheoesophageal anomaly, neuromuscular disorder, congenital anomaly, craniofacial anomaly, and laryngeal neoplasm (Bleile, 1993; Hill & Singer, 1990; Jennings, 1988; Line, Hawkins, Kahlstrom, McLaughlin, & Ensley, 1986; Simon, Fowler, & Handler, 1983). Intellectual impairments are also common. Approximately 50% of children who receive tracheostomies have IQ scores within the range indicating mental retardation. A retrospective study indicated the intelligence of children with IQ scores within the normal range tends to be low average, perhaps resulting from the child's initial medical condition and episodes of asphyxia while tracheostomized (Bleile, 1993; Hill & Singer, 1990).

Absence of vocalizations while cannulated is a necessary inclusion requirement to ascertain whether failure to vocalize influences expressive language development. Vocalization with an in-place tracheostomy may be achieved through one or more of several strategies. Most common is that children physically grow into the ability to vocalize. An infant initially receives a cannula sufficiently large to fill the throat, thus precluding air from flowing upward through the larynx to allow phonation. The large cannula allows all the life-giving air to reach the child's lungs. As the child grows, the cannula becomes smaller relative to the size of the child's throat, permitting phonation to occur as air flows around the cannula and upward across the larynx. If the child's medical condition so requires, a surgeon replaces the cannula with a larger one; otherwise, a smaller cannula is kept in place and the child is able to use the excess air to phonate.

One-way speaking valves provide another phonation option for children with in-place tracheostomies. The valve is placed on the end of the tracheostomy,

Table 1. Minimum requirements for inclusion in studies on the relationship between babbling and the development of expressive language

- Cannulated during babbling period
- Relatively intact oral mechanism
- At least typical cognitive abilities
- Lack of vocal experience while tracheostomized

Table 2. Possible hindrances in meeting minimum inclusion requirements

Common physical impairments: Tracheomalacia, tracheoesophageal anomaly, neuro-muscular disorder, congenital anomaly, craniofacial anomaly, laryngeal neoplasm

Intellectual impairments: Approximately 50% of children who receive tracheostomies have intelligence within the mental retardation range, and the intelligence of children within the typical range tends to be in the low average range

Vocal experiences: Children "grow into" vocalizations; one-way speaking valves; electro-larynx; buccal speech

permitting air to enter during inhalation but blocking air on exhalation, so that speech may occur as the breath exits the body via the mouth and nose. One-way speaking valves typically are introduced for only a few minutes during early phases in treatment but may be worn during most of the child's waking hours after some experience with the device.

Children with in-place tracheostomies may also produce speech without laryngeal vibration in one of two ways. The first method is an electrolarynx that serves as a mechanical vibration source when placed on the child's cheek or neck. The second method, called buccal speech, allows the child to vocalize using the air trapped in his or her cheeks as a vibration source. Buccal speech (also sometimes referred to as *Donald Duck speech*) is discovered by many children with tracheostomies during the course of play.

Children with Bronchopulmonary Dysplasia

The most likely tracheostomized candidates for inclusion in a study of babbling and the development of expressive language are former premature infants who have bronchopulmonary dysplasia (BPD) as their primary medical diagnosis. BPD is an acute, life-threatening neonatal lung injury that may arise indirectly as a consequence of prematurity. To illustrate, a premature infant may initially experience difficulty breathing on his or her own because premature lungs lack surfactant, a secretion usually formed in the last month of pregnancy that helps the lungs to breathe (Metz, 1993). The result of surfactant deficiency is called *hyaline membrane disease*, which in the early months of life may be treated through intubation. However, intubation involves insertion of a tube through the nose and downward through the pharynx and vocal folds, which can cause irritation to tissues and also may be insufficient to treat the disease. For these reasons, mechanical ventilation may be delivered via a tracheostomy tube with or without a trial period of intubation. The most commonly used type of mechanical ventilator helps inflate the lungs, allowing natural recoil to perform the deflation part of the breathing cycle (i.e., positive pressure ventilation). Even while delivering lifesaving oxygen, the pressure exerted on the lungs by the mechanical ventilator may also damage the delicate premature lungs, resulting in BPD.

BPD may require months or even years to resolve. During this time, the child continues to receive mechanical ventilation through a tracheostomy tube. As the condition resolves, the mechanical ventilator supplies oxygen on an intermittent schedule, which allows the child's lungs to practice breathing on their own. Later, the child may be entirely weaned from the mechanical ventilator, even while still receiving assistance through a tracheostomy tube. A child receiving mechanical ventilation and tracheostomy assistance typically lives in a hospital, although home care is an increasingly viable option for selected children and their families (Dougherty, 1993; Hock-Long, Trachtenberg, & Vorters, 1993).

Children with BPD are not different from others with tracheostomies in that they are likely to experience a variety of cognitive, physical, and developmental disabilities. Occasionally, however, a child is encountered whose sole medical difficulty is BPD. Such a child may be entirely healthy but have an in-place tracheostomy for many months while his or her lungs recover. If the child is small or if damage to the lungs is severe, the surgeon may maintain a tight-fitting cannula to avoid precious air from escaping into the oral tract.

STUDIES OF CHILDREN WITH TRACHEOSTOMIES

Three studies have used children with tracheostomies to investigate the relationship between babbling and expressive language development (Bleile et al., 1993; Locke & Pearson, 1990; Simon et al., 1983). The Simon et al. study employed a group design to compare expressive language outcomes of children decannulated prelinguistically with those decannulated after the age at which language is obtained by typically developing children. The other two studies employed case study designs to investigate the period following decannulation. The authors of the case studies reasoned that if babbling did not facilitate the development of expressive language, then their participants' expressive language during the period of the study would not be delayed relative to other areas of cognition and language development. However, as the investigators hypothesized, if babbling facilitated expressive language, then their participants' expressive language development during this period should be delayed relative to other areas of cognition and language development.

Group Design Study

Simon et al. (1983) studied 23 children identified by families and professional medical staff as aphonic or producing only intermittent vocalizations while the tracheostomy was in place. The authors compared the expressive language outcomes of those decannulated prelinguistically with those who were decannulated after the onset of language. Results indicated that those children decannulated prelinguistically experienced better speech outcomes than those decannulated after the age during which babbling typically occurs. The investigators interpreted the findings to indicate that failure to babble results in a poorer expressive language outcome.

Although this study is pioneering in its efforts and provides invaluable descriptive outcome data, design factors limit the conclusions about babbling and expressive language that can be drawn from it. Most important, the two groups of children (those decannulated early and those decannulated late) were likely drawn from different populations. Children decannulated early (before the onset of language) may have had less-intensive medical needs and developmental problems than those decannulated later. Thus, better expressive language outcomes would be expected from those decannulated earlier in development, regardless of hypotheses related to the relationship between babbling and expressive language.

Case Study: Jenny

Locke and Pearson (1990) analyzed the phonetic output of a child identified as Jenny, a nearly full-term infant (37 weeks' gestational age) who was intubated intermittently during the first few months of life secondary to BPD. Jenny received a tracheostomy at age 5 months that remained in place until age 1 year, 8 months. Intubation largely prohibited typical vocalization during the early months of Jenny's life, and clinical records indicated that Jenny produced only sporadic vocalizations while the tracheostomy was in place.

Jenny's communication and cognitive development were assessed near the time of decannulation. At age 18 months, Jenny's cognitive development as measured by the Assessment in Infancy (Uzgiris & Hunt, 1975) approximated that of an infant age 16 months. The Bayley Scales of Infant Development (Bayley, 1969) were administered at ages 20 and 21 months, yielding age-equivalency scores for cognitive development of ages 19 and 21 months, respectively. Jenny's language reception abilities were assessed at age 18 months and were found to approximate those of a child ages 15–17 months based on the Receptive-Expressive Emergent Language Scale (Bzoch & League, 1971). Other assessments related to language development performed near the time of decannulation indicated voice quality and hearing within typical limits. Jenny apparently communicated largely through pointing and eye gaze because, although Jenny's mother listed 19 signs that Jenny knew, the authors reported that Jenny more often mimicked signs rather than signing independently.

The speech that served as the basis of the phonetic analysis occurred spontaneously in both hospital and home settings while Jenny interacted with family members, clinicians, or the investigators. Language samples were collected during eight sessions during the 3 months before decannulation and during four sessions in a 1-month period following decannulation. When possible, the investigators compared Jenny's phonetic development with that of children who were typically developing or deaf or had hearing impairments (Oller & Eilers, 1988; Smith & Oller, 1981; Stoel-Gammon & Otomo, 1986). Children with hearing impairments and deaf children were chosen for comparison because they, like children with tracheostomies, may experience difficulty hearing their own vocalizations.

Analyses   Three phonetic analyses were performed. In the first analysis, the investigators measured canonical syllables, which Oller (1986) defined as syllables containing a supralaryngeal consonant and a vowel. To illustrate, [ba] is a canonical syllable because it contains both a supralaryngeal consonant ([b]) and a vowel ([a]). This is in contrast to noncanonical syllables such as [ha] and [i], the first of which contains a consonant produced at the glottis ([h]) and the latter of which contains no consonant at all. One of the most striking finds of Locke and Pearson's study was that only 2% of Jenny's syllables were canonical when the language samples were averaged over the month postdecannulation. This compares with 20% for typically developing infants ages 6–9 months.

In the second analysis, the investigators calculated the number of different consonants in Jenny's phonetic inventory. Jenny's speech was found to average only 4.5 (range, 3–6) different consonants across the four postdecannulation sessions. Such a consonant inventory size is similar to that found in the language of deaf children of approximately Jenny's age. In contrast, typically developing infants might be expected to have 11 or 12 different segments in their phonetic inventories by age 5 months and to have nearly 30 consonants in their phonetic inventories by age 18 months (Stoel-Gammon & Otomo, 1986).

The investigators' final analysis identified the types of consonants and vowels in Jenny's 14 canonical syllables produced during the 8 weeks before and the 4 weeks after decannulation. The analysis indicated that all the syllables were consonant–vowel (CV) and that vowels were perceived to be [a], [aI], and [E]. Eleven of the consonants were perceived as [b] and three as [j]. The preponderance of labial consonants in Jenny's phonetic inventory is somewhat unusual compared with typically developing children. Although 78% of Jenny's consonants were labials, less than 20% of consonants are produced at that place of production by typically developing children around ages 12–15 months, the oldest ages of typically developing children for which comparable data exist (Smith & Oller, 1981). In contrast, labial consonants are reported to account for almost 100% of the consonant inventories of children with hearing impairments near Jenny's age.

The investigators obtained additional information after the period of the study regarding Jenny's subsequent language development. At 6 weeks after decannulation, Jenny's expressive vocabulary was estimated to consist of six to eight words, which she produced with five consonants and four lexical shapes. At age 4 years, 4 months (several years after the investigation), Jenny's receptive and expressive language was assessed as age 4 years, 7 months, using the Preschool Language Scale (Zimmerman, Steiner, & Pond, 1979). Jenny's speech was judged to be entirely intelligible.

Interpretation Locke and Pearson (1990) interpreted the combined results of their analyses as support for the hypothesis that babbling facilitates the development of expressive language. This interpretation was based on Jenny's limited inventories of canonical syllables, consonants, and vowels during the month following decannulation. These inventories appeared to approximate an infant younger than age 6 months, the age at which typically developing children often begin to babble in syllables. The investigators, observing that labial consonants dominated the consonant inventories of both Jenny and children with hearing impairments at a similar age, hypothesized that visibility of such consonants may make them particularly salient to children who are unable to easily hear their own vocalizations. The investigators also hypothesized that Jenny's notably good expressive language outcome at age 4 years, 4 months, may have resulted because decannulation occurred while Jenny was still within a sensitive phase in language development. Locke and Pearson speculated that Jenny's outcome may not have been so good if decannulation had occurred at some unspecified later age.

Case Study: *E*

Bleile et al. (1993) also analyzed the phonetic output of a child shortly after decannulation. Their participants, a child identified as *E*, had been born at 29 weeks' gestation and had been intubated shortly after birth subsequent to BPD. *E* had been tracheostomized from ages 1–28 months. Because *E* experienced severe BPD, a tight-fitting cannula was maintained.

Reports by *E*'s parents, physicians, nurses, and speech-language pathologists indicated that *E* did not vocalize while cannulated. *E*'s primary means of communication while the tracheostomy remained in place was through pointing, signs, and a few oral words produced without phonation. By parental report, *E* used approximately 30 different signs. The oral words were a voiceless, wet-sounding labiodental sound (e.g., a request for blowing bubbles); a silent, wide-open mouth (e.g., to signify a barking or roaring animal); and a voiceless, bilabial popping sound (e.g., for "Pop Pop," the family name for grandfather).

E received a battery of medical and developmental evaluations near the time of decannulation, and, 1 month before decannulation, granulomas were removed from *E*'s vocal cords. Oral and vocal mechanism examinations performed after the surgery by *E*'s physician and a certified speech-language pathologist indicated normal structure and function of the oral and phonatory mechanisms. *E*'s hearing was assessed by a certified audiologist and found to be normal in one ear and to have a 40-decibel loss in the other ear that later was corrected by pressure equalization tubes (American National Standards Institute, 1969).

Near *E*'s second birthday, a licensed psychologist using the Bayley Scales of Infant Development found *E*'s intelligence to fall within the low-average range. *E*'s language reception abilities were assessed using the Preschool Language Scale (Zimmerman, Steiner, & Pond, 1979) and the Kennedy Developmental Scales, the latter of which is a compilation of developmental milestones derived from published reports and standardized assessment instruments (Bleile, 1987). When *E* was age 2 years, 5 months (6 weeks after decannulation), *E*'s language reception abilities approximated a child near age 2 years, based on the results of both assessment instruments. Testing undertaken using both assessment instruments when *E* was age 2 years, 8 months (4 months after decannulation), indicated that *E*'s language reception approximated a child around age 2 years, 4 months. *E*'s mother estimated *E*'s receptive vocabulary at both ages 2 years, 4 months, and 2 years, 8 months, to contain many hundreds of words. *E*'s mean length of utterance at both ages was 1.0.

The language samples used for the analysis occurred spontaneously or were elicited through naming games involving pictures of objects. All elicitation sessions occurred at the same time of day, and each session lasted approximately 1 hour. Data were collected beginning 5 days after decannulation. Subsequent language samples were collected three times weekly during the first 6 weeks after decannulation and at monthly intervals thereafter for the following 10½ months. *E*'s speech outcome was compared with Stoel-Gammon (1985) and with 11 children matched to *E* on either size of expressive vocabulary or language reception abilities.

E's phonetic development was analyzed at 6 weeks and at 4 months after decannulation. Following Locke and Pearson (1990), the incidence of syllables was calculated using the same procedures as that study. Different procedures were used to analyze *E*'s consonant inventory, making it difficult to compare those aspects of the two studies. Bleile et al. (1993) based their analysis of *E*'s consonant inventory on utterances perceived to have referential content, whereas Locke and Pearson (1990) based their analysis on utterances regardless of their referential nature.

Analyses The analyses indicated that, at 6 weeks after decannulation, *E* was substantially delayed in her development of expressive language compared with both her chronological peers and the age of those with similar language reception abilities. The canonical syllable analysis revealed that only 6% of *E*'s syllables were canonical. As with Locke and Pearson's subject, a high percentage (85%) of the consonants in these syllables were labials. As shown in Table 3, *E*'s entire expressive vocabulary at 6 weeks after decannulation consisted of six words: *bottle, bubble, grandfather, daddy, mom*, and *up*. The inventory of consonants in these words approximates that of children near age 15 months.

Table 3.   *E*'s expressive vocabulary at 6 weeks after decannulation

Word	Gloss
[baba]	bottle
[baba]	bubble
[dada]	grandfather (Pop Pop)
[dada]	daddy
[mam]	mom
[ʌp]	up

E demonstrated somewhat more advanced phonetic abilities 4 months after decannulation. The canonical syllable analysis indicated that 94% of *E*'s
syllables were canonical. Almost 73% of the consonants in the canonical syllables were labial. *E*'s entire expressive vocabulary at 4 months after decannulation is listed in Table 4. Thirteen of *E*'s 17 words began with some type
of labial consonant (e.g., [b p m w]). The consonant inventory of the consonants in these words approximated that of a child near age 15 months.

The investigators obtained additional information on *E*'s speech and language development for up to 1 year after decannulation. At age 3 years, 4
months, *E*'s language reception abilities approximated a child near age 3 years
as measured by the receptive portion of the Preschool Language Scale. *E* produced short sentences ranging in length from two to six words. A measure of
mean length of utterance was not obtained. *E*'s consonantal development at
that age was sufficiently advanced to allow comparison with normative information for preschool- and school-age children (Sander, 1972). Results of these
analyses indicated that *E*'s development in consonants approximated that of a
child between ages 3 and 4 years.

Table 4.   *E*'s expressive vocabulary at 4 months after decannulation

Word	Gloss	Word	Gloss
[dæda]	daddy	[ʌp]	up
[haɪ]	hi	[baɪ]	please
[da]	down	[baɪ]	bye
[mɑm]	mom	[baɪ]	bag
[bɑp]	hop	[bʌ]	bubble
[wɑwɑ]	water	[bɑp]	pop
[bʊk]	book	[bɔ]	ball
[boʊ]	bow	[pɑp pɑp]	Pop Pop (grandfather)
[bʌbʌ]	baby		

Two analyses of *E* were performed subsequent to the publication of the study. The first analysis was of a presleep monologue that occurred 3 weeks after decannulation. *E*'s mother had reported that *E* engaged in monologues before sleep, and the recording was made by *E*'s mother at the request of the investigators. The mother waited outside *E*'s bedroom while the recording was obtained. Other attempts to record these monologues were unsuccessful because of the mother's schedule.

E's presleep monologue lasted 21 minutes, during which time 57 utterances were produced. The utterances were identified and analyzed for canonical syllables using the same procedures as Bleile et al. (1993) and Locke and Pearson (1990). None of the utterances appeared referential. Results of the analysis indicated that 15% of *E*'s utterances consisted of canonical syllables. All the canonical syllables were [ba] or [baba]. The noncanonical utterances consisted primarily of isolated voiced and voiceless vowels, [h], and lip-smacking sounds.

The second analysis occurred 3 years subsequent to the publication of the study, when *E*'s mother was contacted by one of the investigators. *E*'s mother reported that *E* was enrolled in a general first-grade class and was doing well in all subjects. It was reported that *E* was understood by people with whom she was in contact but that she spoke with a lateral lisp for which she received therapy 20 minutes per week. *E* was also reported to receive occupational therapy services once a week for printing.

Interpretation   As with Locke and Pearson (1990), the investigators interpreted their results as supporting the hypothesis that babbling facilitates the development of expressive language. The primary basis for this interpretation was *E*'s reduced phonetic abilities in the weeks and months subsequent to decannulation. The authors noted that their results of the canonical syllable analysis closely approximated that of Locke and Pearson's subject. Approximately 2% of Jenny's syllables were canonical at 3 weeks after decannulation compared with 4% of *E*'s syllables at 6 weeks after decannulation. At the same time after decannulation, 78% of Jenny's syllables were labial compared with 85% of *E*'s syllables.

The two subsequent analyses supported and enriched the findings of the original study. The first analysis indicated that *E*'s limited ability to produce canonical syllables during the period following decannulation extended to her presleep vocalizations. The relatively higher percentage of canonical syllables in *E*'s presleep monologue (15% of her utterances at 3 weeks after decannulation compared with 4% at 6 weeks after decannulation in other contexts) may indicate that presleep monologues served as a practice context for vocal development. The second analysis indicated that *E*'s speech development appeared almost typical at 3 years after decannulation. *E*'s successful placement in a general classroom indicated that she had relatively intact cognitive abilities.

DISCUSSION

This chapter begins by asking if babbling facilitates the development of expressive language. A complete answer to this question awaits more studies and is likely to be slow in coming. Children with tracheostomies are sufficiently rare that opportunities to study them do not arise often. Few among such children meet the inclusion requirements for a study of relationships between babbling and expressive language. Although investigators may develop clever experimental designs to circumvent such problems, it seems more likely that information will accrue by accumulated case studies. Yet, even at this early juncture, a picture of the role of babbling in the development of expressive language is emerging that may provide initial hypotheses to test against future studies.

The results of the studies of Jenny and *E* are compatible with the hypothesis that babbling facilitates the development of expressive language. If this were not so, the children should have sprung into expressive language after decannulation with phonetic inventories appropriate to children of their chronological ages and language reception abilities. Instead, both children experienced a period of a month or longer after decannulation during which less than 5% of their vocalizations contained canonical syllables. *E*'s percentage of canonical syllables approached 15% during presleep monologue, which may have served her as an important practice context for vocal development. By comparison, the vocalizations of infants near 6 or 7 months of age often contain 20% or more canonical syllables.

The children's development of expressive language appeared to be limited by their speech abilities. Although at the time of decannulation Jenny's cognitive development approximated a child ages 19–21 months and *E*'s language reception abilities approximated that of a child near age 24 months, neither child demonstrated expressive vocabularies commensurate with his or her cognitive and language reception abilities. For example, Jenny and *E* did not combine the sounds and syllables in their phonetic inventories to make more words or combine words together to form simple sentences. Instead, the expressive vocabularies of both children consisted of six words nearly 6 weeks after decannulation and were extremely limited in their range of sounds and syllables. In common with children with hearing impairments, the labial place of production dominated the speech of both children, perhaps reflecting a visual bias in the speech of children who are unable to hear their own vocalizations.

A surprise of the studies is that, several years (Jenny) and 1 year (*E*) after decannulation, the children's development of expressive language appeared appropriate for their chronological ages. The developmental picture that emerges is that, in the first weeks after decannulation, the children struggled to pronounce canonical syllables, a building block of expressive language acquired by typically developing children through babbling during the first year of life. Success in acquiring canonical syllables occurred relatively quickly, perhaps accelerated by the children's advanced language comprehension and cognitive abilities. However, learning to produce canonical syllables did not teach the myriad constellations of vowels, consonants, syllable shapes, and stress patterns needed to build words. Thus, even after acquiring the ability to pronounce canonical syllables, the children struggled to acquire, at first slowly, then more rapidly, an expressive vocabulary.

Lenneberg (1967) and others hypothesized that resiliency in language acquisition might be limited to a certain window of time. The cases of Genie and other children raised in extreme circumstances are often cited in support of such a critical (or sensitive) period. Researchers have not suggested a specific age range during which babbling must occur. The case studies of *E* and Jenny suggest that such a window (should it exist) does not close by age 2 years, 4 months. Neither Jenny nor *E* experienced significant long-term articulation and phonological difficulties subsequent to decannulation. *E*, decannulated approximately 8 months later than Jenny, experienced persistent (albeit relatively minor) problems with consonants and consonant clusters in first grade. However, children who never underwent tracheostomies may also experience such problems in similar school grades. Furthermore, approximately 13%–17% of children who had been able to vocalize while tracheostomized experience similar problems relative to other areas of development (Hill & Singer, 1990; Simon et al., 1983).

It is possible that children for whom babbling occurs outside a supposed sensitive period may produce speech errors that cannot be perceived (Bleile et al., 1993; Saletsky Kamen & Watson, 1991). If this is correct, the studies of both Jenny and *E* were conducted at the wrong level of analysis to address this topic. A child for whom babbling occurs outside a supposed sensitive period might experience difficulties that require specialized instrumentation to detect. Spectrographic analysis of the transitions between vowels and consonants seems a particularly important domain within which to test such a possibility.

CONCLUSIONS

Although specific details of the experiences of Jenny and *E* are too unique to be applied to the clinical care of other children, their case studies support the view that facilitating infant vocal development is a reasonable therapeutic goal. As indicated in the first section of this chapter, facilitation of an infant's vocal development is worthwhile if such vocalizations constitute a type of practice activity. The studies of Jenny and *E* support the view that babbling is related to expressive language and plays a facilitating role in its development.

Children with tracheostomies also serve to emphasize the importance of the speech connection in expressive vocabulary development. In typically developing children, the development of expressive vocabularies is probably paced both by maturing speech-motor and phonological systems and by advances in cognitive and language reception abilities. However, the relative influences of speech and language on expressive language development are difficult to isolate because, in typically developing children, both systems develop concurrently. In children with tracheostomies, the influence of speech and language connections on expressive vocabulary development operates somewhat independently, allowing their relative influence to be better studied.

The results of the studies indicate that speech was a limiting factor in the children's expressive vocabulary development. The evidence for this is that, at the time of the children's decannulations, their cognitive and language comprehension abilities were sufficient to support both a large expressive vocabulary and, for E, the production of at least short sentences. Yet, during this period, the children's expressive vocabulary consisted of only a small number of single words.

Although children with tracheostomies provide unique opportunities to study disconnections between speech and language development, a growing body of research strongly suggests that they are not unique in having speech be a limiting factor in expressive vocabulary development (see discussions in Chapters 7 and 8). Children from such large and diverse populations as those with Down syndrome and those with expressive language delays seem limited in expressive vocabulary development by their speech abilities (Miller, 1992; Paul & Jennings, 1992). Such children remind us that the task of acquiring a language is not only learning how to mean but also how to sound to mean (Ferguson & Macken, 1983).

The existence of children with limited expressive vocabularies as the result of speech problems suggests a possible need for intervention approaches focusing on the speech component (Bleile, 1995; Bleile & Miller, 1994). Intervention for children with limited expressive vocabularies typically involves language stimulation with special emphasis on pragmatics and discourse (Greenspan, 1985, 1992; MacDonald, 1989; MacDonald & Carroll, 1992; Wilcox, 1989). Such approaches, although providing an invaluable foundation on which to build intervention, may not focus enough on the development of children's speech abilities. A challenge to the profession is to develop intervention approaches designed specifically to treat the speech impairments of children whose development places them on the very border of language acquisition.

REFERENCES

American National Standards Institute. (1969). *Specifications for audiometers (ANSI S3.6-1969)*. New York: Author.

Bayley, N. (1969). *Manual for the Bayley Scales of Infant Development*. New York: The Psychological Corporation.

Bleile, K. (1987). *The Kennedy Development Scales*. Unpublished assessment instrument, Kennedy Krieger Institute for Handicapped Children, Baltimore, MD.

Bleile, K. (1993). Children with longterm tracheostomies. In K. Bleile (Ed.), *The care of children with longterm tracheostomies* (pp. 3–19). San Diego: Singular Publishing Group.

Bleile, K. (1995). *Manual of articulation and phonological disorders*. San Diego: Singular Publishing Group.

Bleile, K., & Miller, S. (1994). Toddlers with medical needs. In J. Bernthal & N. Bankson (Eds.), *Child phonology: Characteristics, assessment, and intervention with special populations* (pp. 81–109). New York: Thieme.

Bleile, K., Stark, R.E., & Silverman McGowan, J. (1993). Speech development in a child after decannulation: Further evidence that babbling facilitates later speech development. *Clinical Linguistics and Phonetics, 7,* 319–337.

Boysson-Bardies, B., & Vihman, M. (1991). Adaptation to language: Evidence from babbling and first words in four languages. *Language, 67,* 297–319.

Braitenberg, V., & Schüz, A. (1992). Basic features of cortical connectivity and some consideration on language. In J. Wind, B. Chiarelli, B. Bichakjian, & A. Jonker (Eds.), *Language origin: A multidisciplinary approach* (pp. 89–102). Dordrecht, Netherlands: Kluwer Academic Publishers.

Bzoch, K., & League, R. (1971). *Receptive-Expressive Emergent Language (REEL) Scale*. Austin, TX: PRO-ED.

Curtiss, S. (1977). *Genie: A psycholinguistic study of a modern-day "wild child."* New York: Academic Press.

Dougherty, J. (1993). Training caregivers. In K. Bleile (Ed.), *The care of children with longterm tracheostomies* (pp. 223–248). San Diego: Singular Publishing Group.

Ferguson, C., & Macken, M. (1983). The role of play in phonological development. In K. Nelson (Ed.), *Children's language IV* (pp. 262–282). Hillsdale, NJ: Lawrence Erlbaum Associates.

Greenspan, S.I. (1985). *First feelings: Milestones in the emotional development of your child from birth to age 4*. New York: Viking Press.

Greenspan, S.I. (1992). *Infancy and early childhood: The practice of clinical assessment and intervention with emotional and developmental challenges*. Madison, CT: International Universities Press.

Handler, S. (1993). Surgical management of the tracheostomy. In K. Bleile (Ed.), *The care of children with longterm tracheostomies* (pp. 23–40). San Diego: Singular Publishing Group.

Hewes, G. (1992). History of glottogonic theories. In J. Wind, B. Chiarelli, B. Bichakjian, & A. Jonker (Eds.), *Language origin: A multidisciplinary approach* (pp. 3–20). Dordrecht, Netherlands: Kluwer Academic Publishers.

Hill, B., & Singer, L. (1990). Speech and language development after infant tracheostomy. *Journal of Speech and Hearing Disorders, 55,* 15–20.

Hock-Long, L., Trachtenberg, S., & Vorters, D. (1993). In K. Bleile (Ed.), *The care of children with longterm tracheostomies* (pp. 203–222). San Diego: Singular Publishing Group.

Humphrey, G., & Humphrey, M. (1932). *The wild boy of Aveyron*. New York: Appleton-Century-Crofts.

Jakobson, R. (1968). *Kindersprache, Aphasie, und allgemeine Lautgesetze [Child language, aphasia, and phonological universals]* (A. Keiler, trans.). The Hague, Netherlands: Mouton. (Original work published 1941)

Jennings, P. (1988). Nursing and home aspects of the care of a child with tracheostomy. *Journal of Laryngology and Otology, 17*(Suppl.), 25–29.

Kipling, R. (1895). *The jungle book*. Garden City, NY: Doubleday.

Lenneberg, E. (1967). *Biological foundations of language*. New York: John Wiley & Sons.

Line, W.S., Hawkins, D., Kahlstrom, E.J., McLaughlin, E., & Ensley, J. (1986). Tracheostomy in infants and young children: The changing perspective. *Laryngoscope, 96,* 510–515.

Locke, J. (1983). *Phonological acquisition and change.* New York: Academic Press.

Locke, J., & Pearson, D. (1990). Linguistic significance of babbling: Evidence from a tracheostomized infant. *Journal of Child Language, 17,* 1–16.

MacDonald, J. (1989). *Becoming partners with children: From play to conversation.* San Antonio, TX: Special Press.

MacDonald, J., & Carroll, J. (1992). A social partnership model for assessing early communication development: An intervention model for preconversational children. *Language, Speech, and Hearing Services in Schools, 23,* 113–124.

Menn, L. (1980). Phonological theory and child phonology. In G. Yeni-Komshian, J. Kavanagh, & C. Ferguson (Eds.), *Child phonology: Production* (pp. 23–41). New York: Academic Press.

Metz, S. (1993). Ventilator assistance. In K. Bleile (Ed.), *The care of children with longterm tracheostomies* (pp. 41–56). San Diego: Singular Publishing Group.

Miller, J. (1992). Lexical development in young children with Down syndrome. In R. Chapman (Ed.), *Processes in language acquisition and disorders* (pp. 202–216). St. Louis: Mosby–Year Book.

Office of Technology Assessment. (1987). *Technology-dependent children: Hospital v. home care* (Technical Memorandum OTA-TM-H-38). Washington, DC: U.S. Government Printing Office.

Oller, D. (1980). The emergence of the sounds of speech in infancy. In G. Yeni-Komshian, J. Kavanagh, & C. Ferguson (Eds.), *Child phonology: Production* (pp. 93–112). New York: Academic Press.

Oller, D. (1986). Metaphonology and infant vocalizations. In B. Lindblom & R. Zetterstrom (Eds.), *Precursors to early speech.* New York: Stockton Press.

Oller, D., & Eilers, R. (1988). The role of audition in infant babbling. *Child Development, 59,* 441–449.

Paul, R., & Jennings, P. (1992). Phonological behavior in toddlers with slow expressive language development. *Journal of Speech and Hearing Research, 35,* 99–107.

Rymer, R. (1993). *Genie: An abused child's flight from silence.* New York: HarperCollins.

Saletsky Kamen, R., & Watson, B. (1991). Effects of long-term tracheostomy on spectral characteristics of vowel production. *Journal of Speech and Hearing Research, 34,* 1057–1066.

Sander, E. (1972). When are speech sounds learned? *Journal of Speech and Hearing Disorders, 37,* 55–63.

Simon, B.M., Fowler, S.M., & Handler, S.D. (1983). Communication development in young children with long-term tracheostomies: A preliminary report. *International Journal of Pediatric Otorhinolaryngology, 6,* 37–50.

Smith, B., & Oller, D. (1981). A comparative study of pre-meaningful vocalizations produced by normally developing and Down's syndrome infants. *Journal of Speech and Hearing Disorders, 46,* 46–51.

Stark, R. (1980). Stages of speech development in the first year of life. In G. Yeni-Komshian, J. Kavanagh, & C. Ferguson (Eds.), *Child phonology: Production* (pp. 73–92). New York: Academic Press.

Stoel-Gammon, C. (1985). Phonetic inventories, 15–24 months: A longitudinal study. *Journal of Speech and Hearing Research, 28,* 505–512.

Stoel-Gammon, C., & Otomo, K. (1986). Babbling development of hearing-impaired and normally hearing subjects. *Journal of Speech and Hearing Disorders, 51,* 33–41.

Uzgiris, I., & Hunt, J.McV. (1975). *Assessment in infancy: Ordinal scales of psychological development*. Urbana: University of Illinois Press.

Velten, H. (1943). The growth of phonemic and lexical patterns in infant language. *Language, 19,* 440–444.

Vihman, M. (1996). *Phonological development: The origins of language in the child.* Oxford, England: Blackwell Publishers.

Vihman, M., Ferguson, C., & Elbert, M. (1986). Phonological development from babbling to speech: Common tendencies and individual differences. *Applied Psycholinguistics, 7,* 3–40.

Wilcox, J.M. (1989). Delivering communication-based services to infants, mothers, and their families: Approaches and models. *Topics in Language Disorders, 10,* 68–79.

Zimmerman, I.L., Steiner, V.G., & Pond, R.E. (1979). *Preschool Language Scale.* Columbus, OH: Charles E. Merrill.

6

Communicative Development in Augmented Modalities
Language without Speech?

Rhea Paul

CHILDREN WITH SEVERE MOTOR IMPAIRMENTS that limit the use of speech for communication present a case study in the acquisition of language without speech as a primary expressive channel. For children whose speech is seriously limited because of severe speech-motor and physical impairments (SSPI) but who do not have significant cognitive or hearing disabilities, the equipment necessary to master receptive language and to use it as a foundation for literacy appears to be intact. It would seem, then, that all that these individuals need is some form of augmentative or alternative communication (AAC) output system adapted to their physical abilities. However, does this inaccessibility of the speech channel and the necessity of adopting an unnatural output code have effects on the acquisition of language, literacy, and communicative skill, even in children without significant hearing or cognitive limitations? This is the issue that is explored in this chapter: whether language learning is affected in children with pure motor speech disorders. The purpose behind asking this question is to investigate the ways in which speech and language interact in development in cases that exemplify the most severe limits on the ability to learn to speak, in the context of the least severe limits on what is typically thought of as the abilities needed to learn language. In doing so, the focus of the chapter is on the language acquisition of children who use AAC systems as a result of SSPI but who do not have significant cognitive or hearing impairments. To explore this question, though, it is necessary to draw on information gathered on other kinds of children who use AAC: those with cognitive and hearing impairments, both in conjunction with SSPI and without it.

This chapter was supported by a grant from the Medical Research Foundation of Oregon. Portions of this chapter were presented at the 1995 National Convention of the American Speech-Language-Hearing Association. The author would like to thank Jan Bedrosian and Janice Light for their very helpful comments on earlier versions of this chapter.

This necessity is dictated by the dearth of research on language development in particular subpopulations of children who use AAC. Thus, it is necessary to apply information from several different populations of children who use AAC and to extrapolate what this information suggests for the specific population of interest: children with SSPI in the absence of significant cognitive and hearing impairments. In this way, an attempt is made to glean suggestions about how language development is affected in this population of children with severely limited speech. This information, in turn, sheds light on the ways in which speech limitations affect the development of language.

Before turning to the research itself, though, several clarifications are needed. First, what is meant by AAC needs to be clear. According to the American Speech-Language-Hearing Association (ASHA), AAC is an "attempt to compensate (either temporarily or permanently) for the impairment and disability patterns of individuals with severe expressive communication disorders" (1989, p. 107). An AAC system is "an integrated group of components, including the symbols, aids, strategies, and techniques used by individuals to enhance communication" (ASHA, 1991, p. 10). AAC interventions are multimodal and make use of all of the individual's capacities, including residual speech vocalizations, gestures, signs, and aided communication (ASHA, 1991). When discussing AAC use in children with SSPI, it is important to remember that many of these children are neither completely nonspeaking nor completely nonvocal. They may have some degree of speech, such as the ability to say "no" and "hi" intelligibly. In addition or instead, they may use vocalizations to communicate some of their intentions. Children using AAC as an early expressive system may have communicated previously through small amounts of speech or vocalization, and the AAC system may not be either their first or their only expressive modality. Even for children with pure speech disorders, their expressive system is never a pure one; it typically involves some degree of multimodality. Thus, the language of children with SSPI is not truly "without speech" as the subtitle of this chapter might suggest. It is instead associated with severely limited but nonetheless existent speech and vocal behavior. This complication must be remembered when considering the implications of severely limited speech on language development.

Second, the assumption that children with SSPI in the absence of other significant impairments have typical cognitive and related skills that can serve as a basis for language acquisition must be questioned. There is reason to believe that severe motor limitations in and of themselves can affect cognitive development, even in the presence of typical potential. Bruner (1966) discussed the role of motor exploration in the development of the first phase of representational development, the enactive phase. In this form of mental representation, exemplified by motor imitation, the child constructs mental representations in the form of actions. Later, iconic modes of representation are added; iconic modes are those that involve the processing of images that are more or less free of action but still bear some nonarbitrary relation to the referent. Drawing is a primary example of this kind of representational behavior. Only after both of these modalities of representational behavior have been developed does true symbolic behavior emerge, with language serving as one example. Such a sequence of development suggests that children with SSPI could have difficulties with symbolic development beyond their difficulties with the motor act of speech. McNaughton (1993) discussed the ways in which the restriction in motor behavior in children with SSPI would limit the symbolic foundation that they could establish through enactive experiences with objects and actions, thus laying a shaky basis for the development of higher-level representational skills, such as iconic imagery and symbolization.

Moreover, Stoel-Gammon (see Chapter 2) has shown the close connections between lexical and phonological skill in early development. Swank and Larrivee (see Chapter 10) have discussed the relations between speech production and phonological awareness in the acquisition of literacy. These authors suggest that speech is intimately connected to the development of language and serves to facilitate certain aspects of language acquisition. Again, it might be asked in this connection what the effects on language development of very limited speech practice and feedback might be.

In attempting to answer this question, the kinds of conditions that can result in an inability to use speech as a primary mode of communication need clarification. One condition is a severe congenital dysarthria or anarthria associated with a motor impairment, such as cerebral palsy (CP). This condition, referred to in the literature as SSPI, may be present in children without significant impairments in hearing and cognition. However, many children with severe motor disabilities also experience multiple disabling conditions, including cognitive effects. Johnson-Martin, Wolters, and Stowers (1987) addressed the difficulty of doing valid psychological assessments of children with SSPI. Because early cognitive milestones are often evaluated through language and fine motor tasks, finding fair and valid assessments that allow children with SSPI to express their potential is a particular challenge. Still, these authors concluded that it is possible to get a reasonably accurate picture of the mental abilities of children with SSPI through careful collaboration with other professionals regarding ways to get around the child's physical output limits, careful planning of assessment procedures to meet specific goals, cautious interpretation of results, and periodic reassessments. In using such methods, the research reviewed here has generally attempted to report whether typical cognitive potential is present in subjects with SSPI. However, in studying language acquisition through the augmented modalities available to children with SSPI, it cannot be assumed that typical cognitive development is always present.

A second set of conditions associated with lack of functional speech includes severe to profound cognitive impairments without SSPI. Individuals with mental retardation or autism may fall into this category. For these individuals, lack of functional speech cannot be attributed primarily to motor limitations. Nonetheless, many such individuals are provided with AAC systems to facilitate their communication, and some of the research on language development in augmented modes includes such subjects whose primary limitation is cognitive rather than motor. Although the principal purpose of this chapter is to look at the effects of motor-speech limitations as they affect language development, research on nonspeaking individuals with cognitive limitations is also reviewed. In attempting to draw conclusions about the implications of findings on language development in children who use AAC as an early expressive communication system, though, it is important to recall that some of these individuals do not display significant motor limitations; instead, a cognitive factor appears to be primary in limiting their speech production. Caution is necessary in interpreting this research in light of the possibility that some of the effects observed may be the result of cognitive differences in the individuals studied rather than of the interactions of speech and language in development.

In this chapter, knowledge about language development in the augmented modalities provided to children who use AAC, both with and without SSPI, is examined. The ways in which these children communicate, both with and without their AAC devices, are described. The question of how these data can inform understanding of the speech–language connection is then addressed.

TRANSITIONS IN LANGUAGE ACQUISITION

One way to approach the question of how the data described in the preceding section can be used to understand the speech–language connection is to examine certain crucial transitions in language development that appear to be mediated to some extent by the production of speech. In making each of these transitions, the child goes from a more basic form of communication to one with a significantly increased degree of complexity.

Although the motivation to communicate is always present in language development, this motivation alone does not explain why children move from one more or less successful mode of communication to one that is more formally complex. Why, for example, should a child learn the complex rules of tag question formation in English (as every typically developing child does), when putting "right?" at the end of a statement works just as well (deVilliers & deVilliers, 1978)? Paul (1997) identified three major transitions that take place during the first 5 years of life that seem to involve a strong degree of modulation provided by the ability to use speech (see Table 1).

From Illocution to Locution

The first of these transitions takes place in the move from what Bates (1976) called *illocutionary* to *locutionary communication*. That is, children success-

Table 1.   Transitions in child language

Age in typical development	Description	Language domains
12 months	Babbling→Words	Pragmatics→Semantics
18 months	Single-word utterances→ Multiword utterances	Semantics→Syntax
4–6 years	Speaking and listening→ Reading and writing	Phonology→ Metaphonology

fully express communicative intent using gestures and nonlinguistic vocalizations before their first birthday, but at some point around 12 months of age, they begin relying more heavily on vocal forms of communication and shaping their vocalizations into conventional words. These words are one manifestation of the child's emerging ability to use symbols. In children with typical hearing, the particular symbols (i.e., words) used grow out of the repertoire of sounds developed during babbling in the first year of life; in children learning American Sign Language (ASL) as their first language, symbolic gestures evolve into conventional signs. Data from Oller et al. (see Chapter 1) suggest that infants who do not produce canonical babbling by age 10 months are at risk for developing language disorders. Thus, the appearance of speechlike vocalizations seems to be at least one component of the process in the transition to linguistic communication. Many early one-word utterances simply encode the same pragmatic intentions that were expressed earlier by prelinguistic vocalizations and gestures (Chapman, 1981). Thus, in a sense, this transition is from pragmatics to semantics, from communicative intent to a conventional form of expression for the same intention. Children learning sign as a first language make this transition by building conventional signs on the foundation of symbolic gestures that have evolved during their first phase of development. Children learning speech do so through evolving their babbled vocalizations into words. It could be asked, on what foundation do children using AAC as an early expressive system build their first symbols?

From Semantics to Syntax

A second transition typically takes place at about age 18 months. At this time, expressive vocabulary size reaches about 50 words, and two things happen. The rate of vocabulary acquisition increases dramatically, resulting in what has been called a *vocabulary spurt*, and children begin combining words to express many of the same semantic notions that they had been expressing previously with single words (Owens, 1992). This transition is, in a sense, from semantics to syntax. The additional piece of complexity that syntax adds is not only length of the string but also a hierarchical principle: Units must be expressed in a particular order to convey the intended meaning. This reliance on word order constitutes a steppingstone (or bootstrap) to more complex hierarchical relationships in syntax. In the process of this transition, children also learn to encode semantic relationships through the combination of words that were not present in either of the words when expressed alone. They also develop working memory capacity by adding to the number of elements held in mind to be produced (Liberman, Shankweiler, & Liberman, 1989). This memory capacity is also thought to be mediated by the use of phonological codes, based to some extent on subvocal articulatory rehearsal (Baddeley, 1986).

Many of the transitional behaviors that would seem to assist a child in going from single words to word combinations appear to be facilitated by speech. For example, one transitional form is the successive one-word utterance (Owens, 1992). Children often produce two separate one-word utterances, each in a distinct intonation contour but produce them in close temporal proximity and seem to be using the two utterances to encode a single semantic relation, such as "Me. Up," to mean "Pick me up." The ability to build slowly toward the production of a longer string through this transitional form might serve as an additional bootstrap to the developing child. Again, it could be asked how the production of language in an alternative modality could affect this transition to syntax, including its effect on the ability to learn word order as a semantic encoding device and the ability to expand working memory capacity through practice with multisymbol strings.

A second form that modulates the transition from semantics to syntax is the "giant word" or unanalyzed language chunk that the child produces as a gestalt and analyzes later. Typical examples of such giant words include "see you later, alligator," "happy birthday," and "choo-choo train." High frequency of use of these forms helps to automatize them in production, allowing the typical child to articulate an overlearned string that is much longer than the child could articulate as single words that need to be programmed individually for production. In turn, these longer strings build up articulatory ability, preparing the way for the production of longer, less routinized forms.

From Phonology to Metaphonology

A third transition takes place at the end of the preschool period, when children begin to develop skills in metalinguistics and phonological awareness. As shown in research (see Chapter 10; Kamhi & Catts, 1989; Vellutino, 1979), phonological awareness is closely correlated with reading ability. This awareness grows out of familiarity with the sound units of speech that is developed, to some degree, from experience with articulating the sounds of speech (Liberman, Cooper, Shankweiler, & Studdert-Kennedy, 1967). For children who do not develop a phonological encoding system through feedback from speech, it might be asked how such a system can be established. This question becomes especially important when considering that learning to read through a decoding method built on phonological awareness is known to be more successful than other methods of literacy acquisition (Adams, 1990; Chall, 1983) and that children with SSPI are known to have poorer reading ability than their mental ages would predict (Foley, 1993).

It seems that each of these transitions to increased linguistic complexity is modulated to some degree by speech. For example, motor behaviors such as babbling provide the infant with a prelinguistic form of communication that is in many ways analogous to language (e.g., vocal behavior, face-to-face interaction, turn-taking structure). The units of language (i.e., phonemes, syllables) evolve out of babbling and lay the basis for the structural components of language production. When this avenue of linguistic precursor is unavailable, what is the effect on communicative development?

This chapter next reviews what is known about communicative development in children who are provided with AAC devices as an early expressive communication system. These data can then be used to address the questions raised previously in the chapter.

LANGUAGE DEVELOPMENT IN CHILDREN WHO USE AAC

Although little is known about the process and sequence of language acquisition in children who use AAC as their primary communication system, some research is beginning to emerge. The three transitions in language development will be examined to glean what is known about how each is accomplished by children acquiring an early expressive system through AAC.

From Illocution to Locution

The transition from illocution to locution for typically developing children consists of the change in the form of expression of communicative intent from gestures and nonlinguistic vocalizations to vocal forms of communication. This section offers information on this transition in children using AAC systems.

Expressing Communicative Intentions　A good deal of research has looked at the ways in which children who use AAC systems express communicative intentions. Many of these studies look at children of a particular chronological age with a particular medical diagnosis (such as CP) and do not control for mental age or developmental level. Thus, some of the studies included individuals with mental retardation as well as motor impairments, and there is no attempt to predict what kinds of communicative behaviors might be expected, based on mental age. Despite these limitations, there is some preliminary information available on illocutionary behavior demonstrated by children who use AAC.

Light, Collier, and Parnes (1985a, 1985b, 1985c) studied the communicative interaction patterns of children using AAC with their parents. The individuals had no identified cognitive impairments and a symbol vocabulary of at least 100 items. Light et al. (1985a) showed that these children with SSPI engaged in interactional exchanges with their caregivers, with each influencing the other during the discourse. However, the pattern of the discourse was highly asymmetrical, with caregivers controlling the interaction by initiating more topics and demanding specific responses from the children. The children often failed to take all of their optional conversational turns, thus obligating the caregivers to use more summoning power in their utterances to keep the conversations going. Hanzlik (1990) reported that children with CP were more compliant and less responsive in free play interactions with parents than were children of similar mental age without disabilities.

Light et al. (1985b) looked at the range of communication intentions expressed in structured and unstructured contexts by the same children. They reported that, in unstructured situations, the children were limited mostly to yes-or-no responses or to responses of specific information that had been requested by the parent. Although a wider range of intentions was expressed in the structured communication situations, there were a variety of intentions, including requesting information, clarification, and expressing social conventions such as greetings, that these children seldom initiated. Moreover, Glennen and Calculator (1985) showed that children who were able to use AAC symbols to respond to others' questions and labels needed specific instruction to use the same symbols to convey other intentions, such as requests. Thus, it appears that the use of AAC modalities to communicate some intentions does not spontaneously generalize to the use of the same means for expressing additional intents.

Light et al. (1985c) showed that communication with children using AAC is a multimodal process. That is, they found that children used some means other than their AAC device (e.g., gaze, vocalization, gesture) in more than 80% of the communicative turns they expressed. Similarly, Romski and Sevcik (1996) reported that when augmented communication through a voice output device was established in nonspeaking individuals with mental retardation, 37% of communicative expressions used the device, with the remainder being expressed by nonword vocalizations. The rate of vocalization did not decrease with the introduction of the device. This process closely parallels the stage in typical language development in which nonlinguistic vocalizations coexist with word approximations.

For children who use AAC, however, the two modes were used for different purposes. Typically developing children use both nonlinguistic and linguistic utterances to express basically the same range of communicative intents in the transition from the illocutionary to the locutionary period (Chapman, 1981). For children using AAC, though, Light et al. (1985b) found that the mode of communication used was strongly influenced by the communicative function being expressed: Responses to requests for information and clarification were usually expressed by using the AAC device; confirmations and denials were conveyed by vocalizations and gestures. Romski and Sevcik (1996) also reported that vocalizations were used primarily to gain attention and answer yes-or-no questions, whereas the AAC device was used for naming, requesting, and answering other types of questions. In general, vocal modes of communication are used to convey intentions with little semantic content, such as requests for attention or answers to yes-or-no questions. AAC systems are used most often to provide more specific linguistic information. Light (1997) emphasized the importance of analyzing both aided and unaided communication when discussing the types of intentions expressed by children using AAC. Light (1985), for example, reported that negation was almost always expressed in an unaided mode. If only aided communication—for example, through a communication device—had been analyzed, it would have been erroneously concluded that subjects had failed to express negation.

These studies examined the expression of communicative intents in activities involving structured or unstructured play. Another type of interactional situation that is very common in typical development is interactive storybook reading. Snow and Ninio (1986) showed that book reading plays an important role in the development of early language and preliteracy skills. Several investigators (Light, Binger, & Kelford-Smith, 1994; Marvin, 1994; Pierce & McWilliam, 1993) showed that children who use AAC have fewer opportunities to participate in interactive book reading than peers with speech. When parents do read stories to these children, they usually dominate the interaction, with the child being in a relatively passive role.

In general, passivity and lack of communicative initiation is an issue with children who use AAC (Calculator, 1997). Part of the reason for this passivity may have to do with the difficulty these children have in obtaining rewarding responses to their communicative attempts. Guess and Siegel-Causey (1985) and Houghton, Bronicki, and Guess (1987) showed that the communicative attempts of children who use AAC are often ignored or redirected by adults with whom they interact. Their choices, even when made, are also frequently rejected, and their opportunities for communication are severely limited.

In addition to a lack of reward for communicating, children who use AAC experience a severely limited set of opportunities for communication. Light (1985) showed that the content, form, and intents expressed by children who use AAC are frequently defined by their caregivers, who tightly control their communicative interactions. These children typically express the semantic relationships and pragmatic functions they are called on to express. For example, Light's (1985) research revealed that vocal modes of communication predominated over aided AAC responses primarily because children were so frequently asked yes-or-no questions by their caregivers, to which they responded vocally. Along the same lines, the vocabulary available to children for expression consists of only that supplied by the adults designing their AAC systems. Moreover, adults typically respond immediately to an initial symbol communicated by the child, thus cutting off the child's opportunity to produce a longer string. Even access to the AAC system is limited. Caregivers must make an AAC device available to the child for the child to use it, and frequently they do not do so in informal communication situations. Calculator (1997) pointed out that these kinds of experiences must have an effect on these children's motivation to communicate and strongly influence the mode of communication used.

These findings suggest that children who use AAC are not only deprived of speech as an output modality, but their interactive experience is significantly different from that of speaking children. Not only do these children miss the practice accorded by babbling and speech, they also lack interactive experiences that typically support the development of a range of communicative intentions. The lack of opportunities for interactive development that these children experience cannot be ignored in evaluating their needs for communicative intervention and in understanding the effects that their condition has on their language development.

Using Symbolic Communication   An important contributor to the understanding of the ways in which symbolic development can occur in the absence of speech was the work done on nonhuman primates to attempt to develop symbolic communication in these animals. Studies by Gardner and Gardner (1975), Premack (1970), and Savage-Rumbaugh, Rumbaugh, Smith, and Lawson (1980), to cite a few examples, demonstrated that it is possible to develop symbolic communication skills in these animals who were unable to express vocal symbols because of limitations in their anatomical structures. This work has been extended to humans with disabilities. Carrier (1974), for example, showed that nonspeaking youth with mental retardation can be taught to represent concepts using a system of plastic chips similar to that used by Premack (1970) to train symbolic communication in chimpanzees. Other groups, following the lead of Gardner and Gardner's (1975) project with the chimp Washoe, successfully used ASL to teach symbolic communication skills in nonspeaking children with mental retardation and autism (e.g., Fouts, Couch, & O'Neil, 1979). Although ASL might seem like a logical solution to the problem of lack of speech, Paul (1987) and Romski and Sevcik (1996) pointed out that not all nonspeaking children with intact motor skills acquire signs, even when instruction is provided. When they do, they often continue to use the signs they have been taught to encode simple one- and two-word messages. They do not experience either the vocabulary spurt or the transition to multiword utterances that takes place soon after the acquisition of first words in typically speaking children (Owens, 1992). Thus, for children who do not speak because of cognitive limitations, it appears that replacement of an auditory-vocal channel by an apparently more accessible visual-gestural channel does not entirely obviate the communication problem. Nonetheless, these studies do demonstrate that it is not the acquisition of symbols per se that blocks the path to linguistic communication in children with cognitive impairments without functional speech. Even those with mental retardation can learn to use symbols of various kinds to refer to objects in the world. All the studies reviewed thus far employed highly structured teaching approaches and behavioral techniques such as modeling, shaping, and other operant procedures.

Romski and Sevcik (1996) provided perhaps the most detailed account of the transition from illocution to locution in children who use AAC as a primary communication system and were the first to introduce more naturalistic teaching procedures. Their research also was based on the work of Savage-Rumbaugh and colleagues (1980), whose chimps were taught to use arbitrary visual-graphic symbols called *lexigrams* that were composed of combinations of nine basic geometrical forms and linked to a computer keyboard similar to the kind used in many AAC devices. Using discrete trial training and multiple trials to establish semantic connections between the lexigrams and their referents, Savage-Rumbaugh et al. (1980) were able to show that a chimp could be taught to employ such symbols for communication.

A serendipitous finding in the next generation of this work (Savage-Rumbaugh, McDonald, Sevcik, Hopkins, & Rupert, 1986), involving bonobos, revealed that one young bonobo acquired symbols without direct instruction and reinforcement simply by observing the training of her mother. This finding, coming at a time when pragmatic views of language development were in ascendancy, coupled with the known difficulties in generalizing skills taught with structured behavioral procedures to natural environments (Spradlin & Siegel, 1982), led to an attempt to use more naturalistic methods for establishing symbol use in children without functional speech.

Romski and Sevcik (1996) described the development of an augmented language system, using the same computer-linked lexigrams employed by Savage-Rumbaugh et al. (1980), that was taught by naturalistic rather than behaviorist methods. The participants were a group of school-age individuals with mental retardation and no previous spoken language. Romski and Sevcik added a voice output communication device to their visual-graphic symbol system, so that when the individual selected a symbol, its equivalent spoken word was pronounced by the computer. This addition was made to link the visual communication system more immediately with a familiar auditory-verbal signal. It both provided the participants with a multimodal communication system and made it easier for listeners to comprehend the participants' messages.

Romski and Sevcik's (1996) findings revealed that the participants, with mental ages that ranged from younger than age 2 years up to age 5 years, were able to learn abstract symbols to represent lexical items through loosely structured, naturalistic communicative experiences embedded in daily routines in which participants were encouraged but not required to use the lexigrams. The participants were first taught one symbol for food using these methods; later, additional food symbols and symbols for other categories were added. When the individual had mastered 12 referential symbols, some social-regulatory symbols, such as PLEASE and HELP, were added to the repertoire. Romski and Sevcik found that their participants used both their new symbolic communication system and their more familiar vocalizations when communicating with adults in their environment.

Another addition made to this system was to provide, above the symbol itself on the keyboard, the printed version of the word that each symbol represented. No instruction in recognizing the printed words was provided; nonetheless, some of the participants did eventually learn to recognize the printed words associated with the symbols they knew.

An important finding of this study and the others in this tradition is that even these youth with mental retardation and mental ages in the late sensorimotor or preoperational range were able to learn abstract symbols that stood for words. As Light (1997) pointed out, many AAC systems use concrete or iconic symbols to represent messages, such as showing a person pouring more juice into a cup to signify *more*. Such iconic representations are thought to be more easily acquired by children, particularly those with cognitive impairments. As Light pointed out, though, some of the iconicity is from an adult's point of view rather than a child's. For example, some AAC systems use a red cross to signify *help*. Although an adult might meaningfully associate the red cross with the concept of *help* because of its association with the International Red Cross organization, it is unlikely that a young child just learning language would. Thus, the simplification value of these iconic symbols for the child is questionable.

However, from a language-learning point of view, this may be just as well. If the lexemes on AAC devices are to resemble the symbolic nature of words in any way, the signifiers used to encode language concepts will at some point have to include an abstract, symbolic dimension. Only by including abstraction can they lay the basis for higher-level developments, such as literacy, which also rely on abstract symbols and are so important for broadening the scope of communicative possibility for individuals using AAC. The findings of this line of research demonstrate that even individuals with mental retardation and developmental levels in the early representational stage have the capacity to acquire symbolic communication. This suggests that it is not symbolic communication per se that represents the major barrier to linguistic communication in individuals with mental retardation and without functional speech. If this is the case, then it follows that it may be possible to develop abstract, symbolic forms of communication at early developmental stages in children with SSPI. However, unlike children with mental retardation who have more or less intact motor skills, children with SSPI may have special difficulty in acquiring symbols because of their lack of enactive experience, as discussed previously. Systematic research on the symbolic abilities of children with SSPI is needed to determine whether this is the case. If it is, these children may need preliminary training in the use of more iconic symbols before employing abstract ones such as lexigrams. Nonetheless, it is important that AAC devices move toward the inclusion of abstract symbols because these provide the most naturalistic transition to linguistic symbols and the greatest access to written words.

Romski and Sevcik (1996) also reported increases in speech intelligibility in the vocalizations of their participants who used the speech output communication devices. They speculated that the consistent, slow output produced by the speech synthesis program built into the device may have facilitated the participants' ability to parse the speech stream and form a stable auditory image of words that was then available for productive use. The implications of this finding, as well as of the finding on the participants' ability to associate printed words with the symbols they had learned, is addressed when the meaning of the information available on children's language development in augmented modes is discussed in the final section of this chapter.

From Semantics to Syntax

As was shown in the discussion on this transition in typical development, it is usually associated with an expressive vocabulary size of about 50 words and a subsequent spurt in vocabulary production. One difficulty in doing research on this transition in children using AAC is, as Light (1997) pointed out, that children using AAC do not have independent control over vocabulary acquisition. Instead of selecting words for production from the many available in the receptive vocabulary, as typically developing children do (Ferguson & Farwell, 1975), children using AAC are given vocabulary on their devices. Although professionals designing AAC systems exercise much care in selecting this vocabulary, it is the adults, not the child AAC user, who make the selection (Fried-Oken & More, 1992). This limitation in opportunity for vocabulary development may play a crucial role in the transition to multiword utterances.

Some research has focused on the acquisition of multisymbol production in individuals using AAC. Karlan et al. (1982) reported that school-age children with mental retardation who had been taught a small vocabulary of manual signs could be trained to combine two signs. Using a structured behavioral approach, the participants were trained to combine nouns and verbs in systematic combination matrices. They were successful in producing generalized and novel combinations within structured environments using this approach.

Reichle, York, and Sigafoos (1991) reported a similar study in which individuals with severe mental retardation were first taught to use a single symbol for a generalized request function (WANT) and then taught to pair the symbol with a specific item (WANT COOKIE; WANT DRINK). The structured method again was successful in eliciting symbol combinations. In both of these studies and others like them using behavioral methods, the use of the symbols and their combinations is assessed only in structured contexts similar to the training contexts. Even when generalization is evaluated, it is not generalization to daily activities that is measured but only the use of the forms in alternative settings that are still structured to a high degree. Because generalization is construed in this way, it is difficult to know whether more spontaneous development from one- to two-symbol expressions typically occurs in these populations.

Romski and Sevcik (1996) reported that although word combinations were not taught explicitly to individuals in their research program, word combinations did appear spontaneously in some of their participants. Seven of their thirteen participants spontaneously combined social-regulatory words with referential symbols to produce more semantically complex and pragmatically appropriate remarks (MORE MILK PLEASE). Of the combinations expressed, 89% expressed meanings that were similar to the semantic relationships expressed by younger, typically developing children (cf. Braine, 1976). Five of the seven participants who produced symbol combinations showed some consistent ordering rules, indicating that some degree of syntactic ability was being acquired. The maximum number of vocabulary items in the expressive repertoire of any of these individuals was 25, far below the 50-item expressive vocabulary expected in typical development before word combinations appear (Owens, 1992). Like children with typical language development, many of these participants doubtless had larger receptive vocabularies; but multisymbol combinations are usually associated with expressive vocabulary size, and these participants clearly had smaller expressive vocabularies than are usually seen in children who begin producing symbol combinations. Light (1985) found similar evidence of some types of successive one-symbol utterances and vertical construction of two-symbol strings in the communication board messages of preschoolers using AAC.

These findings suggest that although the acquisition of a set of symbols does not consistently result in spontaneous production of multisymbol combinations, at least some children, even those with severe mental retardation, do spontaneously make this transition. What seems clear from these studies is that, like symbols themselves, which can be taught when they are not spontaneously acquired, symbol combinations can be learned by individuals without functional speech, even when they have mental retardation. Furthermore, in some cases, the combinations appear spontaneously once a repertoire of symbols has been acquired. These combinations can appear even when the expressive repertoire is relatively small by the standards of typical development, suggesting that the processes that constrain or facilitate the ability to combine symbols may operate somewhat differently in this population than they do in speaking children. Although it may seem that speech is facilitating the development of language in speaking children through the use of transitional forms such as successive one-word utterances and giant words to move toward true word combinations, the effect could go the other way. In other words, in children learning alternative modes of expression, the language skills they have acquired and stored in receptive modes may facilitate a process usually mediated by speech. If this is the case, it suggests that effects in language development could be multidirectional and that there may be alternative routes to the same outcomes.

To understand the nature of these effects, it is necessary to know more about the cognitive and language behaviors that accompany the spontaneous advances seen in the children who make them. It is important to know what language and cognitive characteristics are present in the spontaneous combiners that might account for why some children make this leap and others with similar exposure and developmental levels do not. More information is also needed on the relation of the production of these combinations to short-term memory performance, the ability to understand syntax, or the ability to produce further syntactic acquisitions. Such research would be useful in elaborating the understanding of the way language development in augmented modalities parallels and diverges from language development in speaking children.

Another important consideration in the transition to syntax in children who use AAC is the multimodal nature of this communication. Light (1997) pointed out that children using AAC often combine an aided form of communication, such as indicating a symbol on a communication board, with an unaided form, such as making a vocalization. The role of these types of combinations, and their relation to the development of syntax, is also an area that needs to be elucidated by research.

From Phonology to Metaphonology

The motor theory of speech perception (Liberman & Mattingly, 1985) holds that speech perceptual capacities are developed at least in part through motor practice achieved through articulation of sounds. This theory suggests that lack of experience with speech production has an impact on speech perception, particularly on higher, more conscious levels of perception. One such higher-level perceptual skill is the awareness of sound segments in words, often referred to as *metaphonology* or *phonological awareness*.

Evidence from children with functional speech impairments reinforces the notion that speaking experience affects the development of phonological awareness. Webster and Plante (1992), for example, showed that school-age children with persistent phonological impairments and poor intelligibility scored significantly lower on measures of phonological awareness than peers with typical speech. Regression analyses revealed that speech intelligibility was the best predictor of phonological awareness performance, independent of mental age.

Phonological awareness, particularly the ability to segment words into component phonemes, is known to be highly related to success in reading. Numerous studies have documented the association of phoneme segmentation skills and early reading achievement (for review, see Chapter 10; Blachman, 1989) and instruction in phoneme segmentation skills has been demonstrated to increase reading ability in typical children (Bradley & Bryant, 1983). Although not all methods of teaching reading rely on instruction in phonological awareness (e.g., whole language; cf. Goodman, 1986), phonologically based methods are known to be the most effective in developing reading skills in children (Adams, 1990; Chall, 1983).

Literacy is well established as an important key to maximal communicative effectiveness in AAC (Blackstone & Cassatt-James, 1988; Koppenhaver, Coleman, Kalman, & Yoder, 1991). Users who can spell out messages are able to have their communications understood by a much wider audience than those who must use symbols or signs that are familiar only to those initiated in their AAC system. Being able to use spelled messages provides the greatest degree of flexibility in the language being expressed; users are not limited to whatever vocabulary was included in the device but can encode any word they wish to express. Thus, the achievement of literacy is an extremely important goal for AAC users.

Yet it is known that children with SSPI have poorer reading skills than would be expected based on their intelligence and educational levels (Foley, 1993). Moreover, reading ability is not significantly correlated with nonverbal intelligence or visual-perceptual ability in this population; instead, it is closely related to the degree of speech and physical impairment (Barsch & Rudell, 1962). This finding would seem to confirm the view advanced by Liberman, Shankweiler, Liberman, Fowler, and Fischer (1977) that the ability to read relies heavily on the phonological codes developed through experience with speaking.

Does this mean that individuals without functional speech must be unable to learn to read because of their impairments in articulatory experience? Clearly, some do learn to read despite this lack of experience. Berninger and Gans (1986) reported that three participants with SSPI and IQ scores in the typical range, although all were underachieving in terms of reading, had each nonetheless acquired at least some reading skill. One of these participants also showed a high level of phonological awareness performance, and the other two had more limited metaphonological skills.

Smith (1989) looked at 10 school-age children with SSPI and found that reading scores were most highly related to scores on a visual matching test, but phonological awareness performance correlated with speech ability. Smith concluded that even limited speech experience helps in the development of phonological awareness skills. Nonetheless, such skills can be developed without speech experience, as demonstrated by errorless performance on the phonological awareness task by one participant with complete anarthria.

A study by Foley (1993) looked further at phonological abilities in 12 adolescents and adults with SSPI, half of whom were dysarthric and half of whom were anarthric. All participants were able to judge whether printed word (e.g., *bear/bare*) and nonword pairs (e.g., *wone/woan*) sounded alike, suggesting that all could access phonological codes from memory. On other phonological coding tasks presented, participants with dysarthria performed better than those with anarthria; however, the two anarthric participants who had significant experience generating written text with voice-output AAC devices performed more similarly to those with dysarthria than to the other anarthric participants. Moreover, the anarthric participants who did not have voice-output AAC experience also had difficulty recognizing printed words. Foley concluded that it is possible for individuals with SSPI to develop phonological coding ability, even with very limited speech experience. Another important finding of this research is that it is possible to develop these abilities, and the word recognition skills with which they are so strongly associated, even with *no* speech experience, as long as experience with a voice-output AAC system is provided.

As reported previously, Romski and Sevcik (1996) found an increase in speech intelligibility following introduction of a voice-output AAC device with their participants with severe mental retardation. Romski and Sevcik suggested that the speech output provided by the AAC device resulted in an immediate, consistent auditory signal at a slow rate of presentation without intonational variation that was closely paired with the participants' own communicative intent. This form of output provided a highly consistent model of the spoken word that seemed to facilitate the development of a stable auditory image of the word that was available to use as a basis for production. These studies suggest that an AAC system equipped with voice output appears to compensate to some degree for limitations in speech production and appears to facilitate the development of mental representations of phonological information.

CONCLUSIONS

These studies on communicative behavior in children without functional speech highlight first that it is not only speech that these children lack. Their severely limited ability to talk leads to a pattern of communicative sparseness and passivity associated with less-than-ideal interactive conditions under which their language learning takes place. Several writers (Bedrosian, 1997; Calculator, 1997; Light, 1997) have emphasized the role that this nonoptimal interactive environment plays in the language development of children without functional speech. When considering the implications of a lack of speech on language development, it is necessary to think not only about intrapersonal effects on the development of a linguistic processing system but also about interpersonal effects and the way in which these influence the substrate of language acquisition. Both research and clinical practice in developing language in children without functional speech need to describe the differences in the interactive environment that these children experience and to develop intensive interventions to address these differences.

Second, although vocal experience would seem to lay a foundation for the acquisition of vocal symbols, it is clearly possible to teach symbolic behavior without this foundation to individuals without functional speech. Although some direct teaching appears to be necessary, instruction may take the form of very structured behavioral intervention or more naturalistic methods. It would appear that once the notion is instilled that nonvocal symbols can be used as a means of communication, representational abilities can be tapped through a variety of modalities. Again, these findings, derived principally from children with mental retardation, need to be extended to those with SSPI.

Third, once some single symbols have been acquired, symbol combinations can be elicited through structured intervention. Using structured behavioral procedures, this can be accomplished without access to transitional forms, such as successive one-word utterances and giant words, available to speaking children. Like other forms taught through behaviorist methods, however, these combinations do not appear either to generalize easily to natural conversation or to evolve into higher levels of syntactic production, at least in children with mental retardation. The finding of Romski and Sevcik (1996) that some though not all nonspeaking individuals with severe mental retardation began to use spontaneous symbol combinations when they had vocabularies in the range of 12–25 symbols is particularly intriguing. Longer-term research is needed to learn whether these combinations will evolve into more elaborated utterances. Similarly, the individuals' characteristics associated with the spontaneous development of word combinations need to be investigated further. Romski and Sevcik reported that performance on a standardized measure of language comprehension did not predict word combination ability. However, relation of word combination ability to vocalization and speech intelligibility was not assessed. Looking at the interactions of these variables with combinatory ability would be a useful contribution to understanding the ways in which speech and language relate. Again, more research is needed in extending these findings to children with SSPI. Studying the early course of expressive development in an augmented modality in children with more or less typical cognitive skills, with particular attention to the ways in which word combinations and syntactic skills emerge, would add greatly to the understanding of the ways in which speech and language support each other.

Fourth, these data indicate that although the development of phonological awareness is more difficult in the absence of speech, some individuals without functional speech do acquire both metaphonological skills and the reading ability with which they are associated. Moreover, these acquisitions appear to be facilitated by AAC devices that employ a voice-output component. This finding suggests that there are alternative routes to the same achievements. Although speech experience is the most natural and efficient way to acquire phonological awareness, other avenues can be used when this route is blocked. Research on methods of enabling these alternative avenues, through the use of voice-output AAC devices and through direct instruction in phonological awareness, is crucial to learning more about how to inculcate this important skill in children without functional speech. Paul (1997) made some suggestions in this area.

Finally, the data on expression of intentions by children without functional speech clearly demonstrate that their communication is a multimodal process. Despite the increased intelligibility that an AAC device provides, all the children studied continued to express the majority of their intentions vocally and to use the AAC device to express a limited range of their intents. These data suggest a powerful drive toward vocal communication, a natural coupling of vocal behavior and communicative expression that persists even when functional speech is not feasible and a more effective communicative method has been supplied. They highlight the connection between speech and language that so many of the chapters in this book have identified: Speech is the modality in which humans are predisposed to express language. Yet, for some human beings with motoric impediments to speech, it is not a viable mode of expression. In these cases, individuals frequently demonstrate the ability to acquire important communication skills by circumventing the speech channel, either spontaneously or with the benefit of instruction. Although these data demonstrate the powerful predisposition toward the use of speech, they also highlight the inherent flexibility of the language-learning system and the robustness of the "language instinct" (Pinker, 1994). Even though speech appears to facilitate a variety of important transitions in typical development and to be a modality strongly preferred for communication, the research on children without functional speech suggests that when speech is unavailable, other avenues can be exploited. This research points out the need to investigate these alternative routes and to characterize the kinds of abilities that make them available to individual children without functional speech. By learning more about how to augment the natural speech channels to linguistic competence, intervention for individuals without functional speech can be optimized.

Implications for Speech-Language Interactions

The data reviewed in this chapter reinforce the theme articulated throughout this volume: Speech and language are closely connected in development, as can be seen in the persistence of vocal communication in children without functional speech and in the difficulties these children encounter in acquiring nonvocal symbols, syntax, and phonological awareness. The data also demonstrate the usefulness of studying disorders as natural experiments that disentangle effects of phenomena that are closely intertwined in typical development. The research on children without functional speech suggests that, although several crucial transitions in language acquisition are closely connected with speech, the transitions are more difficult, more restricted, and less spontaneous but not impossible to accomplish when the speech-language connection is broken. It would appear that speech facilitates but is not absolutely necessary for these accomplishments.

This suggestion closely parallels that of Bleile (see Chapter 5). His data on children who have received tracheostomies suggest that toddlers who are precluded from babbling do experience some delays in lexical production, but these are eventually overcome. Children with SSPI experience more profound and longer-term impediments to language acquisition. Not only are there severe and persistent obstacles to their most natural route to communicative competence, but their motor impairments also significantly affect other abilities on which language depends. Motoric restrictions on the ability to interact with objects affect their cognitive representational abilities. Similar restrictions on the ability to interact with people profoundly affect the linguistic substrate from which they must acquire a language system. Thus, these children are a more extreme and less clear-cut example of the way in which a lack of access to speech affects language development than are tracheostomized children. Nonetheless, the data available tend to support the suggestion derived from tracheostomized children: Speech is the most efficient, helpful, and natural route to the acquisition of full linguistic competence; but when speech is severely limited, a variety of language skills, though more difficult, is not impossible to attain.

Clinical Implications

Although many individuals without functional speech require specific interventions to make the crucial transitions in language acquisition usually facilitated by speech, these interventions appear capable of tapping potential alternative routes to the various linguistic achievements. The challenge for clinicians is to understand more fully how speech facilitates these language acquisitions and to develop interventions that approximate or compensate for the experiences, both interactive and psycholinguistic, provided by speech. In this way, it is feasible to help individuals without functional speech to reach their full potential for linguistic competence. This is just one way in which the study of the relationships between speech and language informs clinical practice.

REFERENCES

Adams, M.J. (1990). *Beginning to read: Thinking and learning about print.* Cambridge, MA: MIT Press.
American Speech-Language-Hearing Association (ASHA). (1989). Competencies for speech-language pathologies providing services in augmentative communication. *Asha, 31,* 107–110.
American Speech-Language-Hearing Association (ASHA). (1991). Report: Augmentative and alternative communication. *Asha, 33*(Suppl. 5), 9–12.

Baddeley, A. (1986). *Working memory.* Oxford, England: Oxford University Press.

Barsch, R., & Rudell, B. (1962). A study of reading development among 77 children with cerebral palsy. *Cerebral Palsy Review, 23,* 3–12.

Bates, E. (1976). *Language in context: Studies in the acquisition of pragmatics.* New York: Academic Press.

Bedrosian, J. (1997). Language acquisition in young AAC system users. *Augmentative and Alternative Communication, 13,* 179–185.

Berninger, V., & Gans, B. (1986). Language profiles in nonspeaking individuals of normal intelligence with severe cerebral palsy. *Augmentative and Alternative Communication, 2,* 45–50.

Blachman, B. (1989). Phonological awareness and word recognition. In A. Kamhi & H. Catts (Eds.), *Reading disabilities: A developmental language perspective* (pp. 133–158). San Diego: College-Hill Press.

Blackstone, S., & Cassatt-James, E. (1988). Augmentative communication. In N. Lass, L. McReynolds, & J. Northern (Eds.), *Handbook of speech-language pathology and audiology* (pp. 986–1013). Toronto: B.C. Decker.

Bradley, L., & Bryant, P. (1983). Categorizing sounds and learning to read: A causal connection. *Nature, 30,* 419–421.

Braine, M. (1976). Children's first word combinations. *Monographs of the Society for Research in Child Development, 41*(1, Serial No. 164).

Bruner, J. (1966). On cognitive growth. In J. Bruner, R. Over, & P. Greenfield (Eds.), *Studies in cognitive growth* (pp. 73–142). New York: John Wiley & Sons.

Calculator, S. (1997). Fostering early language acquisition and AAC use: Exploring reciprocal influences between children and their environments. *Augmentative and Alternative Communication, 13,* 149–157.

Carrier, J. (1974). Nonspeech noun usage training with severely and profoundly retarded children. *Journal of Speech and Hearing Research, 17,* 510–517.

Chall, J. (1983). *Stages of reading development.* New York: McGraw-Hill.

Chapman, R. (1981). Exploring children's communicative intents. In J. Miller (Ed.), *Assessing language production in children: Experimental procedures* (pp. 111–138). Needham Heights, MA: Allyn & Bacon.

deVilliers, J., & deVilliers, P. (1978). *Language acquisition.* Cambridge, MA: Harvard University Press.

Ferguson, C., & Farwell, C. (1975). Words and sounds in early language acquisition. *Language, 51,* 419–439.

Foley, B. (1993). The development of literacy in individuals with severe congenital speech and motor impairments. *Topics in Language Disorders, 13*(2), 16–32.

Fouts, R., Couch, J., & O'Neil, C. (1979). Strategies for primate language training. In R.L. Schiefelbusch & J. Hollis (Eds.), *Language intervention from ape to child* (pp. 295–323). Baltimore: University Park Press.

Fried-Oken, M., & More, L. (1992). A suggested vocabulary source list for the augmentative and alternative communication of 3 to 6 year old, preliterate children: Data from environmental and developmental samples. *Augmentative and Alternative Communication, 8,* 41–56.

Gardner, R., & Gardner, B. (1975). Early signs of language in child and chimpanzee. *Science, 187,* 752–753.

Glennen, S., & Calculator, S. (1985). Training functional communication board use: A pragmatic approach. *Augmentative and Alternative Communication, 1,* 134–142.

Goodman, K. (1986). *What's whole in whole language?* Portsmouth, NH: Heinemann.

Guess, D., & Siegel-Causey, E. (1985). Behavioral control education of severely handicapped students: Who's doing what to whom? and why? In D. Bricker & J. Fuller (Eds.), *Severe mental retardation: From theory to practice* (pp. 230–244). Reston, VA: Council for Exceptional Children, Division on Mental Retardation.

Hanzlik, J. (1990). Nonverbal interaction patterns of mothers and their infants with cerebral palsy. *Education and Training in Mental Retardation, 13,* 333–343.

Houghton, J., Bronicki, G., & Guess, D. (1987). Opportunities to express preferences and make choices among students with severe disabilities in classroom settings. *Journal of The Association for Persons with Severe Handicaps, 12,* 18–27.

Johnson-Martin, N., Wolters, P., & Stowers, S. (1987). Psychological assessment of the nonvocal, physically handicapped child. *Physical and Occupational Therapy in Pediatrics, 7,* 23–38.

Kamhi, A., & Catts, H. (Eds.). (1989). *Reading disabilities: A developmental language perspective.* Needham Heights, MA: Allyn & Bacon.

Karlan, G., Brenn-White, B., Lentz, A., Hodur, P., Egger, D., & Frankoff, D. (1982). Establishing generalized, productive verb–noun phrase usage in a manual language system with moderately handicapped children. *Journal of Speech and Hearing Disorders, 47,* 31–42.

Koppenhaver, D., Coleman, P., Kalman, S., & Yoder, D. (1991). The implications of emergent literacy research for children with developmental disabilities. *American Journal of Speech-Language Pathology: A Journal of Clinical Practice, 1,* 38–44.

Liberman, A., Cooper, F., Shankweiler, D., & Studdert-Kennedy, M. (1967). Perception of the speech code. *Psychological Review, 74,* 431–461.

Liberman, A., & Mattingly, I. (1985). The motor theory of speech perception revised. *Cognition, 21,* 1–37.

Liberman, I., Shankweiler, D., & Liberman, A. (1989). The alphabetic principle and learning to read. In D. Shankweiler & I. Liberman (Eds.), *Phonology and reading disability: Solving the reading puzzle* (IARLD Monograph Series, pp. 1–34). Ann Arbor: University of Michigan Press.

Liberman, I., Shankweiler, D., Liberman, A., Fowler, C., & Fischer, F. (1977). Phonetic segmentation and recoding in the beginning reader. In A. Rober & D. Scarborough (Eds.), *Toward a psychology of reading* (pp. 201–212). Hillsdale, NJ: Lawrence Erlbaum Associates.

Light, J. (1985). *The communicative interaction patterns of young nonspeaking physically disabled children and their primary caregivers.* Unpublished master's thesis, University of Toronto, Ontario, Canada.

Light, J. (1997). "Let's go star fishing": Reflections on the contexts of language learning for children who use aided AAC. *Augmentative and Alternative Communication, 13,* 158–171.

Light, J., Binger, C., & Kelford-Smith, A. (1994). Story reading interactions between preschoolers who use AAC and their mothers. *Augmentative and Alternative Communication, 10,* 255–268.

Light, J., Collier, B., & Parnes, P. (1985a). Communicative interactions between young nonspeaking physically disabled children and their primary caregivers: Part I. Discourse patterns. *Augmentative and Alternative Communication, 1,* 74–83.

Light, J., Collier, B., & Parnes, P. (1985b). Communicative interactions between young nonspeaking physically disabled children and their primary caregivers: Part II. Communicative function. *Augmentative and Alternative Communication, 1,* 98–107.

Light, J., Collier, B., & Parnes, P. (1985c). Communicative interactions between young nonspeaking physically disabled children and their primary caregivers: Part III. Modes of communication. *Augmentative and Alternative Communication, 1,* 125–133.

Marvin, C. (1994). Home literacy experiences of preschool children with single and multiple disabilities. *Topics in Early Childhood Special Education, 4,* 436–454.

McNaughton, S. (1993). Graphic representational systems and literacy learning. *Topics in Language Disorders, 13,* 58–75.

Owens, R. (1992). *Language development.* Columbus, OH: Charles E. Merrill.

Paul, R. (1987). Communication. In D. Cohen, A. Donnellan, & R. Paul (Eds.), *Handbook of autism and pervasive developmental disorders* (pp. 61–84). New York: John Wiley & Sons.

Paul, R. (1997). Facilitating transitions in language development in children who use AAC. *Augmentative and Alternative Communication, 13,* 141–148.

Pierce, P., & McWilliam, P. (1993). Emerging literacy and children with severe speech and physical impairments (SSPI): Issues and possible intervention strategies. *Topics in Language Disorders, 13,* 47–56.

Pinker, R. (1994). *The language instinct: The new science of language and mind.* London: Penguin Books.

Premack, D. (1970). Language in chimpanzees. *Science, 172,* 808–822.

Reichle, J., York, J., & Sigafoos, J. (1991). *Implementing augmentative and alternative communication: Strategies for learners with severe disabilities.* Baltimore: Paul H. Brookes Publishing Co.

Romski, M.A., & Sevcik, R.A. (1996). *Breaking the speech barrier: Language development through augmented means.* Baltimore: Paul H. Brookes Publishing Co.

Savage-Rumbaugh, E., McDonald, K., Sevcik, R., Hopkins, W., & Rupert, E. (1986). Spontaneous symbol acquisition and communicative use by pygmy chimpanzees (*Pan paniscus*). *Journal of Experimental Psychology: General, 115,* 211–235.

Savage-Rumbaugh, E., Rumbaugh, D., Smith, S., & Lawson, J. (1980). Reference: The linguistic essential. *Science, 210,* 922–925.

Smith, M. (1989). Reading without speech: A study of children with cerebral palsy. *Irish Journal of Psychology, 10,* 601–614.

Snow, C., & Ninio, A. (1986). The contracts of literacy: What children learn from learning to read books. In W. Teale & E. Sulzby (Eds.), *Emergent literacy* (pp. 116–138). Norwood, NJ: Ablex.

Spradlin, J., & Siegel, G. (1982). Language training in natural and clinical environments. *Journal of Speech and Hearing Disorders, 47,* 2–6.

Vellutino, F. (1979). *Dyslexia: Theory and research.* Cambridge, MA: MIT Press.

Webster, P., & Plante, S. (1992). Effects of phonological impairment on word, syllable, and phoneme segmentation and reading. *Language, Speech, and Hearing Services in Schools, 23,* 176–182.

7

Down Syndrome
The Impact of Speech
Production on Language Development

Jon F. Miller and Mark Leddy

THE EXPLORATION OF THE RELATIONSHIP between speech production and language development in children with Down syndrome is particularly interesting from a theoretical as well as a practical perspective. Theoretically, researchers are working to identify the causes for the productive language problems consistently associated with this syndrome (Chapman, 1995; Miller, 1987b, 1988). Practically, clinicians and parents are struggling to improve the communication ability of these children, given their persistent speech intelligibility problems. This chapter describes impairments in the speech production mechanism of these children that are associated with the syndrome and discusses their implications for language learning and oral communication.

AN OVERVIEW OF THE DOWN SYNDROME POPULATION

The incidence of Down syndrome is about 1 in 700 births on average, with incidence increasing with increasing maternal and paternal age. Equal numbers of males and females are affected. The most frequent genetic mechanism (accounting for 96% of cases) responsible for Down syndrome is a trisomy of chromosome 21. Two other genetic mechanisms involving chromosome 21 are also responsible for the syndrome: translocation and mosaicism. Translocation of chromosome 21 accounts for about 3% of the population. In *translocation*, the extra copy of the chromosome is attached to another chromosome, usually chromosome 14 or 22. *Mosaicism* refers to a condition in which some of the cells in the body have the extra copy of chromosome 21 and other cells do not. Mosaicism accounts for about 1% of the population. For the majority of these children, about 95%, the causal mechanism is accidental and not inherited. A number of molecular geneticists are actively investigating the specific genes on chromosome 21 responsible for the syndrome and its associated impairments (Korenberg, Paulst, & Gerwehr, 1992).

People with Down syndrome have a number of distinguishing features. They are short in stature, with a distinct facial morphology including a flat facial profile and epicanthal folds. The tongue is large relative to a small oral cavity. Motor function is characterized by generalized hypotonia, which may be mild to severe. Joints are hyperextendable. Mental retardation is common in people with Down syndrome; Down syndrome is the leading genetic cause of mental retardation. About 50% of affected children have hearing impairments, and an almost equal number have a variety of gastrointestinal problems and/or congenital heart disease.

Neurological Characteristics

A variety of differences have been found in the central nervous system of people with Down syndrome. Brain weight, which is normal at birth, increases at a very slow rate, resulting in smaller brain size by 2–3 years of age. There are also differences found in the size, shape, and function of other central nervous system structures, such as the cerebellum and brain stem. At a microscopic level, differences have been found in the density of cortical neuron layers, in the structure of dendrites, and in the number of synapses. Neurochemical abnormalities have been observed in the neurotransmitter systems of both the peripheral and central nervous systems, and neurophysiological studies suggest impairments in synaptic transmission. Reports of seizure activity are higher during infancy and adulthood.

Cognitive Skills

Individuals with Down syndrome range in severity of mental retardation, with anecdotal reports of average intelligence. However, it has been reported that the majority of individuals with Down syndrome evidence mental retardation. It has been suggested that the severity of this intellectual impairment is closely related to the institutionalization and education of individuals with Down syndrome. It has been argued historically that children with Down syndrome proceed through the same developmental stages as typically developing children; but this is questionable given the documented problems these children exhibit with language production relative to comprehension. In addition, given the multifaceted nature of cognition, the vast range of talents exhibited by those with Down syndrome in music, in the visual arts, and in athletics must be considered as unexplored areas of cognitive development.

Speech Skills

Although individual children with Down syndrome may exhibit specific phonological rule impairments or distinct speech-sound error patterns, the most common problem that children with Down syndrome evidence is reduced speech intelligibility. Fluency problems are also exhibited frequently by these children, though it is not clear whether their dysfluency is a speech-based or a language-based difficulty.

Language Skills

Children with Down syndrome have particular trouble acquiring language, particularly productive language skills. These children show an asynchrony in the acquisition of language exhibited by their comprehension of language exceeding their production ability. In a sample of 20 children with Down syndrome that we have followed for several years, from the onset of first words, only 7 children showed appropriate rates of vocabulary acquisition in production. All of these children showed comprehension skills comparable to their nonverbal mental age. The onset of multiword utterances was significantly delayed for the group. The average mean length of utterance (MLU) at a mental age of 30 months was 1.13, with five children not yet combining words. Their rate of progress was very slow for productive syntax, with a predicted MLU of 1.66 for the group by 8 years of age, relative to cognitive skills averaging 4;2 years of mental age. An MLU of 1.66 is generally achieved by 24 months in typical children. Given that chronological age and mental age are equivalent in typical children, the children with Down syndrome in our study are delayed almost 2 years in acquiring productive syntax. Impairments in acquiring syntax are more pronounced than in vocabulary acquisition, though both are impaired relative to nonverbal mental age. Several investigators have documented the difficulties with syntax (Chapman, 1995; Miller, 1987b, 1988), and Fowler (1988, 1990) proposed that syntax is the basis of their language-learning deficit. Impairments in syntactic comprehension appear after mental age 3–4 years, though vocabulary comprehension is better than nonverbal cognitive skills with increased age.

In summary, the majority of research on the communication impairments of children with Down syndrome has focused on their development of language skills. Their language production is significantly delayed compared with their other cognitive skills. Syntax is thought to be more seriously impaired than vocabulary by some researchers. Language comprehension skills are more advanced than language production skills. Several hypotheses have been advanced to explain this language production profile, including a specific linguistic-cognitive theory, a speech–motor-control thesis, a hypothesis that hearing loss associated with otitis media contributes to the problem, and a theory that a lack of environmental responsivity reinforces the delay (Miller, 1987b, 1988). Our research has demonstrated that neither hearing nor environment are responsible for the productive language impairments of these children.

SPEECH PRODUCTION MECHANISMS

Children with Down syndrome are biologically different from typically developing children. Abnormal anatomical structures have been found in all of the body systems of people with Down syndrome, including the skeletal, muscular, nervous, cardiovascular, digestive, respiratory, urogenital, and endocrine systems. Those systems that are thought to have the strongest association with speech production include the skeletal, muscular, nervous, and respiratory mechanisms. Although anatomical-structural abnormalities in the skeletal, muscular, and nervous systems are found in a high percentage of children with Down syndrome, they are not found in every child. In addition, differences in these systems do not always cause speech production impairments or reduced speech intelligibility. Human physiology has a great capacity to accommodate structural deviations, and some children with Down syndrome may adapt to system anomalies to produce acceptably intelligible speech. Other children with Down syndrome who have more serious nervous system anomalies may have greater difficulty accommodating these skeletal, muscular, and respiratory structural differences. We hypothesize that neurological impairments influence motor speech production in people with Down syndrome and that these impairments affect a child's ability to adapt to his or her unique vocal tract structures.

Skeletal System

Anomalies in the skeletal systems of people with Down syndrome include absent or deficient bone growth. These differences are found in the bones of the head and face, in those structures designed to support speech articulators, and in their associated muscles. These structures also contribute to the shape and size of the resonant cavities for speech production. People with Down syndrome often have a smaller skull; missing or poorly developed midfacial bones; and a smaller, wider mandible than typically developing people (Frostad, Cleall, & Melosky, 1971; Kisling, 1966; Roche, Roche, & Lewis, 1972; Sanger, 1975). Although not directly influencing speech production, these anomalies create a smaller oral cavity and pharynx (Ardran, Harker, & Kemp, 1972), which may influence speech-sound resonance and the unique voice quality of those with Down syndrome (Pentz, 1987).

These structural differences in the skeletal system contribute to the smaller oral cavity of people with Down syndrome, a characteristic that may limit the distance and range of movements for a normal-size tongue. Clinicians have reported observing a high palate in children with Down syndrome; but careful examination of the palate reveals that it is actually equal in height to the palate of typically developing children, though it is short and very narrow (Redman, Shapiro, & Gorlin, 1965; Shapiro, Gorlin, Redman, & Bruhl, 1967; Shapiro, Redman, & Gorlin, 1963). Given that individuals with Down syndrome have difficulty producing alveolar and palatal fricatives and palatal affricate speech sounds (Borghi, 1990; Van Borsal, 1988), it is quite plausible that these speech production difficulties stem from tongue articulation restrictions in the presence of a narrow palate.

Information about tongue position in the oral cavity is obtained when the vowel productions of individuals with Down syndrome are analyzed using acoustic measures, specifically first (F1) and second (F2) formant frequency data. Rosin, Swift, Khidr, and Bless (1992) found lower F1 and F2 values for the /i/ productions of adolescent males with Down syndrome. These findings suggest a lower and more posterior tongue carriage for production of the /i/ vowel, which might be an indirect result of the smaller oral cavity and narrower palate. However, people with Down syndrome have multiple neuromuscular anomalies that probably contribute to tongue control and positioning for vowel production.

Muscular System

People with Down syndrome are known to have absent and extra muscles throughout their bodies (Bersu, 1976, 1980). In the facial region, this includes poorly differentiated midfacial muscles and an additional muscle, the platysma occipitalis, running from the corner of the mouth to the back of the head. Fusion of the midfacial muscles probably limits the elevation of the upper lips and the corners of the mouth for facial expressions such as sneering or smiling. However, the platysma occipitalis likely contributes to lateral labial retraction, and its presence may assist in smiling and speech. This may serve to increase the oral opening for facial expression, feeding, and sound radiation during speech, but it likely has minimal effects on speech production.

People with Down syndrome have a relatively larger muscular tongue that protrudes from the oral cavity (Ardran et al., 1972). Clinicians have suspected for many years that the relatively larger tongue interferes with articulatory placements for both vowel and consonant production, thus contributing to reduced speech intelligibility (Gibson, 1978; Miller, 1992). These observations have resulted in some children with Down syndrome undergoing partial tongue resections to reduce tongue size. Carefully conducted research studies show almost no speech improvement as a result of this procedure (Katz & Kravitz, 1989; Parsons, Iacono, & Rozner, 1987). These findings suggest that improved speech function does result from alterations in structure in those with Down syndrome and that the underlying neuromuscular influences affecting speech-motor control may have a greater impact.

Nervous System

Anatomical differences in the central and peripheral nervous system of individuals with Down syndrome likely influence motor speech production, probably disrupting the sequence and timing of speech movements. Researchers examining the gross morphology of the central nervous system in individuals with Down syndrome have found reduced brain size and weight, smaller and fewer sulci and gyri, a narrower superior temporal gyrus, and a smaller cerebellum (see Flórez, 1992). Kemper (1988) reported that people with Down syndrome have fewer cortical neurons and decreased neuronal density. In addition, investigators have found that those with Down syndrome have delayed neural myelination, abnormal dendrite structures, and altered cellular membranes (see Flórez, 1992; Scott, Becker, & Petit, 1983). These anatomical differences may affect motor speech production, probably disrupting the accuracy, speed, consistency, and economy of speech movements, thus altering the sequencing and timing of speech.

Variations in speech-motor function, specifically in speech-timing characteristics, are evident in the dysfluent productions of people with Down syndrome. Additional examples of motor problems include voicing errors (Borghi, 1990), highly variable formant transition patterns (Kimelman, Swift, Rosin, & Bless, 1985), and difficulties maintaining adequate intraoral pressure for speech (Swift, Rosin, Khidr, & Bless, 1992). Hesselwood, Bray, and Crookston (1995) described speech prosody and rhythm errors of an adult with Down syndrome; these investigators suggested that the speech intelligibility problems stem from speech-planning deficits. Such impairments may stem from the underlying nervous system dysfunction in those with Down syndrome and all may contribute to reduced speech intelligibility.

DYSFLUENT SPEECH PRODUCTION: A MOTOR OR LINGUISTIC DYSFUNCTION?

There is a higher prevalence of stuttering, or dysfluent speech, found in the population with Down syndrome when comparing this group with other people with developmental disabilities or with typically developing individuals (Van Riper, 1982). Whereas stuttering occurs in approximately 1% of the typically developing population and in about 10% in those with developmental disabilities, it occurs in about 45%–53% of people with Down syndrome (see Devenny & Silverman, 1990; Preus, 1990). Although there is a higher prevalence of dysfluent speech production in individuals with Down syndrome, there is disagreement about whether the speech behaviors they exhibit are the same as those observed in typically developing speakers with dysfluent speech. These speech behaviors primarily include sound prolongations; interjections; pauses; and repetitions of sounds, syllables, parts of words, and whole words (Devenny & Silverman, 1990; Evans, 1977; Willcox, 1988).

There are two competing views of the dysfluent speech of people with Down syndrome. The first is that this behavior resembles the classic stuttering behavior in the speech pathology literature and is characterized by blocks, tremors, and vocal spasms and that these events are the result of speech-motor dysfunction. The second view is that the disfluencies of this group are language based, associated with an utterance formulation or word-finding impairment. Investigators have attributed the higher dysfluency prevalence to linguistic influences (Preus, 1973; Willcox, 1988), to the point of calling the disorder *cluttering* instead of *stuttering* (Cabanas, 1954), and to impairments in the speech-motor control system (Devenny & Silverman, 1990; Farmer & Brayton, 1979; Van Riper, 1982).

A Speech-Motor Basis for Stuttering

The argument that dysfluent speech is due to a motor-control impairment gains support from other investigations that addressed nonspeech motor coordination and timing deficits in people with Down syndrome (Frith & Frith, 1974; Henderson, Morris, & Frith, 1981; Henderson, Morris, & Ray, 1981). In addition, the results of several studies on laryngeal reaction time and vocal-tracking behavior involving dysfluent speakers suggest that stutterers have specific speech-motor control impairments that could be the result of neural processing difficulties that negatively influence early stages of preparatory speech-motor control programming (Dembowski & Watson, 1991; Nudelman, Herbich, Hess, Hoyt, & Rosenfield, 1992). When Otto and Yairi (1974) compared the dysfluent speech patterns of people with Down syndrome with those of typically developing individuals, the investigators found that besides repeating parts of words and whole words more frequently, speakers with Down syndrome also had more "dysrhythmic phonations." These disruptions might be due to speech-motor control impairments secondary to different neurophysiological mechanisms.

Because people with Down syndrome have cognitive-linguistic impairments as well as gross, fine, and speech-motor impairments, it is unlikely that only one specific and atypically functioning system explains the underlying basis for their dysfluent speech behavior. Theories and models of stuttering recognize multifactorial influences, or the combined effects of several factors including cognitive-linguistic and motor-control parameters, on dysfluent speech production (Conture, 1990; Nudelman et al., 1992; Smith, 1990).

The Cluttering or Language-Based Hypothesis

There is a history of research and clinical reports contrasting stuttering as a speech production–based fluency problem with cluttering, which is a language-based fluency problem. The behaviors defining each disorder have been debated with more heat than light. The classical definition of *stuttering* includes sound and syllable repetitions and blocking (i.e., lack of vocalization associated with tension in the speech system, tremors, facial tics). Cluttering is associated with rapid speech rate, word repetition, and phrase revision and repetition.

Since the mid-1980s, word and phrase repetition and revision behaviors have been cited as evidence for word-finding problems in children with language-learning disabilities (German, 1992). Work aimed at defining different types of language disorders among children classified as having specific language impairment suggests that these dysfluent behaviors may be indicative of two different language production impairments, word finding and utterance formulation (Miller, 1987a; Miller & Leadholm, 1992). For some children, the repetitions and revisions are primarily of phrase units, indicating that they are struggling with units longer than single words. These children may be struggling with learning complex syntax to express more than one proposition at a time or are having difficulty coordinating utterance content, either within the utterance or with previous utterances. Word-level repetitions and revisions are more likely associated with word-finding problems.

There are measures that reflect a general class of verbal fluency behaviors as an index of language formulation load (Miller, 1991). These measures, referred to as *mazes*, were first described by Loban in 1976. Mazes were characterized as false starts, repetitions, and reformulations and Loban used them to describe children's progress toward adult language competence. Miller (1991) documented that mazes are an index of formulation load in that the number of mazes children produce in utterances increases in narrative-speaking contexts compared with conversational contexts. Narratives place a greater burden on utterance formulation and discourse cohesion for the speaker than does conversation, in which these duties are shared. Mazes also increase when children attempt longer utterances rather than shorter utterances, supporting the hypothesis that formulation load is greater when message content is increased.

These data suggest that mazes can be used to differentiate between stuttering and language-based fluency impairments. Mazes are the key to identifying the nature of the fluency problems in children with Down syndrome. Recording and transcribing a language sample provide the data needed to document the nature of the disfluencies in an individual child. Valuable indices of dysfluent speech are provided when a sample is analyzed for several maze measures, including the nature of the maze (e.g., filled pause, repetition, revision), the size of the maze (e.g., part word, word, phrase), and the proportion of words in mazes to the total words in the sample. Further analysis of where the mazes occur in the utterance will help to identify specific linguistic features with which the child is having difficulty.

When maze data are combined with the visual observation of tension, facial tics, and/or other blocking behaviors associated with stuttering, then investigators and clinicians will have the information necessary to differentiate speech-based stuttering from language-based fluency problems. Speech-based problems probably result from the same causal mechanisms as stuttering in typical children. Chief among these is the environmental pressure to speak that children who stutter feel is being thrust upon them. Real or imagined, this pressure must be reduced so that children feel that their speech is accepted at any level.

SPEECH INTELLIGIBILITY

Reports in the literature strongly suggest that individuals with Down syndrome have speech intelligibility problems (Horstmeier, 1990; Miller, 1987b, 1988, 1992). However, relatively few investigators have examined speech intelligibility in people with Down syndrome, and those who have were investigating other issues, that is, linguistic factors influencing dysfluency (Willcox, 1988) and the communication pattern of adolescent speakers with Down syndrome (Rosin, Swift, Bless, & Vetter, 1988). Nonetheless, both Rosin et al. (1988) and Willcox (1988) found poor speech intelligibility performance (averaging 65% speech intelligibility) in groups of older children and adolescents with Down syndrome. Rosin et al. hypothesized that the intelligibility performance may be related to possible impairments in sequential information processing.

The majority of speech studies in the literature on Down syndrome have not investigated speech intelligibility but have instead examined speech-sound articulation, speech-sound and distinctive feature error patterns, and the phonological skills of individuals with Down syndrome. Investigations in the 1950s and 1960s found a prevalence rate of 95%–100% for deviant, or defective, articulation among individuals with Down syndrome (Blanchard, 1964; Schlanger & Gottsleben, 1957), a significantly higher prevalence rate than that found among individuals with other developmental disabilities or typically developing individuals. However, others have argued that the phonological errors of children with Down syndrome are consistent with typical development (Dodd, 1976; Willcox, 1988). This view is contested by Stoel-Gammon (1980) and Van Borsal (1988), who consider phonological development in people with Down syndrome to be deviant.

The articulation impairments and speech error patterns of people with Down syndrome have been attributed to a variety of influencing factors: cognitive impairments, muscle hypotonia, cerebellar abnormalities, fine motor coordination deficits, and oral anatomical–structural abnormalities (Blager, 1980; Miller, Leddy, Miolo, & Sedey, 1995; Miller, Stoel-Gammon, Leddy, Lynch, & Miolo, 1992; Yarter, 1980). Whether the cause of these impairments is neurological in nature or due to a combination of anatomical and physiological differences, they affect language production and ultimately communication.

SPEECH PRODUCTION IMPAIRMENTS
INFLUENCE LANGUAGE AND COMMUNICATION
PERFORMANCE: PROSPECTS FOR FUTURE RESEARCH

The two prominent speech production impairments observed in individuals with Down syndrome, reduced speech intelligibility and dysfluency, have been discussed relative to possible neurological limitations, in the context of anatomically different vocal tract structures, that may affect sequencing and speech timing. The association between the anatomical and physiological differences and speech intelligibility or fluency impairments can only be speculated upon. There is, however, a great deal of support for future research to test several hypotheses put forward in this chapter.

Speech Intelligibility

The relationship between speech intelligibility impairments and language and communication performance among people with Down syndrome requires some discussion, as does the relationship between verbal fluency impairments and communication proficiency. Is the impact of speech intelligibility impairments on productive language development and communicative efficiency any different in individuals with Down syndrome than in typical individuals? Can intervention improve speech intelligibility in this population? There are three areas in which the impact of speech intelligibility on language learning and communication can be demonstrated. First, impairments in speech intelligibility interfere with message understanding, which may cause the child with Down syndrome to reduce speaking attempts, which limits the language production practice required for learning language.

A second effect of unintelligible speech is increased frustration resulting from messages not being understood. This frustration can lead to behavior problems if not addressed early (Reichle & Wacker, 1993). Interventions to limit frustration and improve communicative effectiveness include the introduction of gestural communication by teaching 20–50 signs for frequently used vocabulary when children begin to indicate wants and needs through vocalizations and gestures at 12–18 months of age. Children with Down syndrome use signs until speech becomes more intelligible, at 3–4 years of age for many children, and then the signs fade from use. Signs should be taught as augmenting speech and not as a second language. Children always opt for speech as the most efficient method of communicating their wants and needs.

The third effect of unintelligible speech on language and communication is on the complexity of messages attempted. Children choose to produce short, intelligible messages rather than long, unintelligible messages. This trade-off between length and intelligibility and message complexity may be a resource allocation limitation; that is, if the child is focusing on the articulation of sounds and the clarity of speech, the available resources for language formulation and message construction are reduced. Alternatively, the lack of practice with productive language may have limited language learning to simple sentence patterns. There are some data to support this hypothesis (Fowler, 1990).

Verbal Fluency Deficits

What do the prevalence data of dysfluent speech in people with Down syndrome show? The data do not differentiate stuttering from language-based fluency impairments. Thus, there is no clear understanding of how frequent dysfluent behaviors can be considered "stuttering." Our experience with several hundred children with Down syndrome suggests that the frequency of stuttering behaviors is far too high and that these observations are probably contaminated with typical developmental dysfluencies. (See Chapter 9 for a more detailed discussion of disfluency.) Data from typical children document that 20%–25% of utterances contain mazes in children 3–13 years of age in conversational contexts. In narrative samples, the percentages increase to 30%–45% over the same age range (Miller, 1994). Given these high rates of dysfluent behavior, it is conceivable that the majority of these children were exhibiting typical nonfluent behavior. Do children with Down syndrome have similar rates of language-based dysfluencies?

Are mazes the cause or a consequence of productive language disorder? If mazes were the cause of productive language disorder, it would be argued that somehow the dysfluent behavior prevented the child from practicing or trying new language forms to express increasingly complex messages. This certainly could happen. However, it is far more likely that mazes are the consequence of a specific linguistic impairment such as word-finding or utterance formulation problems.

If related behaviors are considered when evaluating this hypothesis, there is support for this point of view. Two types of behavior suggest themselves: pauses, which can occur either between or within utterances, and abandoned utterances, which occur when the child makes repeated attempts to repair an utterance, producing several mazes in succession, and fails to complete the utterance. Pauses may be simply a silent version of a maze resulting from the same source; that is, the child cannot find the right word or utterance form to express a thought. Pauses may be substituted for mazes, which is one method a child may use to gain time to sort the message. Therefore, mazes and pauses may not be distributed together. The authors' data on 256 children with specific language impairment confirm this view: Children usually produced mazes or pauses, but rarely both.

Abandoned utterances can be considered unresolved mazes in which the child could not pull enough of the utterance together to finish it. Abandoned utterances should increase as the number of mazes increases, particularly where the mazes are predominant at the phrase level. This is exactly the pattern found in children with specific language impairment. A high frequency of mazes in children with Down syndrome may be associated with their limited syntactic skills or their short-term memory impairments, making finding the right word difficult. These disfluencies provide a valuable insight into the productive language deficits of this group, and further research is necessary to document their impact on language development and communication proficiency.

CONCLUSIONS

We suggest that both unintelligible and dysfluent speech have adverse effects on language and communication performance in children with Down syndrome. It is important to continue investigating these speech behaviors to determine whether they are causing or contributing to specific language or communication problems and whether they are the result of cognitive-linguistic impairments. Both behaviors are amenable to intervention in children and adults with Down syndrome. Leddy and Gill (1996) reported that, as a result of clinical speech and language treatment, adults with Down syndrome make significant improvements in speech intelligibility and use this to repair communication breakdowns. These findings provide hope for improving the communication skills of individuals with Down syndrome and suggest the need for intervention studies in this population.

REFERENCES

Ardran, G.M., Harker, P., & Kemp, F.H. (1972). Tongue size in Down syndrome. *Journal of Mental Deficiency Research, 16,* 160–166.

Bersu, E.T. (1976). *An analysis of the anatomic variations in human trisomy based on dissections of 21- and 18-trisomies.* Doctoral dissertation, University of Wisconsin–Madison.

Bersu, E.T. (1980). Anatomical analysis of the developmental effects of aneuploidy in man: The Down syndrome. *American Journal of Medical Genetics, 5,* 399–420.

Blager, F.B. (1980). Speech and language development of Down's syndrome children. *Seminars in Speech, Language, and Hearing, 1,* 63–72.

Blanchard, I.B. (1964). Speech patterns and etiology in mental retardation. *American Journal of Mental Deficiency, 68,* 613–617.

Borghi, R.W. (1990). Consonant phoneme, and distinctive feature error patterns in speech. In D.C. Van Dyke, D.J. Lang, F. Heide, S. van Duyne, & M.J. Soucek (Eds.), *Clinical perspectives in the management of Down syndrome* (pp. 147–152). New York: Springer-Verlag.

Cabanas, R. (1954). Some findings in speech and voice therapy among mentally deficient children. *Folia Phoniatrica, 6,* 34–37.

Chapman, R. (1995). Language development in children and adolescents with Down syndrome. In P. Fletcher & B. MacWhinney (Eds.), *Handbook of child language* (pp. 641–663). Cambridge, England: Basil Blackwell.

Conture, E.G. (1990). *Stuttering* (2nd ed.). Englewood Cliffs, NJ: Prentice-Hall.

Dembowski, J., & Watson, B.C. (1991). Preparation time and response complexity effects on stutterers' and nonstutterers' acoustic LRT. *Journal of Speech and Hearing Research, 34,* 49–59.

Devenny, D.A., & Silverman, W.P. (1990). Speech dysfluency and manual specialization in Down's syndrome. *Journal of Mental Deficiency Research, 34,* 253–260.

Dodd, B.J. (1976). A comparison of the phonological systems of mental age matched, normal, severely subnormal and Down's syndrome children. *British Journal of Communication, 11,* 27–42.

Evans, D. (1977). The development of language abilities in mongols: A correlational study. *Journal of Mental Deficiency Research, 21,* 103–117.

Farmer, A., & Brayton, E.R. (1979). Speech characteristics of fluent and dysfluent Down's syndrome adults. *Folia Phoniatrica, 31,* 284–290.

Flórez, J. (1992). Neurologic abnormalities. In S.M. Pueschel & J.K. Pueschel (Eds.), *Biomedical concerns in persons with Down syndrome* (pp. 159–173). Baltimore: Paul H. Brookes Publishing Co.

Fowler, A. (1988). Determinants of rate of growth with Down syndrome. In L. Nadel (Ed.), *The psychobiology of Down syndrome* (pp. 217–246). Cambridge, MA: MIT Press.

Fowler, A. (1990). Language abilities in children with Down syndrome: Evidence for a specific syntactic delay. In D. Cicchetti & M. Beeghly (Eds.), *Children with Down syndrome: A developmental perspective* (pp. 302–328). Cambridge, England: Cambridge University Press.

Frith, U., & Frith, C.D. (1974). Specific motor disabilities in Down's syndrome. *Journal of Child Psychology and Psychiatry, 15,* 293–301.

Frostad, N.A., Cleall, J.F., & Melosky, L.C. (1971). Craniofacial complex in the trisomy 21 syndrome (Down's syndrome). *Archives of Oral Biology, 16,* 707–722.

German, D. (1992). Diagnosis of word finding disorders in children with learning disabilities. *Journal of Learning Disabilities, 17,* 353–358.

Gibson, D. (1978). *Down's syndrome: The psychology of mongolism.* Cambridge, England: Cambridge University Press.

Henderson, S.E., Morris, J., & Frith, U. (1981). The motor deficit in Down's syndrome children: A problem of timing? *Journal of Child Psychology and Psychiatry, 22,* 233–245.

Henderson, S.E., Morris, J., & Ray, S. (1981). Performance of Down syndrome and other retarded children on the Cratty Gross-Motor Test. *American Journal of Mental Deficiency, 85,* 416–424.

Hesselwood, B.C., Bray, M., & Crookston, I. (1995). Juncture, rhythm and planning in the speech of an adult with Down's syndrome. *Clinical Linguistics and Phonetics, 9,* 121–137.

Horstmeier, D. (1990). Communication. In S.M. Pueschel, *A parent's guide to Down syndrome: Toward a brighter future* (pp. 233–257). Baltimore: Paul H. Brookes Publishing Co.

Katz, S., & Kravitz, S. (1989). Facial plastic surgery for persons with Down syndrome: Research findings and their professional and social implications. *American Journal on Mental Retardation, 94,* 101–110.

Kemper, T.L. (1988). Neuropathology of Down syndrome. In L. Nadel (Ed.), *The psychobiology of Down syndrome* (pp. 266–289). New York: Academic Press.

Kimelman, M., Swift, E., Rosin, M.M., & Bless, D.M. (1985, October). *Spectrographic analysis of vowels in Down's syndrome speech.* Paper presented at the 110th Meeting of the Acoustical Society of America, Nashville, TN.

Kisling, E. (1966). *Cranial morphology in Down's syndrome: A comparative roentgenocephalometric study in adult males.* Copenhagen: Munksgaard.

Korenberg, J., Paulst, S., & Gerwehr, S. (1992). Advances in the understanding of chromosome 21 and Down syndrome. In I. Lott & E. McCoy (Eds.), *Down syndrome: Advances in medical care* (pp. 3–12). New York: John Wiley & Sons.

Leddy, M., & Gill, G. (1996, July). *Speech and language skills of adolescents and adults with Down syndrome: Enhancing communication.* Paper presented at the National Down Syndrome Congress Annual Convention, Miami Beach, FL.

Loban, W. (1976). *Language development: Kindergarten through Grade 12* (Research Report No. 18). Urbana, IL: National Council of Teachers of English.

Miller, J. (1987a). A grammatical characterization of language disorder. *Proceedings of the First International Symposium on Specific Speech and Language Disorders in Children.* London: AFASIC Press.

Miller, J. (1987b). Language and communication characteristics of children with Down syndrome. In S. Pueschel, C. Tingey, J.E. Rynders, A.C. Crocker, & D.M. Crutcher (Eds.), *New perspectives on Down syndrome* (pp. 233–262). Baltimore: Paul H. Brooks Publishing Co.

Miller, J. (1988). The developmental asynchrony of language development in children with Down syndrome. In L. Nadel (Ed.), *The psychobiology of Down syndrome* (pp. 167–198). New York: Academic Press.

Miller, J. (1991). Quantifying productive language disorder. In J. Miller (Ed.), *Research on child language disorders: A decade of progress* (pp. 211–220). Boston: College-Hill Press.

Miller, J. (1992). Lexical acquisition in children with Down syndrome. In R.S. Chapman (Ed.), *Child talk* (pp. 202–216). St. Louis: Mosby–Year Book.

Miller, J. (1994, April). *Documenting rate and verbal facility deficits in children with language disorders.* Paper presented at the University of Amsterdam, Netherlands.

Miller, J., & Leadholm, B. (1992). *Language sample analysis guide: The Wisconsin guide for the identification and description of language impairment in children.* Madison: Wisconsin Department of Public Instruction.

Miller, J., Leddy, M., Miolo, G., & Sedey, A. (1995). The development of early language skills in children with Down syndrome. In L. Nadel & D. Rosenthal (Eds.), *Down syndrome: Living and learning in the community* (pp. 115–120). New York: John Wiley & Sons.

Miller, J., Stoel-Gammon, C., Leddy, M., Lynch, M., & Miolo, G. (1992, November). *Factors limiting speech development in children with Down syndrome.* Miniseminar presented at the annual American Speech-Language-Hearing Association Convention, San Antonio, TX.

Nudelman, H.B., Herbich, K.E., Hess, K.R., Hoyt, B.D., & Rosenfield, D.B. (1992). A model of the phonatory response time of stutterers and fluent speakers to frequency-modulated tones. *Journal of the Acoustical Society of America, 92,* 1882–1888.

Otto, F.M., & Yairi, E. (1974). An analysis of speech disfluencies in Down's syndrome and in normally intelligent subjects. *Journal of Fluency Disorders, 1,* 26–32.

Parsons, C.L., Iacono, T.A., & Rozner, L. (1987). Effect of tongue reduction on articulation in children with Down syndrome. *American Journal of Mental Deficiency, 91,* 328–332.

Pentz, A.L. (1987). Formant amplitude of children with Down syndrome. *American Journal of Mental Deficiency, 92,* 230–233.

Preus, A. (1973). Stuttering in Down's syndrome. In Y. LeBrun & R. Hoops (Eds.), *Neurologic approaches to stuttering* (pp. 90–100). The Hague, Netherlands: Mouton.

Preus, A. (1990). Treatment of mentally retarded stutterers. *Journal of Fluency Disorders, 15,* 223–233.

Redman, R.S., Shapiro, B.L., & Gorlin, R.J. (1965). Measurement of normal and reportedly malformed palatal vaults: III. Down's syndrome (trisomy 21, mongolism). *Journal of Pediatrics, 67,* 162–165.

Reichle, J., & Wacker, D. (Eds.). (1993). *Communication and language intervention series: Vol. 3. Communicative alternatives to challenging behavior: Integrating functional assessment and intervention strategies.* Baltimore: Paul H. Brookes Publishing Co.

Roche, A.F., Roche, J.P., & Lewis, A.B. (1972). The cranial base in trisomy 21. *Journal of Mental Deficiency Research, 16,* 7–20.

Rosin, M.M., Swift, E., Bless, D., & Vetter, D.K. (1988). Communication profiles of adolescents with Down syndrome. *Journal of Childhood Communication Disorders, 12,* 49–64.

Rosin, M., Swift, E., Khidr, A., & Bless, D. (1992, November). *Acoustic manifestations of voice production in adult males with Down syndrome.* Poster presented at the annual convention of the American Speech-Language-Hearing Association, San Antonio, TX.

Sanger, R.G. (1975). Facial and oral manifestations of Down's syndrome. In R. Koch & F.F. de la Cruz (Eds.), *Down's syndrome (Mongolism): Research, prevention and management* (pp. 32–46). New York: Brunner/Mazel.

Schlanger, B.B., & Gottsleben, R.H. (1957). Analysis of speech defects among the institutionalized mentally retarded. *Journal of Speech and Hearing Disorders, 22,* 98–104.

Scott, B.S., Becker, L.E., & Petit, T.L. (1983). Neurobiology of Down's syndrome. *Progress in Neurobiology, 21,* 199–237.

Shapiro, B.L., Gorlin, R.J., Redman, R.S., & Bruhl, H.H. (1967). The palate and Down's syndrome. *New England Journal of Medicine, 276,* 1460–1463.

Shapiro, B.L., Redman, R.S., & Gorlin, R.J. (1963). Measurements of normal and reportedly malformed palatal vaults: I. Normal adult measurements. *Journal of Dental Research, 42,* 1039.

Smith, A. (1990). Factors in the etiology of stuttering. *American Speech-Language-Hearing Association Reports, Research Needs in Stuttering: Roadblocks and Future Directions, 18,* 39–47.

Stoel-Gammon, C. (1980). Phonological analysis of four Down's syndrome children. *Applied Psycholinguistics, 1,* 31–48.

Swift, E., Rosin, M., Khidr, A., & Bless, D. (1992, November). *Aerodynamic properties of speech in adult males with Down syndrome.* Poster presented at the annual convention of the American Speech-Language-Hearing Association, San Antonio, TX.

Van Borsal, J. (1988). An analysis of the speech of five Down's syndrome adolescents. *Journal of Communication Disorders, 21,* 409–421.

Van Riper, C. (1982). *The nature of stuttering.* Englewood Cliffs, NJ: Prentice-Hall.

Willcox, A. (1988). An investigation into non-fluency in Down's syndrome. *British Journal of Disorders of Communication, 23,* 153–170.

Yarter, B.H. (1980). Speech and language programs for the Down's population. *Seminars in Speech, Language and Hearing, 1,* 49–60.

8

Progress in Multiple Language Domains by Deaf Children and Hearing Children

Discussions within a Rare Event Transactional Model of Language Delay

Keith E. Nelson and Janet A. Welsh

SPEECH AND LANGUAGE IN DEAF children have often been discussed in relative isolation from literature on hearing children with and without language delay. This chapter instead places deaf children's development of speech, spoken language, sign language, and text under a common theoretical framework that also covers hearing children's development in each of these domains. Three themes are stressed: 1) Understanding development in any aspect of language requires consideration of multiple learning conditions interacting in a dynamic, transactional fashion; 2) deaf children with moderate to profound hearing losses usually exhibit a form of specific language impairment (SLI), serious speech delay, and language delay in the absence of cognitive impairments other than hearing loss, and thus insights into their development may be aided by examining development in hearing children with SLI; and 3) new theoretically based intervention strategies are needed to support communicative development in hearing children and deaf children with demonstrated communicative delays or with evident risks for such delays.

The question of speech–language connections that is central to all chapters in this volume is incorporated as part of a larger series of questions. These questions concern how first-language strengths in either speech or sign at the levels

Considerable background research underpinning the development of ideas presented in this chapter was provided by grants to the first author from the National Science Foundation (BNS-8013767), National Institute on Deafness and Other Communication Disorders (RO1-NS26437 and 2R01DC00508), U.S. Department of Education (G008302959, G008430079, G0008300361), and Hasbro Children's Foundation.

In addition, the first author thanks Leilani and the second author thanks Will for their lasting contributions to our lives and to our attempts to understand children's development.

of phonology, intelligibility, production speed, comprehension speed, and complexity influence acquisition and performance at other levels in communicative repertoires: syntax, conversation, phonological, narrative, semantic, and metalinguistic domains. Discussion ranges across three modes of language: text, sign language, and spoken language. Related questions concern possible ways of facilitating progress in each mode and each domain. These questions are examined using the theoretical framework of the next two sections. The first section presents the core ideas of the Rare Event Transactional Model of Language Delay. The second spells out Rare Event Learning (REL) conditions more fully and places the REL theory in relation to other theoretical work.

RARE EVENT TRANSACTIONAL MODEL OF LANGUAGE DELAY

The Rare Event Transactional Model of Language Delay is an integrative account of language delay in hearing children, in deaf children, and in children with other disabilities (Nelson, Welsh, Camarata, Heimann, & Tjus, 1996). It draws on transactional theory (e.g., Sameroff & Chandler, 1975) and REL theory with its associated tricky mix framework of learning conditions. Following are the eight central components of the model:

1. All forms of language delay are produced by multiple factors but with somewhat different factors operating in different children.
2. Individual children's strengths and weaknesses in diverse processing capacities are important contributors to how interactions with language partners dynamically unfold across developmental periods and produce indirect effects on language delay or language acceleration.
3. Strengths and weaknesses in diverse processing capacities also are important contributors directly to the success of processing some input well enough to trigger language advances. Among the most relevant cognitive processes are working memory abstractions of phonological, syntactic, lexical, and pragmatic structures; regulation of working memory contents; long-term memory encoding and retrieval; and "hot spot" tracking of discrepancies between input and the child's current language structure representations.
4. Input conditions negatively affect language delay when there are relatively few stage-relevant challenges, when there are relatively few discourse facilitators of processing (e.g., placement of challenges in recasts), and when few favorable social-emotional conditions are mixed into conversational learning opportunities.
5. Motor encoding and planning abilities directly affect developmental progress in production of language and may indirectly affect comprehension progress as well. As Bates, Bretherton, and Snyder (1988), Smith and Thelen (1993), and Thelen and Smith (1994) argued, there are rich interrelations among phonological, syntactic, lexical, and contextual factors in production.

6. Complex interrelations arise among underlying representations of language (in all domains) and both on-line production and on-line comprehension in varied contexts. Across children, there are tremendous differences, especially during the early periods of language development, in the relationships among representational status, realized comprehension, and realized production.

7. Progress in language depends on dynamic transactions between the child and interactional partners over time, influenced by all of the factors in items 2–6 in this list. In addition, emotional, social, and cognitive sophistication may influence transactional patterns. For example, in some cases of SLI, as the hearing child approaches ages 5–7 years and shows typical cognitive, social, and physical developmental levels, dynamic transactions may evolve toward fewer and fewer processing facilitators because interactional partners find these characteristics of the child more salient than the child's delayed language level. The impact of any of the factors previously specified depends on complex transactional patterns that often either diminish or potentiate the predicted impact from an isolated measurement. For example, subtle perceptual impairments in a child and some relatively low frequencies of certain syntactic structures in samples of input might both prove to be no serious brake on acquiring those particular syntactic structures if the few exemplars that do occur are richly scaffolded by multiple processing facilitators. For deaf children, in contrast, there typically are serious risks that input conditions in both speech and sign will be less optimal, that speech processing will be very limited, and that a transactional pattern may evolve in which neither the child's parents nor his or her teachers provide rich scaffolding or high expectancies of normative rates of language progress in speech, sign, or text.

8. For language progress to continue in deaf or hearing children with language delays, tricky mixes of cognitive, motor, strategic, input, and social-emotional conditions need to converge. Many language advances are rare events, based on fairly rare instances in which such tricky mix convergences occur. Some clues on how to create such tricky mixes for syntax acquisition are provided in this chapter. However, more innovations are needed to help language therapists, parents, and other interested adults become better at finding the particular procedures and contexts that help individual children with language delays experience the tricky mixes that strongly boost their language progress.

TRICKY MIX CONDITIONS WITHIN RARE EVENT LEARNING

REL theory is summarized in this section according to multiple conditions required for significant developmental steps forward, for acquisition of significant new structures of comprehension and/or expression. Significant new structures are those that represent definite additions to the complexity and flexibility of the child's repertoire. Across domains and across developmental levels, the broad terms *performance* and *deployment* of a significant new structure are used to allow for a variety of advances in literacy, first-language communication in speech or sign language, problem solving, mathematics, music, art, and other complex domains. The central characteristics of the REL theory presented in this section were laid out in previously published presentations of the model (Nelson, 1980, 1981, 1982, 1987, 1989, 1991a, 1991b; Nelson, Heimann, Abuelhaija, & Wroblewski, 1989; Nelson, Heimann, & Tjus, 1997; Nelson, Loncke, & Camarata, 1993; Nelson, Welsh, et al., 1996). The following are the five categories of learning conditions, abbreviated as LEARN, which are organized under REL theory:

1. **L:** *Launching conditions* lead to initial engagement with new challenges. These conditions include attention to challenging structures; priming of multiple relevant prior representations; and abstraction and storage in long-term memory of some information, however incomplete, about the challenges. For example, learners might encode into long-term memory some partial representation of structures that are challenges for their current developmental levels; for readers or speakers, these might include relative clauses in text, such as "The monkey with the white foot rode the pony." Launching of learning can be delayed in any or all domains of text or spoken language learning for many months or years if settings are not chosen or created in which the child feels comfortable and engaged and in which the child holds positive expectancies of support and learning.

2. **E:** *Enhancing conditions* The probability of learning increases dramatically when luck or planning provides multiple catalysts (e.g., challenge-carrying recasts, rapid interplay of multiple information channels) that limit competing processing demands and that specifically scaffold comparison and abstraction processes in working memory. Other examples of enhancers are learner strategies that fit the current context of learning. In combination with good launching, readiness, and adjustment conditions, other important enhancers include fun and humor. In addition, for many school-age children, learning is enhanced by cues and strategies that bring out the child's planfulness, monitoring of plans, and other metacognitive processes.

3. **A:** *Adjustment conditions* concern ongoing adjustments during learning so that positive emotion, self-esteem, and motivation conditions converge with other conditions. The learner and supporting partners often need to take regulatory steps to ensure that emotional, motivational, and attentional levels support sustained processing and learning (Campos, Mumme, Kermoian, & Campos, 1994; Cole, Michel, & Teti, 1994; Fox, 1994; Newby, 1994). Expectancies that effort will lead to new learning need to be adjusted so that positive expectancy contributes to engagement

but also so that target rates of learning do not lead to disappointment. According to tricky mix transactional theorizing, each new episode of learning or attempted learning has its own pattern and, depending on the initial states of the learner (e.g., mood, knowledge, fatigue, strategy, expectancy), different adjustments need to be made to ensure engagement and learning. In areas as different as tutoring in mathematics (Lepper, Woolverton, Mumme, & Gurtner, 1993), language therapy at the syntactic level (Haley, Camarata, & Nelson, 1994), and reading multimedia teaching for children with autism (Nelson, Heimann, & Tjus, 1997), it has been shown that the same basic instructional procedure can be far more effective when tutor–child adjustments are made that enhance the child's positive emotion, self-esteem, and depth of motivational engagement.

4. **R:** *Readiness conditions* are illustrated by preparedness (i.e., prior knowledge, interest, motivation) for new challenges and by degree of intactness of learning mechanisms (which are hard to estimate for many children with deafness or other disabilities). It is also essential that a child have some appropriate strategies available. For deaf children or hearing children with very low language skills, it should be determined whether a child has the fundamental strategy of making communicative attempts as opposed to rather passive observation (Koegel & Koegel, 1995). After several years of limited communicative progress in any modality, it is not unusual to see deaf children with quite low rates of communicative attempts (e.g., Goldin-Meadow, 1985).

5. **N:** *Network conditions* refer to the need for representations of new structures that are well integrated into representational networks. Convergent learning conditions that support such integration often include multiple modes of representation and at least a few separate occasions of active processing before newly abstracted structures are consolidated. In addition, powerful effects on developmental progress can be seen if particular episodes of learning stimulate multiple levels of processing of challenging new structures. The consolidation of effective representational networks for first language appears to extend well beyond the preschool years, with increasing levels of speed, sophistication, and flexibility arising with further learning and maturation (Biddle, 1996; Bowerman, 1985; Nelson & Nelson, 1978).

Learning of new language structures and fluent, rapid language performance using already acquired structures are enhanced in multiple ways when language networks are redundant and overlearned. As speed and accuracy of access (Catts, Hu, Larrivee, & Swank, 1994; Kamhi & Catts, 1989) to network representations increase with practice, processing capacity is freed for better planning and monitoring of ongoing text or speech or sign output. Likewise, these changes allow challenges to learning to receive more attentional and abstraction resources (cf. Paul, 1992; Wolf, Bally, & Morris, 1986, on automatization). In addition, for both language performance and language advances, highly consolidated and redundant networks help limit errors due to background noise and other potential distractors (Case, 1985; Fox, 1994; Mandler, 1962; Thelen & Smith, 1994). Striking individual differences occur in the relationships between underlying representations as indexed by comprehension and frequency, accuracy, and speed of language expression. For example, a minority of children at 16–24 months of age show production rates (for comprehended lexical items) that are at least five times lower than normative rates (Fenson, Dale, Reznick, Bates, & Thal, 1994; Nelson & Bonvillian, 1973, 1978). A reasonable speculation is that for many such children there will be little fluent productive expression (in sign, speech, or text) until relevant language representations have reached normative levels of consolidated, redundant network status.

Over a period of years, typically developing children with typical language change dramatically in their language network efficiency. Nelson and Kosslyn (1977) found that speed of comprehending simple English sentences such as "A lion has a mane" dropped from about 2.3 seconds at age 8 years to about 1.3 seconds at age 13 years. In terms of how rapidly individual words and sentences already known by a child can be retrieved and used to name pictures or objects or scenes, there are similar notable speed increases as age increases across the age range from 3 to 14 years (Kail, 1991; Wolf, 1982; Wolf et al., 1986). These trends are exemplified by a decline in reaction time for deciding that two different pictures match the same word (e.g., *umbrella*), from 1.6 seconds at age 8 years to .8 second at age 14 years (Kail, 1986). There is little doubt that, in typically developing children, these increases in network efficiency for all domains of language depend both on continued brain maturation and on the cumulation of extensive experience with language. For deaf children and other children with disabilities, teaching benchmarks should be set that include advances in network efficiency in addition to expansions of language repertoires.

The importance of the favorable convergence of multiple facilitating conditions can be seen in other sections of this chapter. Such convergence also can be partly represented as the joint probability that the child will encounter one or more favorable conditions in each LEARN category. If, for a particular learning episode, the probability of favorable conditions under **L, E, A, R,** and **N** categories were each a respectable .8, then the joint probability would be considerably less at .33 (.8 × .8 × .8 × .8 × .8). However, the practical problem of creating effective tricky mixes of LEARN conditions is even more vividly demonstrated if, for any combination of reasons, the probability of favorable conditions in each LEARN category falls to .5 (let alone below that); then the joint probability would be .5 × .5 × .5 × .5 × .5 for a mere .03.

In comparison with related developmental theories, REL theory provides greater emphasis than most on understanding the conditions under which new structures are initially acquired and then consolidated. It has many common-alities with cognitive orientations in accounts of growth of language and conceptual knowledge (cf. Bohannon & Stanowicz, 1989; Bowerman, 1985; Case, 1985; Demetriou, 1988; Elman et al., 1996; Maratsos & Chalkley, 1980; Plunkett, Karmiloff-Smith, Bates, Elman, & Johnson, in press; Slobin, 1985). However, because REL looks at social, emotional, and self-concept conditions as integrally mixing together with traditionally more cognitive and linguistic components of learning, it has the heuristic value of suggesting new kinds of observations on how learning is hindered or supported. In this respect, REL theory has much in common with dynamic systems accounts of how multiple systems (i.e., perceptual, motor, emotional, social, linguistic) couple or inter-act to support skilled performance and learning (e.g., Csikszentmihalyi, 1990, 1993; Csikszentmihalyi & Csikszentmihalyi, 1988; Karmiloff-Smith, 1981; Thelen, 1988; Thelen & Smith, 1994). Within language development theoriz-ing, Paul (1992) presented a related framework for discussing learning and consolidation of new structures in multiple language domains. REL discus-sions have left open the possible future identification of maturationally based neural components specific to language but stress that any such components would affect language progress only when other conditions in the child's ac-tual interactions with conversational partners are favorable. In common with theorizing by Bates et al. (in press), Bowerman (1985), Fey (1986), Fischer and Pipp (1984), Lieven (1978), Lieven and Pine (1996), Nelson and Nelson (1978), Ninio (1996), Pizzuto and Caselli (1994), Plunkett et al. (in press), Siegler (1991), and Smith and Thelen (1993). REL theory suggests that the path to eventual mastery of new complex skills can be highly varied across in-dividual children.

LANGUAGE DOMAIN RELATIONS IN DEAF
CHILDREN IN PRIMARILY ORAL ENVIRONMENTS

Children with greater hearing losses are at greater risk than those with lesser hearing losses for severe delay in spoken language, even when nearly all lan-guage input is in the form of speech. In addition, as degree of hearing loss in-creases, it becomes increasingly difficult for children to achieve useful levels of literacy (i.e., reading, writing, spelling, narrative). These conclusions have been documented by many different investigators in many countries (Bonvil-lian, Nelson, & Charrow, 1976; Conrad, 1970; Cross, Nienhuys, & Kirkman, 1985; de Villiers, 1991; Harris & Beech, 1995; Hudgins & Numbers, 1942; Leybaert, 1993; Moores, 1978; Nelson, Loncke, et al., 1993). Discussion of how speech and other domains interrelate is organized by the tricky mix cate-gories of learning conditions summarized in Table 1.

Table 1. Tricky mixes for learning

Dynamically contributing conditions within five central categories:

L   Launching conditions
> Challenges to learner
> Prior primes
> Settings
> Initial expectancies
> Initial abstractions, however incomplete

E   Enhancing conditions
> Attentional catalysts
> Motivational catalysts
> Abstraction catalysts
> Background processing strategies
> Foreground mindfulness and monitoring
> Feedback elicitors
> Fun, humor, and entertainment

A   Adjustment conditions
> Abstractions revised and adjusted
>> New structures fully abstracted
>> New fits of available structures to contexts
> Inhibition regulation
> Emotional regulation
> Self-esteem regulation
> Expectancy/Confidence regulation
> Cultural-social processes
> Motivational cycles
> Attributional processes
> Ongoing strategy adjustments

R   Readiness conditions
> Domain engages learner identity
> Motivational and attributional dispositions
> Intactness of learning mechanisms
> Learner strategies
> Learner preparedness for challenging new structure or new performance occasion

N   Network conditions
> Parallel processing and multiple buffers
> Multiple recasting–facilitated comparisons
> Follow-through opportunities
> Sustained processing rounds until new structures are consolidated
> Redundant and overlearned networks

Readiness and Enhancers

Hearing losses in the severe to profound range make the young child far less ready than hearing children to process and express speech. Many children simply do not process most spoken language input around them; thus, the potential challenges and facilitators in that input have little or no impact on their learning. In consequence, speech is multiply impaired: There is not a full phonological repertoire in either production or comprehension, speed is slow when accessing those phonemes that are available, and intelligibility is very poor. Moores (1985) provided a representative study in which, after 4 years of oral schooling between 3 and 7 years of age, intelligibility of children with severe hearing impairments averaged only 30%. These speech impairments in an oral environment typically are linked to severely impaired language levels. As Harris and Beech, for example, observed,

> We encountered children with very little language at age 5. By contrast, we found that the children who had learned to sign had a much more even distribution of language ability: None of the signing children had language ability that was as impoverished as that of some children whose experience had been exclusively oral. (1995, p. 201)

Similar observations made by Goldin-Meadow (1985) stressed the extremely low developmental levels and the low rates of meaningful speech production (less than 4% of communication attempts) by deaf children in oral home environments.

Launching Conditions for Literacy

For deaf children orally educated during preschool years, there are multiple complications in teaching literacy when primary school begins. According to tricky mix analyses, ideally the child is placed in settings where learning expectancy is high, where relevant prior language representations are easily primed, and where text challenges are meaningfully encountered. However, for a child with very low speech skills and very low semantic and syntactic levels, there is a paucity of language representations available to map to text. Expectancies by the child and by teachers are not likely to be high in settings where previous classes of similar children have had limited success in learning to read and write. There is the risk that text exercises guided by teacher speech that continues to be very inadequately processed will not make much sense; that no special catalysts for facilitating abstraction of text will be provided; and that, over the course of an instructional year, adjustments may proceed poorly. Thus, self-esteem, expectancy, and motivational engagement may all decline. Self-attributions may be made by such children that they do not have a language brain (cf. Koegel & Koegel, 1995, for children with autism).

Research documents that many orally educated deaf children experience all of these difficulties. Even by fifth grade, some children are able to read only a few isolated words, such as the frequent English functor *the* (Nelson & Camarata, 1996). This is made easier to understand, though no easier to accept, by research showing that, in some first-grade classes, more than half of the children failed to achieve any reading progress by the end of the school year (Harris & Beech, 1995). Cumulated across school years to age 16, the no-progress and slow-progress years put the typical deaf child far behind in literacy; at age 16, less than 5% of children are at age norms (Bonvillian et al., 1976; deVilliers, 1991; de Villiers, de Villiers, & Hoban, 1994; Gaines, Mandler, & Bryant, 1981). At age 17, average reading grade levels in most studies are about 8 years behind the levels for hearing students (Gentile, 1972;

Moores, 1978). Expressed in rare event, tricky mix terms, these outcomes demonstrate that despite the best of intentions, many deaf children with good cognitive abilities fail year after year to encounter the complex mixes of learning conditions needed to make text learnable and motivating.

Common Transactional Processes
Across Language Domains and Modes

In the field of children's language delay and disorders, scientific fragmentation has occurred just as in other fields of science. For deaf children, largely separate fields of inquiry have arisen around literacy, spoken language, and sign language. For hearing children, similar fragmentation can be seen in instructional approaches, theories, journals, and networks of professional contact that are largely separate for communication disorders and children without disabilities, as well as for the language domains of speech, semantics and syntax, pragmatics and narrative, literacy, and first-language versus second-language acquisition. However, there are some countervailing attempts to look at common processes and shared insights about pathways to effective intervention and instruction. The remaining sections of this chapter examine a few of these latter cross-domain contributions.

Returning to the issues of why deaf children usually show such significant language delay in every language mode—spoken language, sign language, and literacy—the transactional model presented previously is heuristic in thinking along certain common lines, regardless of language mode or language domain. For example, learning in speech or in sign always requires much more than simple exposure to a lot of language from social partners. Instead, understanding language advances requires a close look at the learner's characteristics as well as at the structural details of input challenges, the availability of processing facilitators within the input, and the pattern of emotional and self-esteem regulation or dysregulation that occurs in potential learning situations. The details of child–environment transactions that support progress in phonology are different from the detailed transactions for syntax and for each other language domain. Thus, the basic learning process and the *kinds* of REL tricky mix conditions contributing are highly similar across language modes and domains, but the successful embedding of particular challenges within cognitive-emotional-social transactions requires *many distinct transactional patterns* to ensure that all relevant components of text, spoken language, and sign language are supported in their acquisition.

CONSIDERATION OF LANGUAGE DOMAIN
RELATIONSHIPS FOR HEARING AND DEAF CHILDREN

This section broadens the discussion to look at language learning in deaf children in primarily signing environments or in mixed oral-sign environments and also to look at some related aspects of how spoken language and literacy progress for hearing children. A key goal is that every year a child should make significant progress in one or more modes of language. When this goal is not met, as is evident in the previous examples for some deaf children in oral environments, the transactional REL model suggests monitoring multiple characteristics of differing settings to find some dynamic mix of conditions that works for a child. By the same token, when excellent progress is being made by a child in a particular mode, then examination of the detailed learning conditions may yield useful hypotheses about ways to help other children. In the selected observations in this section, language domain relations are again organized under the five central LEARN categories of tricky mix theorizing: launching, enhancers, adjustments, readiness, and networks.

Launching and Readiness Conditions

Between 1 and 6 years of age, for a small minority (less than 2%) of deaf children, significant progress is launched in the multiple domains of sign, speech, fingerspelling, and text. These atypical children appear to succeed because there is a rich combination of challenges, positive expectancies of learning, and supportive settings. Consider the case of Alice (Maxwell, 1983). Between ages 12 and 24 months, Alice began to use language first in the form of simple signs and sign combinations based on American Sign Language. By age 24 months, she also was using some speech and speech-sign combinations. Another form of language for Alice was fingerspelling, which she used, for example, in spelling people's names or as one part of reading English text. Her skills in fingerspelling, reading text, and printing text all grew between 2½ and 6 years of age. Finally, Alice learned to use a lot of a special form of signing, Sign English, that includes signs that overlap with components of English, such as *s* in dogs or *ing* in barking. This pattern of learning shows the high potential for positive cycles of transactions with parents and other language partners, so that steps forward in one language domain aid another language domain, which in turn aids the first, and so forth (cf. Conte, Rampelli, & Volterra, 1996).

In contrast, deaf children are often expected to progress in speech but fail to meet that expectation. A majority of deaf children studied by Moores (1985) across varied educational approaches, from oral only to combinations of sign and fingerspelling or sign and speech, had quite low speech intelligibility by 7 years of age. They averaged less than 35%, with a range across individual children from 8% to 57%.

Launching significant levels of syntax and narrative and conversational skills is difficult when speech skills are very limited, and all of these skills develop more slowly in children with high rather than low degrees of hearing loss. Language levels at ages 5–7 years in sign language appear to be independent of degree of hearing loss if some reasonable input in sign has been provided (e.g., Moores, 1985). This conclusion fits a view of children as cognitively prepared, flexible learners who can process a fluently provided visual language as efficiently as a spoken language.

Visual processing also is essential in launching progress in spelling, read-ing, and writing. In these domains, there is compelling evidence that complex interactions occur between language domains. Such patterns of interaction vary according to the deaf child's skills in sign language and spoken language. In multiple testing contexts—reading, word and sentence memory, and spelling—it has been demonstrated that encoding strategies and processing pathways depend on the detailed levels of competence that the child has achieved in speech phonology, sign phonology, spoken language lexicon and syntax, and sign language lexicon and syntax. A particular deaf child may have too few skills in any of these areas to support any significant literacy progress or may have moderate skills in speech or sign but not both, or even (though least frequently) may have moderate to high skills in all of these domains (cf. Prinz & Strong, 1997).

Research by Bonvillian and Folven (1993) on 20 hearing children, each with one or two deaf parents, also is of relevance. The children studied all en-countered sign language as their primary language mode with their parents but also had fluent spoken language input in other contexts as well as somewhat variable speech fluency levels at home. All of these children acquired their first signs before their first words. Bonvillian and Folven argued that learner readiness for sign develops early, with visual and motor systems for signing maturing more rapidly than the auditory and motor systems central in speech.

Adjustment Conditions

An additional example of the ways in which learner-processing strategies inter-act with degree of hearing loss and speech or sign skills was provided in the re-search by Leybaert (1993). Older deaf and younger hearing children were matched on overall reading levels so that strategies could be compared. When spelling errors were made, sensible phonological substitutions were the basis less often for children who were both low in speech intelligibility and pro-foundly deaf compared with other deaf children. Leybaert's broader research on literacy, along with that of Hanson and Fowler (1987), Harris and Beech (1995), Orlansky and Bonvillian (1984), and others, indicated the importance of encod-ing strategies for reading, comparing words, and remembering words and sen-tences. Orthographic (e.g., whole word, letter sequence) strategies were used es-pecially by those profoundly deaf children with considerable sign language skill. In contrast, phonological strategies were used especially by those deaf children with the least hearing loss and the highest relative speech skills. For deaf children with significant skill in both speech and sign, the interactions with text skills appear quite complex and in need of more refined research.

Enhancer and Network Conditions

In each language mode and domain, completion of any round of progress de-pends on the presence of some challenges accompanied by a mixture of con-ditions that make those challenges interesting and processible. To advance in any language domain, new challenge structures must pass through the limited processing window of working memory. In typical conversational contexts, any single challenge in syntax must compete for processing resources with multiple other challenges, (i.e., other syntactic challenges, phonological challenges, lexical challenges, pragmatic-narrative challenges). In addition, challenges attract or receive processing resources only if there is efficient processing of already known components of input messages. In the case of a child with profound hearing loss, significant progress in spoken language domains is unlikely unless the child has encounters to help overcome the following multiple disadvantages relative to hearing children: 1) Acoustic processing uses more processing resources yet yields more errors in speech perception, 2) fewer lexical items are known at any given age, 3) access to network representations of those lexical items that are known is slower, 4) more resources are used to maintain phonological loop and other representations in working memory, 5) there are fewer lexicalized components of syntax (e.g., *ing*, *ed*), and 6) there are fewer intonational cues for sentence structure.

FACILITATING COMMUNICATIVE DEVELOPMENT FOR HEARING CHILDREN WITH AND WITHOUT LANGUAGE DELAY

Children with impairments in language but with no other obvious impairments in cognition, perceptual and motor abilities, or social-emotional competence have presented a puzzle for developmental theorists and speech-language pathologists. However, it is only in studies in the 1990s that any reasonably differentiated accounts have been provided of either the actual input typically available to such children with SLI or of pathways to acquiring new language structures under well-controlled experimental interventions. This research appears to hold insights for language intervention with deaf as well as hearing children.

Hearing children with SLI have demonstrated a remarkable and heretofore largely unrecognized strength in their language-learning capacity: Advanced morphological and syntactic targets that are noticeably absent in multiple baseline preintervention samples can be acquired if they are presented within linguistically rich training opportunities. This suggests that these children with SLI are capable of typical learning patterns (cf. also Curtiss, Katz, & Tallal, 1992; Rice, Buhr, & Nemeth, 1990; Rice & Wilcox, 1995) when appropriate input is available and when rigorous matching of typical children and children with SLI is achieved for the level and type of intervention input and for the language levels preceding intervention. However, in most previous studies, these conditions have not been jointly achieved. In the absence of clear demonstrations of how to achieve effective learning rates, for children with SLI as well as for deaf children, it appears that many schoolteachers and clinicians and theorists have underestimated the children's potential for communicative development. There are several replications of the finding that children with SLI are capable of learning previously absent syntactic targets through conversational treatment. This is important in clinical treatment because operating assumptions in most clinical settings have steered treatment away from targets that are totally absent from pretreatment assessments because they were deemed too difficult to treat.

In Nelson, Camarata, Welsh, Butkovsky, and Camarata (1996), seven children with SLI were compared with regard to conversational growth recasting and imitative within-subject treatments. The imitative treatment avoided recasting but emphasized adult modeling of specific absent targets and child imitation. Recasting focused on specific syntactic targets also, as when a passive target was created in an adult recast:

Child: Horse jumped the fence.
Adult recast: Yep, the fence was jumped by the horse.

Additional varied recast examples are provided in this chapter's appendix. Syntactic progress was higher for recasting versus imitation, and the result patterns of the children with SLI were highly similar to result patterns for their younger control individuals with typical language. Across the children in both groups, generalized spontaneous use of acquired targets in at least two utterances at home occurred for 77% of the conversational recasting targets but for only 31% of didactive-imitative targets (chi-square = 5.52, $df = 1$, $p < .02$). Such generalization of acquired syntactic structures to home conversations with the child's parent shows strong evidence of acquisition because correct spontaneous use in this context involves not only a new place but also a new conversational partner and new activities compared with the treatment context.

Camarata, Nelson, and Camarata (1994) reported on 21 children with SLI, each of whom received two treatments on difficult targets, absent in all preintervention sampling and testing. The targets were acquired to spontaneous use after fewer clinician presentations in the conversational growth-recasting condition than in the imitative condition. Spontaneous productions were more frequent in the conversational ($M = 16.4$) than in the didactic-imitative treatment ($M = 5.5$). These treatment differences were highly significant. Similar results were shown in Camarata and Nelson (1992).

By looking across all the treatment studies, it is fully evident that children with SLI actually learned as rapidly as their younger matches without delays. Thus, these findings suggest strongly that the abilities of children with SLI to efficiently acquire genuinely new language structures often may have been underestimated in both prior theorizing and prior practice.

Rare Event Learning Interpretation of Treatment Effects

REL theory stresses how powerful cognitive mechanisms support rapid learning of complex structures in many domains. In syntax acquisition, there may also be language-specific learning mechanisms (not yet documented) that support rapid learning. However, for any learning by a child to proceed, REL theory argues that the child's powerful mechanisms need at least a few highly processible exemplars of the to-be-acquired structure. Processibility is determined by a fairly hard-to-achieve (and thus typically rare) convergence of the challenge with cognitive and linguistic readiness, with interactive scaffolding (e.g., enhancers, catalysts), and with favorable levels of the child's emotional and motivational regulation (cf. Cicchetti & Beeghly, 1987; Cicchetti, Ganiban, & Barnett, 1991; Nelson, 1987, 1989, 1991a, 1991b; Nelson, Heimann, & Tjus, 1997; Nelson, Loncke, et al., 1993; Nelson, Perkins, & Lepper, 1997). Rarely occurring but highly processible exemplar sets in the natural environment or in the experimental studies previously reviewed have proved sufficient to support rapid acquisition of complex syntactic structures. However, frequently occurring exemplars of a structure (e.g., relative clause) do not lead to acquisition unless some of the exemplars are highly processible.

REL theory helps to interpret language delay in both deaf and hearing children. Children who are 2 or more years behind their peers with typical language may have failed to learn many syntactic structures because these structures have never occurred in highly processible conditions, such as the child pursuing a topic of interest and receiving parental recasts on the missing syntactic structures. These highly processible conditions are created in our experimental work, with recasts carrying individualized targets for each child as interested responses to the child's own utterance; limited nontarget processing demands, salience of the target, and emotional engagement of the child should all favor processing of the language targets. In line with this theoretical analysis, passives, gerunds, relative clauses, and other natural language syntactic structures are acquired with equal facility by the hearing children with SLI and their younger language-level matches (for lexical acquisition, cf. Rice et al., 1990). The treatment research implied that learner readiness for processing could be very similar in children with SLI and children with typical language and that it would be revealing to subject home input samples to detailed analyses of frequency of recasts as possible enhancers of processing and learning of new grammatical structures. Background for such research is now presented, and the input studies and their interpretation follow.

Highly Differentiated Data on Input in Each Language Domain and on Uptake of Input

To understand how conditions converge to support children's learning from available input, it is crucial to have some empirical and theoretical characterization of what input opportunities are available to which children. Among linguists, psychologists, and philosophers who have argued for universal acquisition of language by virtually all children, stress has been placed repeatedly on the universal adequacy of children's input to support full mastery of language (e.g., Bickerton, 1984; Chomsky, 1968, 1986). This stress now appears to have been incorrect in several key respects. First, data from research of the 1980s and 1990s show unmistakably that, in addition to children with SLI, there are a substantial number of cognitively typical hearing children who do not achieve full mastery of language; therefore, the adequacy of the input sets for these children also appears doubtful. Second, the data presented elsewhere in this chapter indicate that many children with serious delays—for example, those at age 7 speaking at age 4 levels—learn readily from experimentally provided input that mimics conversational input qualities shown to be related to relatively rapid progress of syntax. These observations remind us that it is all too easy to couple assumptions from universalist perspectives and a documented serious delay in language and conclude prematurely that a particular child with language delays has experienced fully supportive input conditions at home but has subtle or flagrant cognitive and linguistic impairments that prevent the child learning from conversational input.

Third, to gain solid information on the abilities of the child with language delays or with typical language to learn from specified input conditions, there is no substitute for convergent work that examines how well children learn under varied naturalistic and experimental input sets. Highly differentiated looks at input are needed to evaluate a wide range of models of what counts in input toward the child's uptake and learning of new language structures and what different children bring to language acquisition in terms of profiles of cognitive and linguistic strengths and weaknesses. The need for such differentiated studies of input applies equally to deaf and hearing children. However, in much prior work, the input to children has been described at levels so global as to be useless or misleading. By providing details on how effective input variations trigger syntactic acquisition, the program of research reported in this chapter provides a new and richer foundation for theoretical accounts of syntactic acquisition; an essential part of the research is differentiated coding of input.

Fourth, on the theoretical and applied levels we need to know what input details are adequate to support full mastery of language, what aspects of input are necessary, and what aspects are facilitative even if not necessary (Baker & Nelson, 1984; Bohannon, Padgett, Nelson, & Mark, 1996; Cross, 1978; Cross et al., 1985; Furrow, Nelson, & Benedict, 1979; Kaiser, 1993; Nelson, 1977, 1980, 1982, 1987, 1989, 1991a, 1991b; Nelson, Denninger, Bonvillian, Kaplan, & Baker, 1984; Pinker, 1985; Snow, Perlmann, & Nathan, 1987). The latter, the enhancers or catalysts, are especially important if a child with intact cognitive and linguistic mechanisms falls behind schedule because of prior input conditions; catching up may require extensive facilitators beyond the necessary interactional components to support acquisition. All of these needed differentiations of input are relevant for speech in deaf children and sign in deaf children, but the literature is almost silent on these questions for deaf children and only modestly extensive for hearing children.

If children at particular language levels are richly scaffolded in their syntactic progress by very highly specific kinds of recasts and other replies that carry specific targets, then reliable procedures for differentiated coding of the input should be shared across investigators. The appendix to this chapter presents a brief version of the coding system we have found both useful and reliable in multiple published reports. The coding system also provides concrete examples of the kinds of differentiated conversational behaviors under discussion. Within this coding system, recasts and other potential facilitators can be coded for sign language as well as for spoken language. The following section addresses differentiated data on input to children with SLI and typical language at home and the theoretical implications thereof.

Language Input at Home and its Theoretical Implications

To understand how hearing children with SLI achieve rates of acquiring absent syntactic structures equal to or exceeding rates for children without delays, as reviewed previously, yet enter our research with significant language delay, another piece of the puzzle concerns the input that parents are providing to children with typical language and with SLI. The input samples were coded into the categories specified in the coding manual. The results are clear. Children with SLI at preintervention home samples received a lower frequency of conversational recasts in their parents' speech than occurred in parents' speech to younger children with typical language development of matched language stages. Nelson, Welsh, Camarata, Butkovsky, and Camarata (1995) found that the children with typical language without delays received 73% more recasts ($t = 2.69$, $df = 11$, $p < .02$), even though, for both groups of children, recasts on average comprised a minority of parental replies.

By comparison, most prior studies of children with SLI have failed to consider closely either the quality of the input available to the child in his or her language-learning environments or the nature of the interactions between the child and this environment. Yet, when detailed input and interactions have been analyzed, the results have been consistent in indicating, relative to children with typical language or accelerated language, that children with SLI on average encounter fewer maternal recasts (Conti-Ramsden, 1990; Conti-Ramsden, Hutcheson, & Grove, 1995; Cross et al., 1985; Nelson et al., 1989). Any such differential availability of enhancers of processing across a period of months or years could be an important factor in language delay. Conversely, accelerated pace of language acquisition has been related repeatedly to above-average availability of enhancing recasts (e.g., Cross, 1978; Hoff-Ginsberg, 1986; Nelson, 1981, 1989; Nelson et al., 1984; Scherer & Olswang, 1984).

Observations on input to children with SLI also need to be placed in the perspective of the history of ways in which theories of language impairment and observations of children with SLI have addressed input. It has traditionally been assumed that the reason that children with SLI fail to acquire language in a typical fashion is that they have cognitive and/or linguistic impairments that make them inefficient, delayed learners (e.g., Lahey, Liebergott, Chesnick, Menyuk, & Adams, 1992; Leonard, 1981; Paul, 1992; Tager-Flusberg, 1994; Tallal, Stark, & Curtiss, 1976; Tallal, Stark, & Mellits, 1985a, 1985b). The data presented here on acquisition of new syntactic natural language structures by both children with SLI and with typical language under controlled input conditions suggest that the assumption that a deficit in the child with SLI is responsible for language delay may be for many such children incorrect or incomplete. Learner readiness conditions look surprisingly good for many children with SLI under well-specified learning conditions in treatment research. Not only do these children often learn as well as or better than children without impairments under equivalent learning conditions, but the child impairment models fail to explain the children's individual variations (in both groups) in acquisition rate within the same treatment conditions. In our project, target-specific conversational recasting constitutes an environmental intervention that frequently triggers acquisition of new syntactic structures; the fact that a small percentage of children with typical language development and children with SLI fail to learn from particular rounds of recasting treatment is not best explained by any existing model. Rather, it may be more helpful to conceptualize SLI within more complex, multidirectional frameworks relevant to successes or failures in acquisition of specific structures at home and at clinic. One such framework is the transactional model introduced previously in this chapter (Cicchetti et al., 1991; Sameroff & Chandler, 1975). Transactional theory assumes that developmental outcomes are the result of dynamic interactions between the child and the environment and that developmental disorders such as language delays in hearing and deaf children are multiply determined and must always be viewed in context. The frequently persistent nature of delay in one or more communicative modes might then be reconceptualized as a long-term series of transactions in which the environment (at preschool and school as well as at home) commonly fails to provide appropriate language-learning experiences for the child and in which the child contributes also by quite often failing to elicit appropriate support or to focus available learning mechanisms (possibly including some component processes with subtle weaknesses) on whatever useful input is available.

Given these arguments, it is important for future work to examine longitudinally the nature of social and linguistic interactions between particular children with SLI and conversational partners. We now know from a handful of detailed studies that mothers of hearing children with SLI typically provide fewer growth recasts in daily conversation than do mothers of younger children without delays of comparable language level. What remains to be determined are the child and parent and contextual characteristics that contribute to the development and persistence of these different conversational patterns. By acknowledging and attending more closely to these dynamic transactions between children and environments, it might be possible to develop intervention programs that simultaneously approach the problem of language delay from many angles. For example, it might be possible to improve the developmental trajectory of children with language delays by training parents and teachers to adjust their levels of recasting in speech or sign to the children's language levels rather than their chronological ages. Children could also be taught to elicit richer, more processible input from their environments (cf. Hadley & Rice, 1991; Rice & Wilcox, 1995). Further potential strategies and further discussion compatible with transactional theory are provided in the following section, where multiple learner conditions and multiple cognitive, social-motivational, and emotional conditions of the tricky mixes contributing to language learning in deaf children are discussed in reference to implications from the research on hearing children with SLI.

Long-Term Language and Achievement Levels in Children with SLI

If it is hypothesized that many but not all hearing children with SLI have sufficiently intact learning mechanisms to learn language to normative levels if circumstances of learning include many enhancers for engagement and processing, then identifying and replicating significant enhancers is essential. Refined research on such catalysts and other related tricky mix conditions is important in terms of human potential; it could lead to treatment regimes allowing these children the best chances of using their intact cognitive capabilities not only to enjoy more fluent communication but also to have reduced risk for the frequent academic difficulties and social and behavioral disabilities (see Aram, Ekelman, & Nation, 1984; Aram & Nation, 1980; Baker & Cantwell, 1982; Griffiths, 1969; Hadley & Rice, 1991; Records, Tomblin, & Freese, 1992). Such difficulties, along with language impairments that continue into adulthood, have been shown to persist despite language intervention treatment; but the treatments in these studies have been applied usually to language structures already in the children's repertoires (i.e., partially mastered targets). If children were more often given conversational recasting intervention on more difficult targets, absent in all samples and testing before intervention begins, the data here suggest the distinct possibility that many children with language delays would acquire most of the targets and achieve normative language. In line with this observation, one long-term goal should be to determine powerful ways to both improve the language skills and reduce the academic and social risks for children with language delays. Progress in these directions will require at least some longitudinal research that examines treatments comparatively not only for their short-term effects but also for maintenance of acquired language structures.

GAPS IN THE KNOWLEDGE OF DEAF CHILDREN'S COMMUNICATIVE DEVELOPMENT IN VARIED DOMAINS

Moores wrote about information needed to achieve effective communicative development in deaf children:

> The field cries out for theoretical and applied investigations into the acquisition of speech, language, speechreading, and listening skills of deaf children as developmental processes. The efforts of innovative and creative minds must be brought to bear on these processes if we are to take advantage of advances in linguistics and in speech and hearing science. (1978, p. 241)

However, the field has come only a small distance between 1978 and 1998 in providing differentiated understanding of the conditions at home and at school that support or fail to support progress in communicative development.

One strategy that will be helpful in increasing understanding of deaf children's communicative development is to test some of the replicated outcomes on input effects in hearing children with deaf children and their conversational partners. What kinds of recasts, for example, are enhancers of processing and learning in spoken language and sign language? What other interactional tricky mix components are needed to ensure that recasts have a strong effect? There are only a few studies that venture into this territory. Prinz and Masin (1985) found that teachers and parents can be taught to do recasting in sign language and that this recasting boosted the rate of syntactic progress in preschool deaf children. Naturalistic analyses of what hearing mothers provide in input to their deaf children at 2 and 5 years of age by Cross et al. (1985) converged in the sense that the children have language delays and are receiving fewer recasts than children without delays. This result again implicates recasts as one important potential facilitator, such that a relative gap in recast availability is associated in deaf children, as in hearing children, with slower language progress.

Another important dimension for future work is the need for more integrated consideration of the many flexible ways that children with and without disabilities can gradually put together effective communication domains. Historically, understanding human flexibility in organizing language domains has been discouraged by the beliefs that the human brain is innately organized into domains of syntax, phonology, semantics, and pragmatics and that within each of these domains production systems are separate from comprehension systems. Mental representations of text for reading and writing usually are seen as a new domain that must build on spoken language representations. However, strong arguments have been pressed for a view of the brain as remarkably flexible and dynamic. How language domains are organized, how production and comprehension interrelate, and how literacy and first language interrelate are considered to depend on what physiological systems are intact and on the history of dynamic transactions between an individual and his or her multiple social partners (Bates, Elman, et al., 1996; Bates, Thal, et al., in press; Fogel, 1992; Nelson, 1980, 1989, 1991a, 1991b; Ratner, 1996; Thelen, 1988; Thelen & Smith, 1994). None of these theorists deny that there are some built-in biases for organizing language information, but all argue that the strengths of such biases have been exaggerated and that the precise nature of the biases remains to be established.

In seeking better educational interventions and better theoretical understanding of communicative development, there needs to be a continual process of comparing and contrasting pathways to development in varied children under varied interactional conditions. As has been stressed throughout this chapter, discussions of individual differences among deaf and among hearing children should be part of this approach. The next section reviews some of the strongest individual differences among deaf children with an emphasis on multiple pathways to successful development and multiple, complex patterns of delayed development.

Individual Differences Among Deaf Children

A small minority of deaf children encounter year after year an excellent tricky mix of fully fluent sign language embedded in enhancing social, emotional, and discourse patterns. Early attachment relationships and preschool peer relationships are positive, contributing to conversational interactions that frequently make processing and learning of new sign structures efficient (e.g., Bonvillian & Folven, 1993). The fluency of peer as well as adult partners contributes to excellent sign formational, phonological structures that are used with considerable automaticity, thus freeing processing resources for complex syntax and pragmatic structures. In turn, strength in all sign domains by school age supports mapping text to sign and normative rates of progress in literacy (Prinz & Strong, 1997).

The majority of deaf children instead show very mixed levels of developmental progress. Sign language input is not fluent; speech is processed very poorly; and, during the preschool years, slow progress in both speech and sign contributes to less positive attachment and social relationships. Weaknesses in social-emotional development make successful processing of new language structures within the flow of social interaction even less likely. In school years, literacy acquisition proceeds at fairly slow rates because neither spoken language and its phonological codes nor sign language are sufficiently mastered to support text skills. Difficulties in understanding teachers' attempts at instruction also limit text progress. Such teacher–child communication difficulties further work against a supportive tricky mix for school learning, making positive mood and expectancy of success more difficult to sustain.

Finally, there is the minority of deaf children who make extremely limited progress in any mode of communication. These children are most likely to have profound hearing loss combined with no exposure to sign language and slow social-emotional development. Tricky mixes very rarely are experienced for these children. Challenges in language that they can process at all are not frequently available. There are few enhancers to support the challenges that are available. The dynamics of child–parent interaction also do not provide a normative level of support in terms of emotional adjustment, social skills, and self-esteem. Often there is a kind of downward transactional spiral in which low communication progress, poor child–adult relationships (e.g., Greenberg, Calderon, & Kusche, 1984), low confidence and initiative on the child's part, and low expectations of future progress dynamically contribute to less and less satisfactory outcomes across time. Compared with typical hearing children, the deaf children in dyads that have developed relatively low levels of communicative exchange are, at 3–6 years of age, less happy and less socially skilled (Lederberg, 1993; Meadow, Greenberg, Erting, & Carmichael, 1981; Schlesinger & Meadow, 1976). Progress in reading and writing and other school subjects proceeds very slowly.

From the tricky mix transactional framework of this chapter, it is important to see that if a child has been very low in expressive language over an extended period, then communicative strategies will reflect this low language. For example, after extended language delay for the period of 3–7 years of age, the child at age 7 has certain well-established expectancies about social situations, communicative strategies, self-revelation, and the probability that new language learning will occur. If language comprehension has developed to a point well ahead of expressive language, the child also will rely heavily on comprehension clues and contextual clues to guide choices of when to say something (within the limited productive repertoire) and when to let nonverbal actions signify interest and comprehension. This imbalance between comprehension and production levels may fundamentally shift the kinds of transactions that are likely with peers, teachers, parents, speech-language pathologists, and others. Stable, tightly organized patterns for a child's social approaches to others may work for a while against the likelihood of precisely the kinds of interactions needed to scaffold language progress. To establish effective tricky mixes that successfully support the child's analysis and learning and deployment of new expressive skills, particular attention may be required by an intervention team to transactional dynamics that support the child's expressive attempts. For example, within a multiple-goal preschool language plan with overall significant impact on language progress by children with SLI, there was little impact on expressive development for those children with normal typical speech but low initial levels of both expression and comprehension (Rice & Hadley, 1995). Close monitoring of more than one intervention context should help determine if any single context strongly supports both the abstraction of new levels of language structure and the on-line conversational display of newly learned structures. If not, then different contexts and different tricky mixes may be required to support different components of language abstraction, language expression, and language comprehension. It can be hoped that awareness of the range of individual differences, along with theoretical frameworks emphasizing considerable flexibility in developmental pathways, helps to spur new innovations in programs for helping deaf children, their parents, and their teachers.

PROVIDING DEAF CHILDREN LEARNING EPISODES WITH TRICKY MIXES FAVORING GROWTH IN MULTIPLE, INTERACTING LANGUAGE DOMAINS

The arguments and evidence discussed to this point set the stage for a theoretically grounded integrated approach to communicative interaction with deaf children. Although this integrated approach has not yet received any empirical test, prior research does document feasibility and effectiveness of many of the suggested components. It is assumed here that many of the findings on hearing children with SLI and language delays do have implications, along with research directly on the deaf, for innovations in communicative programs for deaf children.

Individualized, Monitored Plans

Deaf children need individualized plans for communicative development because, across deaf children of the same age, there are highly variable profiles of skill in sign, speech, and text and for subdomains in each mode. Well-monitored, individualized plans also are required because it is even trickier to mix an effective set of learning conditions for a deaf child with language delays than for a hearing child with language delays. Even more complexities arise for the minority of deaf children (estimated to be more than 10%; Moores, 1978) with motor, visual, intellectual, or other added disabilities. Continued monitoring once learning has been established is advisable because it usually is difficult to arrange sufficient, sustained human resources to support progress in multiple language domains.

Planned Input Patterns

Research on input with hearing children demonstrates that well-tailored input can be powerful enough to raise language-learning rates of children with serious language delays to those of children with typical language. In addition, among the very few detailed investigations of adult input in speech to deaf children, there are indications that, for the same language level as in matched hearing children, the deaf children receive fewer challenges and fewer recasts and related challenge-processing facilitators (Cross et al., 1985). Accordingly, rather than assuming that adults will spontaneously deploy conversational patterns in either speech or sign that are highly supportive of learning, there should be systematic planning. Each week in each language mode, a plan should be made that ensures that an individual deaf child has multiple conversational partners who use recasts and other established catalysts for language learning and who also use a full range of language challenges. Some partners can be chosen who already display these characteristics when samples of child–partner conversation are analyzed. However, to join these communicative development plans, other partners need to receive training.

As part of input planning in tricky mixes, research has provided a framework for potential enhancers. In place of general conversation strategies, Table 2 shows some recommended kinds of highly differentiated growth recasts placed well in discourse in sign and text, as well as in speech.

Multiple Targets in Each Teaching Episode

Teaching episodes should bring in multiple targets from multiple language domains. During an hour of teaching, there are strong reasons to combine learning targets from mixed modes. For example, when teaching literacy as a central focus, sign and/or speech targets can be an essential part of the dialogue concerning text. This provides the child with choice, so that if conditions at first do not mix quite right for learning in one mode, they may still come together and produce learning in another mode. Any learning achieved in turn enhances self-esteem, motivation, and expectancy, and over the hour progress in each mode provides a boost for learning in other modes. Some demonstrations of the effectiveness of these sorts of literacy or language teaching episodes in multimedia contexts have been provided by Heimann, Nelson, Tjus, and Gillberg (1995); Nelson, Heimann, and Tjus (1997); and Nelson, Prinz, Prinz, and Dalke (1991).

Other kinds of multiple-target episodes also have been demonstrated in prior research. During a single hour of interaction, mothers sometimes bring in recasts that carry quite varied challenges, such as multiple phonological structures, multiple syntactic structures, multiple pragmatic devices, and multiple lexical items, all of which are beyond the child's current language repertoire (Bohannon & Stanowicz, 1989; Conti-Ramsden, 1990; Nelson et al., 1989). At

Table 2.   Successively more differentiated transaction reply strategies to child's spoken, signed, or text message

1. Be responsive to the child's message.
2. Follow the child's basic meaning (semantic contingency).
3. #2 reply, but also elaborate within the child's current language level.
4. Recast: #2 reply plus structural changes through adding, deleting, and rearranging.
5. Growth recast: Recast by specifically displaying structural challenges to this child today relative to the child's current language domains.
6. Sensitive growth recasts: #5 chosen to mix moderate challenges with the child's "best," easiest-to-process, already known structures.
7. Sensitive growth recasts (#6) well placed in the larger narrative or conversational flow.
8. Well-placed, sensitive growth recasts (#7) accompanied by more tricky mix components: Positive affect, self-esteem support, high expectancies of meaningful communication and learning, good learner strategies, and so forth.

the intervention level, clinicians have been trained to use in a single session procedures that for some children range across multiple syntactic targets (Camarata et al., 1994; Nelson et al., 1995) and for some children mix phonological recasts and syntactic recasts (see Chapter 11). However, multiple-target episodes may have to be carefully designed to be effective. It is a tricky mix indeed to provide rich, varied challenges in a teaching episode and to do so in a way that allows for the processing demands for each individual challenge.

Tailored Combinations of Recommended Structures and New Challenges Imagine that some growth recast has just been provided to a child's comment in sign or in speech. By definition, this growth recast carries a challenge to linguistic growth and also follows the basic meaning of the child's original comment. Beyond that, though, there may be a lot of variability in how well consolidated or automatic (cf. Nelson, 1991a; Nelson & Nelson, 1978; Paul, 1992; Wolf et al., 1986) the already known structures happen to be. That is, some growth recasts may bring together challenges with particular known lexical items and particular known syntactic structures that are among the top 10% of the child's repertoire in terms of retrieval speed, ease of maintenance in working memory, and flexibility. Theoretically, the REL tricky mix perspective strongly points to heightened probability of processing of the recast challenge components in such transactions where processing demands for the nonchallenging sentence components are minimized. This prediction appears well worth testing. Moreover, preinstruction assessment can identify a set of well-consolidated structures in the child's repertoire and thus allow selection of materials, settings, and so forth to increase the frequency with which these structures occur in both the child's productions and in the growth recasts of conversational partners.

Related investigations are needed on how to improve the child's network representations. Where research is available, it strongly indicates that, for already known language structures, hearing and deaf children with communicative delays also have network deficiencies; compared with children without delays, they use more processing resources and are slower and less efficient in accessing structures (Biddle, 1996). Practice in production over multiple years may be one route to long-term network improvements over time (cf. Paul, 1992), and even children with focal brain injury show such changes during the preschool and primary school years (Reilly, Bates, & Marchman, 1995). However, suppose that for an 8-year-old deaf child a true "bottleneck" is in place that blocks effective learning of new text, sign, and speech structures; that is, suppose that already known structures in a message are accessed so inefficiently that not enough processing resources are available to allow abstraction of new language structures even in the presence of overall good learning conditions. In such situations, the intervention strategy might be to try to improve network efficiency in a matter of months rather than years.

Innovations on how to improve and assess network efficiency also are needed. Programs to increase practice in using language structures in the rapid-fire context of ordinary conversations, rather than more receptive, passive classroom encounters, would be one route worth considering. If such conversational practice were combined with some episodes of challenge and with other tricky mix interventions, then multiple goals might be achieved from the same episodes of intervention. Other highly speculative and weakly documented approaches are to target improved efficiency in particular components of the information-processing system, such as working memory phonological loops (Gathercole & Baddeley, 1993), word retrieval speed (Wolf et al., 1986), or rapid auditory processing (Tallal et al., 1985a, 1985b). Related work might identify ways of strengthening representations that are specific to planning and execution of communicative expression. In deaf children, sign rehearsal loops, speed of sign retrieval, and other long-term memory storage and retrieval components presumably might also receive selective training. Tracking of any advances in network proficiency is essential for understanding and revising many communicative interventions for deaf children, yet no reported research has included such data as part of systematic instructional programs for deaf children.

Opportunistic Mining of Transactional Patterns   Even for children without language delay or hearing loss, it has been argued that communicative progress depends on quite tricky convergences of multiple cognitive, linguistic, social, and emotional conditions. For deaf children who at ages 3–12 have already demonstrated substantial delay in communicative development, it is even harder to mix conditions to produce significant progress. Successes, therefore, should be mined for optimum impact. If particular conversational partners, settings, materials, and procedures are demonstrated to produce greater child engagement and rapid learning, then in the short term new challenges in multiple modes should be planned around these successful tricky mixes. In the longer run, these successful mixes should be analyzed and attempts should be made to create new but similar patterns that are likely to work for this individual child. Monitoring would then determine whether the new mixes of partners, materials, setting, and so forth are really effective.

Parallel Monitoring Across Competing Mixes   It is always tempting to create one preferred instructional plan that takes into account everything that is known about a child. However, it is argued in this chapter that, even when there is very rich information about a child, modesty is in order—it is tricky to create the right mix of conditions for effective learning. Further modesty is usually appropriate because resources will not have been provided to give rich assessment information about a child. This leaves the position of making many guesses both about the child's characteristics and about what will happen when this child is interacting in a particular setting with parents, teachers, and others who may or may not be able to mix challenges and other learning conditions.

Accordingly, for any domain of communication, each child should always be receiving instruction in more than one mix. This allows determination of whether the best-guess, most preferred plan is working as predicted. If not, then the child can be shifted toward more transactional time in one of the competing mixes of conditions. When that shift is made, new competing mixes should also be provided part of the time and carefully monitored. This parallel, multiple instructional plan approach recognizes from the beginning that creating effective mixes of learning conditions is complex, that there are likely to be surprises in when and where a child learns well, and that what was working well a few months ago may no longer be the best mix. By combining ongoing monitoring with multiple plans, each plan under trial serves as a check and comparison point for the relative effectiveness of other plans. The "mining" of any highly effective instructional mixes should also be conducted as part of the choice of each new phase of comparative, competing instructional plans.

Mixes that Violate Typical Developmental Sequences and Typical Expectations for Learners with Delays The previous discussion has shown that most deaf children have language delays in multiple language modes. At the same time, the profiles of skill in each mode and each subdomain of language are highly variable. Included in this variability are instances in which developmental steps that have been considered prerequisites have often been skipped. Another characteristic of many deaf children's development is greater-than-usual asynchronies between language domains (for hearing children, cf. Bates & Thal, 1991; Bates et al., in press) and asynchronies between usual maturity levels and the stages of development in many language domains (cf. Locke, 1995; Chapter 3).

In trying out potential tricky mixes, these observations should be used to support trial of some plans that intentionally violate usual developmental sequences. If a deaf child is making no progress in phonemic awareness but is learning new levels of reading and writing, then planning mixes that move the child into quite complex text without phonemic awareness components should be considered. Similarly, if no effective tricky mix has been identified for triggering productive skill but comprehension is proceeding well in specified transactional patterns, then comprehension target levels should be set higher without waiting for production to keep pace. For some deaf children, gains in text skills may lead to a "cart before the horse" situation in which mastered text complexity far outpaces either speech or sign. Higher-order language achievements would thus hold the potential to facilitate phonological, lexical, syntactic, and metalinguistic progress in other modes. In other words, this situation would allow the possibility that known text could be mixed together with appropriate sign or speech input to help in tricky mixes for learning new spoken or signed levels of language. Again, any such unconventional planned mixes should be compared and monitored for relative effectiveness within the multiple-plan approach.

INDIVIDUAL VARIABILITY AND
TRANSACTIONAL INTERVENTION STRATEGIES

A small minority of young preschool hearing children and deaf children show combinations of language modes that are atypical for their age. Flexibility of developmental paths is again illustrated. In spoken languages, bilingual and trilingual fluency can be achieved by 5 years of age with documented metalinguistic skills arising from the multiple languages (Galambos & Goldin-Meadow, 1990; Leopold, 1947). Some hearing children exposed to fluent sign input become sign and speech bilinguals by age 5 years (Bonvillian & Folven, 1993; Paul & Quigley, 1994; Prinz & Prinz, 1981). Also, among both deaf (Maxwell, 1983; van der Lem & Timmerman, 1995) and hearing children (Soderbergh, 1977), early high literacy has been combined with a first spoken or signed language. These demonstrations of flexibility in development should be encouraging for new transactional attempts at tricky mixes to mutually facilitate literacy in varied combinations with sign, speech, or simultaneous communication for a broad range of deaf children. Similarly adventurous explorations of new tricky mixes to facilitate first-language, literacy, and second-language acquisition are needed for hearing children with and without disabilities.

Individual variability of many kinds needs to be more forcefully addressed in theorizing and intervention. The literature on language acquisition, communication disorders, and literacy development has, for the most part, underestimated the degrees of individual variability. It is worthwhile to have a few concrete reminders of how much children differ and how flexible developmental pathways can be. For example, in children with early (before age 6 months) focal brain injury (Bates et al., in press), at 27 months of age, mean length of utterance (MLU) (longest utterances) ranges from 1 to 12 morphemes. Children with early (before age 6 months) focal brain injury (Reilly et al., 1995) overlap in their syntactic complexity in narratives with children with no physiological damage, and the children mix complex syntax into their narratives at rates varying from less than 10% to more than 60%. Another example is 1½- to 4-year-olds with no disabilities, in whom the percentage of lexical items acquired (as shown in both production and expression) varies from 10% to 100% and at speeds varying also by a factor of 10 (Bonvillian & Nelson, 1978; Nelson, 1982), even when given the same controlled pattern of examples. In predominantly English-speaking preschools, the minority (about a third or a quarter) of children who speak another first language at home vary in their progress in English after 9 months, from only a handful of single words to complex Stage IV or Stage V sentences (Bunce, 1995; Fillmore, 1989). Also in children with no disabilities, at age 28 months, longest-utterance lengths were at 12 morphemes for the top 10% but still were at 3 morphemes for the slowest-developing 10% of a large normative sample (Fenson et al., 1994). Similarly wide variability is seen in the rapid accessing and speaking of already known names for objects among 9-year-olds, ranging from less than 15% to more than 75% of items (Wolf & Obregon, 1992). Among 5-year-olds, speed of accessing known object names is three times faster in some children compared with the children who retrieved the slowest (Wolf et al., 1986).

Consider in more detail the work by Fillmore (1989) on English progress in preschools mixing children from monolingual English homes with a minority of children who speak another language, such as Spanish, Chinese, or Korean, at home. None of the latter had any significant English at the outset of the 9-month preschool experience. By the end of the preschool year, some had become as fluent as their monolingual English peers, whereas others in the same classroom had learned only a few words of English. These outcome contrasts occurred despite highly similar language-learning opportunities, if these are defined in terms of available English-fluent teachers and peers for conversational partners. The REL transactional model predicts and explains this type of individual variability. It is not the set of teachers, the curriculum, or the peer group per se that stimulates and supports language learning; rather, it is the particular dynamic transactions that evolve between the child and these environmental elements.

One implication of the tricky mix REL perspective is that by remixing conditions for any child, with or without disabilities, strong shifts in learning rates and in the display of already available representations can be created. Another implication is that for optimal performance, differently mixed conditions are required for different children varying along the individual difference continua previously illustrated. Some clues about intervention routes for children with language delays may be generated by examining the kinds of conditions that lead typically progressing children to temporarily shut down their language learning or their language expression. It is not too difficult to shut down the usual Stage IV (Brown, 1973), excited, eight-word sentences of a child to the level of one-word expressions only. This can be achieved by pairing an inner-city minority child with a well-meaning, middle-class Caucasian interviewer asking question after question about the child's recent experiences (Hall & Cole, 1978). The same restriction of expressed language may also occur in a situation with many new perceptual and motor demands, such as a child's first experience of sledding or skating, where the strategies and goals are new, the mix of perception of snow and wind and vibrating sled or skates is new, new words are introduced, and emotional regulation also is taken for a ride. Many talkative Stage IV children not only restrict their language but actually become mute while they dynamically cope with the new frontier of skates or sleds!

In treating children with expressive language delays, there is the risk that some similar effects may be fostered inadvertently. A child may be removed from familiar settings, introduced to new routines and clinicians, and asked to answer far more questions than ordinary conversations present. Children in such treatments should be monitored and their performance should be compared with that in settings where new perceptual, strategic, and conversational demands are minimized. In line with previous discussions on monitoring across multiple comparison contexts, some treatment plans for a child with expressive delays should build treatment into particular already available daily activities and settings that have been identified as best elicitors of expressive language for the child. In some cases of delayed language in deaf or hearing children, strong emphasis may be needed on improving the retrievability and fluency of already established representations so that on-line expressive behavior has more automaticity and frees more processing resources for abstraction and storage of new structural language information. This is largely unexplored territory, but some work by Wolf and Segal (1997) indicated that direct training can improve expressive naming rates in preschool children. Further clues to facilitating faster, more automatic expressive behavior come from research indicating that repeated telling or reading routines, as in rereading and rereading a favorite story, may scaffold children's expressive development (Conti-Ramsden & Freil-Patti, 1987; Snow et al., 1987). It remains to be seen whether a series of activities can be organized that support children with language delays or reading disabilities in establishing more fluent, expressive representational systems that in turn increase the rate at which children learn new first-language and new text structures.

Treatment plans also need to consider the possibility that already organized representational networks for a school-age child (e.g., an 8-year-old) with severe language delay will be resistant to change unless innovative tricky mixes are formulated. According to the theoretical framework of this chapter and also that of some dynamic systems theories (Thelen & Smith, 1994) and connectionist theories (Plunkett et al., in press), perception, language, action, and self-concepts are represented together in complex interrelations that change dynamically between the ages of 2 and 8. For a child with language delays throughout this period, the limited language repertoire available at each point is integrated into action plans and strategies. For language to play a more central role in the child's plans and activities, tricky mixes need to be encountered that not only make learning new language structures possible but also challenge the established networks in which perception, action, emotion, and language have been corepresented. In extreme cases such as preverbal children of school age with autism, finding effective tricky mixes may require especially persistent exploration of varied components.

Because the particular tricky mixes that stimulate learning in a particular child at any given moment are difficult to anticipate, it is often desirable when working with children who demonstrate delays in many areas of language (e.g., intelligibility, syntax, semantics, pragmatics) to develop multiple-purpose interventions. These treatments would be designed to facilitate social-emotional process enhancers and to address multiple communication goals in each session at a clinic, preschool, school, or home. The expectation would be that, during any given few hours, effective mixes of learning conditions might come together for one domain, even when other domains do not progress on that occasion. With a multiple-purpose approach, treatment time may be most effectively used and the probability that some kinds of learning occur frequently may be maximized. Furthermore, interventions that simultaneously address multiple goals may provide bootstrapping opportunities for the child whereby early advances in one domain (e.g., syntax) facilitate later advances in another (e.g., intelligibility). As with all interventions, however, multiple-purpose interventions that simultaneously address a number of communication goals need to be carefully designed to provide multiple challenges without overtaxing children's processing capabilities. In addition, multiple-purpose strategies require careful monitoring to track which treatments are promoting language growth and which are ineffective. Clinicians and educators should adopt a flexible, problem-solving approach that allows assessment of new tricky mix combinations of conditions when children have not been showing excellent progress. Encouragement of this approach is provided by some outcomes in multiple communicative domains such as Blissymbolics and oral comprehension and metalinguistic skills (Hjelmquist, Sandberg, & Hedelin, 1994), or sign language and text (Bonvillian & Nelson, 1978), or speech and text (Nelson, Heimann, & Tjus, 1997) for children with autism, developmental delay, or cerebral palsy who had shown persistent and severe communicative delays. In addition, very few programs with documented outcomes have taken a multiple-domain communication intervention approach at the preschool (Rice & Wilcox, 1995) and primary grade levels.

CONCLUSIONS

As long as children with communicative delays are treated as if they have learning readiness or learning rate limitations tied to biological makeup, they are unlikely to encounter rich transactional learning conditions and high expectations. Catch-22 circumstances may arise in which learners with delays are given no exposure to the best teachers, computer materials, and communication therapists because their history of poor learning is taken as proof that rapid learning even under new conditions would not be possible. Yet the research reviewed in this chapter on treatment of children with SLI shows that when equally rich conversational therapy was provided, these children learned as quickly as children with typical language (cf. Rice & Hadley, 1995). Similar effective rates of learning matching those of children without disabilities have been shown for new literacy skills acquired from multimedia presentations by autistic and deaf and dyslexic children (Nelson, Heimann, & Tjus, 1997). In addition, tremendous flexibility in developmental pathways, even in the face of serious brain injury, has been demonstrated. As Reilly et al. observed,

> Language acquisition and language use may draw on a large number of different neural systems . . . . In some respects, this may make language more vulnerable— especially in the early stages. But in the long run, there may be more alternative ways to deal with the challenges of language learning and language use. (1995, p. 17)

The combination of these observations should lead us in the direction of adventurous testing of rich new mixes of learning conditions. Over time, efforts in this direction may lead to documented tricky mixes that are effective because they provide a dynamic mix of more challenges, more enhancers, more supports for good adjustments in self-esteem and emotional regulation, and more fun than children with language and language-related disabilities usually encounter in instructional contexts.

REFERENCES

Aram, D.M., Ekelman, B.L., & Nation, J.E. (1984). Preschoolers with language disorder: 10 years later. *Journal of Speech and Hearing Research, 27,* 232–244.

Aram, D., & Nation, J. (1980). Preschool language disorders and subsequent language and academic difficulties. *Journal of Communication Disorders, 13,* 159–170.

Baker, L., & Cantwell, D.P. (1982). Language acquisition, cognitive development, and emotional disorder in childhood. In K.E. Nelson (Ed.), *Children's language* (Vol. 3, pp. 286–321). Hillsdale, NJ: Lawrence Erlbaum Associates.

Baker, N.D., & Nelson, K.E. (1984). Recasting and related conversational techniques for triggering syntactic advances by young children. *First Language, 5,* 3–22.

Bates, E., Bretherton, I., & Snyder, L. (1988). *From first words to grammar: Individual differences and dissociable mechanisms.* New York: Cambridge University Press.

Bates, E., Elman, J., Johnson, M., Karmiloff-Smith, A., Parisi, D., & Plunkett, K. (1996). *On innateness* (Tech. Rep. No. 9602). San Diego: University of California, Center for Research in Language.

Bates, E., & Thal, D. (1991). Associations and dissociations in child language development. In J. Miller (Ed.), *Research on child language disorders: A decade of progress* (pp. 147–168). Austin, TX: PRO-ED.

Bates, E., Thal, D., Trauner, D., Fenson, J., Aram, D., Eisele, J., & Nass, R. (in press). From first words to grammar in children with focal brain injury. *Developmental Neuropsychology.*

Bickerton, D. (1984). The language biogram hypothesis. *Behavioral and Brain Sciences, 7,* 173–221.

Biddle, K.R. (1996). *Timing deficits in impaired readers: An investigation of visual naming speed and verbal fluency.* Unpublished doctoral dissertation, Tufts University, Medford, MA.

Bohannon, J.N., Padgett, R.J., Nelson, K.E., & Mark, M. (1996). Useful evidence on negative evidence. *Developmental Psychology, 33,* 551–555.

Bohannon, N., & Stanowicz, L. (1989). Bidirectional effects of imitation and repetition in conversation: A synthesis within a cognitive model. In G.E. Speidel & K.E. Nelson (Eds.), *The many faces of imitation in language learning* (pp. 121–150). New York: Springer-Verlag.

Bonvillian, J.D., & Folven, R. (1993). Sign language acquisition: Developmental aspects. In M. Marschark & D. Clark (Eds.), *Psychological perspectives on deafness* (pp. 229–268). Hillsdale, NJ: Lawrence Erlbaum Associates.

Bonvillian, J.D., & Nelson, K.E. (1978). Development of sign languages in autistic children and other language-handicapped individuals. In P. Siple (Ed.), *Understanding language through sign language research* (pp. 187–212). New York: Academic Press.

Bonvillian, J.D., Nelson, K.E., & Charrow, V.R. (1976). Language and language-related skills. *Sign Language Studies, 12,* 211–250.

Bowerman, M. (1985). Beyond communicative adequacy: From piecemeal knowledge to an integrated system in the child's acquisition of language. In K.E. Nelson (Ed.), *Children's language* (Vol. 5, pp. 369–398). Hillsdale, NJ: Lawrence Erlbaum Associates.

Brown, R. (1973). *A first language: The early stages.* Cambridge, MA: Harvard University Press.

Bunce, B.H. (1995). A language-focused curriculum for children learning English as a second language. In M.L. Rice & K.A. Wilcox (Eds.), *Building a language-focused curriculum for the preschool classroom: Vol. I. A foundation for lifelong communication* (pp. 91–103). Baltimore: Paul H. Brookes Publishing Co.

Camarata, S., & Nelson, K.E. (1992). Treatment efficiency as a function of target selection in the remediation of child language disorders. *Clinical Linguistics and Phonetics, 6,* 167–178.

Camarata, S., Nelson, K.E., & Camarata, M. (1994). A comparison of conversation based to imitation based procedures for training grammatical structures in specifically language impaired children. *Journal of Speech and Hearing Research, 37,* 1414–1423.

Campos, J.J., Mumme, D.L., Kermoian, R., & Campos, R.G. (1994). A functionalist perspective on the nature of emotion. In N.A. Fox (Ed.), *The development of emotion regulation: Biological and behavioral considerations. Monographs of the Society for Research in Child Development, 59*(Serial No. 240), 284–303.

Case, R. (1985). *Intellectual development: Birth to adulthood.* San Diego: Academic Press.

Catts, H.W., Hu, C.F., Larrivee, L., & Swank, L. (1994). Early identification of reading disabilities in children with speech-language impairments. In R.V. Watkins & M.L. Rice (Eds.), *Communication and language intervention series: Vol. 4. Specific language impairments in children* (pp. 145–160). Baltimore: Paul H. Brookes Publishing Co.

Chomsky, N. (1968). *Language and mind.* New York: Harcourt Brace Jovanovich.

Chomsky, N. (1986). *Knowledge of language: Its nature, origin and use.* New York: Praeger.

Cicchetti, D., & Beeghly, M. (1987). Symbolic development in maltreated youngsters: An organizational perspective. *New Directions for Child Development, 36,* 47–68.

Cicchetti, D., Ganiban, J., & Barnett, D. (1991). Contributions from the study of high-risk populations to understanding the development of emotion regulation. In J. Garber & K.A. Dodge (Eds.), *The development of emotion regulation and dysregulation* (pp. 15–48). Cambridge, England: Cambridge University Press.

Cole, P.M., Michel, M.K., & Teti, L.O. (1994). The development of emotion regulation and dysregulation: A clinical perspective. In N.A. Fox (Ed.), *The development of emotion regulation: Biological and behavioral considerations. Monographs of the Society for Research in Child Development, 59*(Serial No. 240), 73–100.

Conrad, R. (1970). Short-term memory processes in the deaf. *British Journal of Psychology, 81,* 179–195.

Conte, M.P., Rampelli, L.P., & Volterra, V. (1996). Deaf children and the construction of written texts. In C. Pontecorvo, M. Orsolini, B. Burge, & L. Resnick (Eds.), *Children's early text construction* (pp. 303–320). Mahwah, NJ: Lawrence Erlbaum Associates.

Conti-Ramsden, G. (1990). Maternal recasts and other contingent replies to language-impaired children. *Journal of Speech and Hearing Disorders, 55,* 262–274.

Conti-Ramsden, G., & Freil-Patti, S. (1987). Situational variability in mother–child conversations. In K.E. Nelson (Ed.), *Children's language* (Vol. 6, pp. 43–64). Hillsdale, NJ: Lawrence Erlbaum Associates.

Conti-Ramsden, G., Hutcheson, G.D., & Grove, J. (1995). Contingency and breakdown: Specific language impaired children's conversations with their mothers and fathers. *Journal of Speech and Hearing Research, 38,* 1290–1302.

Cross, T. (1978). Mothers' speech and its association with rate of syntactic acquisition in young children. In N. Waterson & C. Snow (Eds.), *The development of communication* (pp. 199–216). New York: John Wiley & Sons.

Cross, T., Nienhuys, T.G., & Kirkman, M. (1985). Parent–child interaction with receptively disabled children: Some determinants of maternal speech style. In K.E. Nelson (Ed.), *Children's language* (Vol. 5, pp. 247–296). Hillsdale, NJ: Lawrence Erlbaum Associates.

Csikszentmihalyi, M. (1990). *Flow: The psychology of optimal experience.* New York: HarperCollins.

Csikszentmihalyi, M. (1993). *The evolving self.* New York: HarperCollins.

Csikszentmihalyi, M., & Csikszentmihalyi, I. (1988). *Optimal experience.* New York: HarperCollins.

Curtiss, S., Katz, W., & Tallal, P. (1992). Delay versus deviance in the language acquisition of language impaired children. *Journal of Speech and Hearing Research, 35,* 373–383.

Demetriou, A. (Ed.). (1988). *The neo-Piagetian theories of cognitive development: Toward an integration.* Amsterdam: Elsevier Science Publishers.

de Villiers, P. (1991). English literacy development in deaf children: Directions for research and intervention. In J. Miller (Ed.), *Research on child language disorders* (pp. 349–378). Austin, TX: PRO-ED.

de Villiers, J., de Villiers, P., & Hoban, E. (1994). The central problem of functional categories in the English syntax of oral deaf children. In H. Tager-Flusberg (Ed.), *Constraints on language acquisition: Studies of atypical children.* (pp. 9–47). Hillsdale, NJ: Lawrence Erlbaum Associates.

Elman, J.L., Bates, E.A., Johnson, M.H., Karmiloff-Smith, A., Parisi, D., & Plunkett, K. (1996). *Rethinking innateness.* Cambridge, MA: MIT Press.

Fenson, L., Dale, P.A., Reznick, J.S., Bates, E., & Thal, D. (1994). Variability in early communicative development. *Monographs of the Society for Research in Child Development, 58*(Serial No. 242[5]).

Fey, M. (1986). *Language intervention with young children.* San Diego: College-Hill Press.

Fillmore, L.W. (1989). Teachability and second language acquisition. In M.L. Rice & R.L. Schiefelbusch (Eds.), *The teachability of language* (pp. 311–332). Baltimore: Paul H. Brookes Publishing Co.

Fischer, K.W., & Pipp, S.L. (1984). Processes of cognitive development: Optimal level and skill acquisition. In R.J. Sternberg (Ed.), *Mechanisms of cognitive development* (pp. 45–80). New York: W.H. Freeman.

Fogel, A. (1992). *Developing through relationships.* Chicago: University of Chicago Press.

Fox, N.A. (1994). Dynamic cerebral processes underlying emotion regulation. In N.A. Fox (Ed.), *The development of emotion regulation: Biological and behavioral considerations. Monographs of the Society for Research in Child Development, 59*(Serial No. 240), 152–186.

Furrow, D., Nelson, K., & Benedict, H. (1979). Mothers' speech to children and syntactic development: Some simple relationships. *Journal of Child Language, 6,* 423–442.

Gaines, R., Mandler, J.M., & Bryant, P.E. (1981). Immediate and delayed recall by hearing and deaf children. *Journal of Speech and Hearing Research, 24,* 463–469.

Galambos, S.J., & Goldin-Meadow, S. (1990). The effects of learning two languages on levels of metalinguistic awareness. *Cognition, 34,* 1–56.

Gathercole, S.E., & Baddeley, A. (1993). *Working memory and language.* Hillsdale, NJ: Lawrence Erlbaum Associates.

Gentile, A. (1972). *Further studies in achievement testing, hearing impaired students: 1971.* Washington, DC: Gallaudet College, Office of Demographic Studies.

Goldin-Meadow, S. (1985). Language development under atypical learning conditions: Replication and implications of a study of deaf children of hearing parents. In K.E. Nelson (Ed.), *Children's language* (Vol. 5, pp. 197–246). Hillsdale, NJ: Lawrence Erlbaum Associates.

Greenberg, M.T., Calderon, R., & Kusche, C. (1984). Early intervention using simultaneous communication with deaf infants: The effect on communicative development. *Child Development, 55,* 607–616.

Griffiths, C.P.S. (1969). A follow-up study of children with disorders of speech. *British Journal of Disorders of Communication, 4,* 46–54.

Hadley, P.A., & Rice, M.L. (1991). Conversational responsiveness of speech- and language-impaired preschoolers. *Journal of Speech and Hearing Research, 34,* 1308–1317.

Haley, K., Camarata, S., & Nelson, K.E. (1994). Positive and negative social valence in children with specific language impairment during imitation based and conversation based language intervention. *Journal of Speech and Hearing Research, 37,* 141–148.

Hall, W.S., & Cole, M. (1978). On participants' shaping of discourse through their understanding of the task. In K.E. Nelson (Ed.), *Children's language* (Vol. 1, pp. 445–466). Hillsdale, NJ: Lawrence Erlbaum Associates.

Hanson, V.L., & Fowler, C.A. (1987). Phonological coding in word reading: Evidence from hearing and deaf readers. *Memory and Cognition, 15,* 199–207.

Harris, M., & Beech, J. (1995). Reading development in prelingually deaf children. In K.E. Nelson & Z. Reger (Ed.), *Children's language* (Vol. 8, pp. 181–202). Hillsdale, NJ: Lawrence Erlbaum Associates.

Heimann, M., Nelson, K.E., Tjus, T., & Gillberg, C. (1995). Increasing reading and communication skills in children with autism through an interactive multimedia computer program. *Journal of Autism and Developmental Disorders, 25,* 459–480.

Hjelmquist, E., Sandberg, A.D., & Hedelin, L. (1994). Linguistics, AAC, and metalinguistics in communicatively handicapped adolescents. *Augmentative and Alternative Communication, 10,* 169–183.

Hoff-Ginsberg, E. (1986). Function and structure in maternal speech: Their relation to the child's development of syntax. *Developmental Psychology, 22,* 155–163.

Hudgins, C., & Numbers, F. (1942). An investigation of the intelligibility of the speech of the deaf. *Genetic Psychology Monographs, 25.*

Kail, R. (1986). Sources of age differences in speed of processing. *Child Development, 57,* 969–987.

Kail, R. (1991). Developmental change in speed of processing during childhood and adolescence. *Psychological Bulletin, 109,* 490–501.

Kaiser, A. (1993). Parent-implemented language intervention: An environmental system perspective. In A. Kaiser & D. Gray (Eds.). *Communication and language intervention series: Vol. 2. Enhancing children's communication: Research foundations for intervention* (pp. 63–84). Baltimore: Paul H. Brookes Publishing Co.

Kamhi, A.G., & Catts, H.W. (Eds.). (1989). *Reading disabilities: A developmental language perspective.* Boston: College-Hill Press.

Karmiloff-Smith, A. (1981). The grammatical marking of thematic structure in the development of language production. In W. Deustsch (Ed.), *The child's construction of language* (pp. 121–147). London: Academic Press.

Koegel, R.L., & Koegel, L.K. (Eds.). (1995). *Teaching children with autism: Strategies for initiating positive interactions and improving learning opportunities.* Baltimore: Paul H. Brookes Publishing Co.

Lahey, M., Liebergott, J., Chesnick, M., Menyuk, P., & Adams, J. (1992). Variability in children's use of grammatical morphemes. *Applied Psycholinguistics, 13,* 373–398.

Lederberg, A. (1993). The impact of deafness on mother–child and peer relationships. In M. Marschark & D. Clark (Eds.), *Psychological perspectives on deafness* (pp. 93–121). Hillsdale, NJ: Lawrence Erlbaum Associates.

Leonard, L.B. (1981). Facilitating linguistic skills in children with specific language impairment. *Applied Psycholinguistics, 2,* 89–118.

Leopold, W. (1947). *Speech development of a bilingual child: A linguist's record: Volume II. Sound learning in the first two years.* Evanston, IL: Northwestern University Press.

Lepper, M., Woolverton, M., Mumme, D.L., & Gurtner, J.L. (1993). Motivational techniques of expert human tutors: Lessons for the design of computer-based tutors. In S.P. Lajoie & S.J. Derry (Eds.), *Computers as cognitive tools* (pp. 75–105). Hillsdale, NJ: Lawrence Erlbaum Associates.

Leybaert, J. (1993). Reading in the deaf: The roles of phonological codes. In M. Marschark & D. Clark (Eds.), *Psychological perspectives on deafness* (pp. 269–310). Hillsdale, NJ: Lawrence Erlbaum Associates.

Lieven, E.V.M. (1978). Conversations between mothers and young children: Individual differences and their implications for the study of language learning. In N. Waterson & C. Snow (Eds.), *The development of communication* (pp. 173–187). New York: John Wiley & Sons.

Lieven, E., & Pine, J. (1996, August). *Developing the English verb category.* Paper presented to the International Association for the Study of Child Language, Istanbul, Turkey.

Locke, J. (1995). The co-development of brain and language. *Newsletter of the AILA Child Language Scientific Commission, 4*, 7–8.

Mandler, G. (1962). From association to structure. *Psychological Review, 69*, 415–427.

Maratsos, M.P., & Chalkley, M. (1980). The internal language of children's syntax: The ontogenesis and representation of syntactic categories. In K.E. Nelson (Ed.), *Children's language* (Vol. 2, pp. 127–214). Hillsdale, NJ: Lawrence Erlbaum Associates.

Maxwell, M. (1983). Language acquisition in a deaf child of deaf parents: Speech, sign variations, and print variations. In K.E. Nelson (Ed.), *Children's language* (Vol. 4, pp. 283–314). Hillsdale, NJ: Lawrence Erlbaum Associates.

Meadow, K., Greenberg, M.T., Erting, C., & Carmichael, H. (1981). Interaction of deaf mothers and deaf preschool children: Comparisons of three groups of deaf and hearing dyads. *American Annals of the Deaf, 126*, 454–468.

Moores, D.F. (1978). *Educating the deaf*. Boston: Houghton Mifflin.

Moores, D.F. (1985). Early intervention programs for hearing impaired children: A longitudinal assessment. In K.E. Nelson (Ed.), *Children's language* (Vol. 5, pp. 159–196). Hillsdale, NJ: Lawrence Erlbaum Associates.

Nelson, K.E. (1977). Facilitating children's syntax acquisition. *Developmental Psychology, 13*, 101–107.

Nelson, K.E. (1980). Theories of the child's acquisition of syntax: A look at rare events and at necessary, catalytic, and irrelevant components of mother–child conversation. *Annals of the New York Academy of Sciences, 345*, 45–67.

Nelson, K.E. (1981). Toward a rare-event cognitive comparison theory of syntax acquisition. In P.S. Dale & D. Ingram (Eds.), *Child language: An international perspective* (pp. 229–240). Baltimore: University Park Press.

Nelson, K.E. (1982). Experimental gambits in the service of language acquisition theory. In S.A. Kuczaj (Ed.), *Language development, syntax and semantics* (pp. 159–199). Hillsdale, NJ: Lawrence Erlbaum Associates.

Nelson, K.E. (1987). Some observations from the perspective of the rare event cognitive comparison theory of language acquisition. In K.E. Nelson (Ed.), *Children's language* (Vol. 6, pp. 289–331). Hillsdale, NJ: Lawrence Erlbaum Associates.

Nelson, K.E. (1989). Strategies for first language teaching. In M.L. Rice & R.L. Schiefelbusch (Eds.), *The teachability of language* (pp. 263–310). Baltimore: Paul H. Brookes Publishing Co.

Nelson, K.E. (1991a). On differentiated language learning models and differentiated interventions. In N.A. Krasnegor, D.M. Rumbaugh, & R.L. Schiefelbusch (Eds.), *Language acquisition: Biological and behavioral determinants* (pp. 399–428). Hillsdale, NJ: Lawrence Erlbaum Associates.

Nelson, K.E. (1991b). Varied domains of development: A tale of LAD, MAD, SAD, DAD, and RARE and surprising events in our RELMs. In F.S. Kessel, M.H. Bornstein, & A.J. Sameroff (Eds.), *Contemporary constructions of the child: Essays in honor of William Kessen* (pp. 123–142). Hillsdale, NJ: Lawrence Erlbaum Associates.

Nelson, K.E., & Bonvillian, J.D. (1973). Concepts and words in the two-year-old: Acquisition of concept names under controlled conditions. *Cognition, 2*, 435–450.

Nelson, K.E., & Bonvillian, J.D. (1978). Early language development: Conceptual growth and related processes between 2 and 4½ years of age. In K.E. Nelson (Ed.), *Children's language* (Vol. 1, pp. 467–556). New York: Gardner Press.

Nelson, K.F., & Camarata, S.M. (1996). Improving English literacy and speech-acquisition learning conditions for children with severe to profound hearing impairments. *Volta Review, 98*, 17–41.

Nelson, K.E., Camarata, S.M., Welsh, J., Butkovsky, L., & Camarata, M. (1996). Effects of imitative and conversational recasting treatment on the acquisition of grammar in children with specific language impairment and younger language-normal children. *Journal of Speech and Hearing Research, 39,* 850–859.

Nelson, K.E., Denninger, M.M., Bonvillian, J.D., Kaplan, B.J., & Baker, N.D. (1984). Maternal adjustments and non-adjustments as related to children's linguistic advances and to language acquisition theories. In A.D. Pellegrini & T.D. Yawkey (Eds.), *The development of oral and written language: Readings in developmental and applied linguistics* (pp. 31–56). Norwood, NJ: Ablex.

Nelson, K.E., Heimann, M., Abuelhaija, L., & Wroblewski, R. (1989). Implications for language acquisition models of children's and parents' variations in imitation. In G.E. Speidel & K.E. Nelson (Eds.), *The many faces of imitation in language learning* (pp. 305–324). New York: Springer-Verlag.

Nelson, K.E., Heimann, M., & Tjus, T. (1997). Theoretical and applied insights from multimedia facilitation of communication skills in children with autism, deaf children, and children with other disabilities. In L.B. Adamson & M.A. Romski (Eds.), *Communication and language acquisition: Discoveries from atypical development* (pp. 295–325). Baltimore: Paul H. Brookes Publishing Co.

Nelson, K.E., & Kosslyn, S.M. (1977). Semantic retrieval in children and adults. *Developmental Psychology, 11,* 811–813.

Nelson, K.E., Loncke, F., & Camarata, S. (1993). Implications of research on deaf and hearing children's language learning. In M. Marschark & D. Clark (Eds.), *Psychological perspectives on deafness* (pp. 123–151). Hillsdale, NJ: Lawrence Erlbaum Associates.

Nelson, K.E., & Nelson, K. (1978). Cognitive pendulums and their linguistic realization. In K.E. Nelson (Ed.), *Children's language* (Vol. 1, pp. 223–286). Hillsdale, NJ: Lawrence Erlbaum Associates.

Nelson, K.E., Perkins, D., & Lepper, M. (1997). *Rare event learning theory.* Manuscript in preparation.

Nelson, K.E., Prinz, P.M., Prinz, E.A., & Dalke, D. (1991). Processes for text and language acquisition in the context of microcomputer-videodisc instruction for deaf and multihandicapped deaf children. In D.S. Martin (Ed.), *Advances in cognition, education, and deafness* (pp. 162–169). Washington, DC: Gallaudet University Press.

Nelson, K.E., Welsh, J., Camarata, S.M., Butkovsky, L., & Camarata, M. (1995). Available input and available language learning mechanisms for specifically language-delayed and language-normal children. *First Language, 15,* 1–17.

Nelson, K.E., Welsh, J., Camarata, S., Heimann, M., & Tjus, T. (1996, August). *A rare event transactional model of language delay.* Paper presented to the International Association for the Study of Child Language, Istanbul, Turkey.

Newby, K. (1994). *The relationship between social valence and target acquisition in two types of language intervention.* Honors bachelor's thesis, Pennsylvania State University, University Park.

Ninio, A. (1996, August). *Pathbreaking verbs in syntactic development—English and Hebrew.* Paper presented to the International Association for the Study of Child Language, Istanbul, Turkey.

Orlansky, M.D., & Bonvillian, J.D. (1984). The role of iconicity in early sign language acquisition. *Journal of Speech and Hearing Disorders, 49,* 287–292.

Paul, R. (1992). Speech-language interaction in the talk of young children. In R. Chapman (Ed.), *Processes in language acquisition and disorders* (pp. 235–254). St. Louis: Mosby–Year Book.

Paul, R., & Quigley, S. (1994). *Language and deafness* (2nd ed.). Austin, TX: PRO-ED.

Pinker, S. (1985). Language learnability and children's language: A multifaceted approach. In K.E. Nelson (Ed.), *Children's language* (Vol. 5, pp. 339–442). Hillsdale, NJ: Lawrence Erlbaum Associates.

Pizzuto, E., & Caselli, M.C. (1994). The acquisition of verb morphology in a cross-linguistic perspective. In Y. Levey (Ed.), *Other children, other languages: Issues in the theory of language acquisition* (pp. 137–188). Hillsdale, NJ: Lawrence Erlbaum Associates.

Plunkett, K., Karmiloff-Smith, A., Bates, E., Elman, J.L., & Johnson, M.H. (in press). Connectionism and developmental psychology. *Journal of Child Psychology and Psychiatry.*

Prinz, P.M., & Masin, L. (1985). Lending a helping hand: Linguistic input and sign language acquisition. *Applied Psycholinguistics, 6,* 357–370.

Prinz, P.M., & Prinz, E.A. (1981). Acquisition of ASL and spoken English by a hearing child of a deaf mother and a hearing father: Phase II. Early combinatorial patterns. *Sign Language Studies, 30,* 78–88.

Prinz, P.M., & Strong, M. (1997, April). *The synchronic and diachronic relationships between ASL and English literacy.* Paper presented to the Society for Research in Child Development, Baltimore.

Ratner, N.B. (1996). From "signal to syntax": But what is the nature of the signal? In J. Morgan & K. Demuth (Eds.), *From signal to syntax* (pp. 135–150). Mahwah, NJ: Lawrence Erlbaum Associates.

Records, N., Tomblin, J., & Freese, P. (1992). The quality of life of young adults with histories of specific language impairment. *American Journal of Speech-Language Pathology, 1,* 44–53.

Reilly, J.S., Bates, E., & Marchman, V. (1995). *Narrative discourse in children with early focal brain injury* (Tech. Rep. CND-9504). San Diego: University of California.

Rice, M.L., Buhr, J., & Nemeth, M. (1990). Fast mapping word learning abilities of language delayed preschoolers. *Journal of Speech and Hearing Disorders, 55,* 33–42.

Rice, M.L., & Hadley, P. (1995). Language outcomes of the language-focused curriculum. In M.L. Rice & K. Wilcox (Eds.), *Building a language-focused curriculum for the preschool classroom: Vol. I. A foundation for lifelong communication* (pp. 155–170). Baltimore: Paul H. Brookes Publishing Co.

Rice, M.L., & Wilcox, K. (Eds.). (1995). *Building a language-focused curriculum for the preschool classroom: Vol. I. A foundation for lifelong communication.* Baltimore: Paul H. Brookes Publishing Co.

Sameroff, A.J., & Chandler, M. (1975). Reproductive risk and the continuum of caretaker casualty. In F. Horowitz & M. Hetherington (Eds.), *Review of child development research* (Vol. 4. pp. 187–243). Chicago: University of Chicago Press.

Scherer, N.J., & Olswang, L.B. (1984). Role of mother's expansions in stimulating children's language production. *Journal of Speech and Hearing Disorders, 27,* 387–396.

Schlesinger, H.S., & Meadow, K. (1976). *Studies of family interaction, language acquisition, and deafness.* San Francisco: University of California.

Siegler, R.S. (1991). *Children's thinking.* Englewood Cliffs, NJ: Prentice-Hall.

Slobin, D.I. (1985). Crosslinguistic evidence for the language-making capacity. In D.I. Slobin (Ed.), *The crosslinguistic study of language acquisition* (pp. 1157–1256). Hillsdale, NJ: Lawrence Erlbaum Associates.

Smith, L.B., & Thelen, E. (1993). *A dynamic systems approach to development: Applications.* Cambridge, MA: MIT Press.

Snow, C.E., Perlmann, R., & Nathan, D. (1987). Why routines are different: Toward a multiple-factors model of the relation between input and language acquisition. In

K.E. Nelson (Ed.), *Children's language* (Vol. 6, pp. 65–98). Hillsdale, NJ: Lawrence Erlbaum Associates.

Soderbergh, R. (1977). *Reading in early childhood: A linguistic study of a preschool child's gradual acquisition of reading ability.* Washington, DC: Georgetown University Press.

Tager-Flusberg, H. (Ed.). (1994). *Constraints on language acquisition.* Hillsdale, NJ: Lawrence Erlbaum Associates.

Tallal, P., Stark, R.E., & Curtiss, S. (1976). The relation between speech perception impairment and speech production impairment in children with developmental dysphasia. *Brain and Language, 3,* 305–317.

Tallal, P., Stark, R.E., & Mellits, P. (1985a). Identification of language impaired children on the basis of rapid perception and production skills. *Brain and Language, 25,* 314–322.

Tallal, P., Stark, R.E., & Mellits, E.P. (1985b). The relationship between auditory temporal analysis and receptive language development: Evidence from studies of developmental language disorder. *Neuropsychologia, 23,* 527–534.

Thelen, E. (1988). Dynamic approaches to the development of behavior. In J.A. Kelso, A.J. Mandell, & M.F. Schlesinger (Eds.), *Dynamic patterns in complex systems* (pp. 348–369). Singapore: World Scientific.

Thelen, E., & Smith, L.B. (1994). *A dynamic systems approach to the development of cognition and action.* Cambridge, MA: MIT Press.

van der Lem, G.J., & Timmerman, D.E. (1995). Joint picture book reading in signs: An interaction process between parent and deaf child. In K.E. Nelson & Z. Reger (Eds.), *Children's language* (Vol. 8, pp. 171–180). Hillsdale, NJ: Lawrence Erlbaum Associates.

Wolf, M. (1982). The word-retrieval process and reading in children and aphasics. In K.E. Nelson (Ed.), *Children's language* (Vol. 3, pp. 437–493). Hillsdale, NJ: Lawrence Erlbaum Associates.

Wolf, M., Bally, H., & Morris, R. (1986). Automaticity, retrieval processes, and reading: A longitudinal study in average and impaired readers. *Child Development, 57,* 988–1000.

Wolf, M., & Obregon, M. (1992). Early naming deficits, developmental dyslexia, and a specific deficit hypothesis. *Brain and Language, 42,* 219–247.

Wolf, M., & Segal, D. (1997). *An intervention program for reading disabled children.* Manuscript in preparation.

Appendix: Coding Manual for Utterance Pairs in Conversation

1. Exact Imitations

This category includes exact, immediate imitations, both complete and partial. Imitations contain no structural changes or new words but may contain minor pronunciation adjustments or corrections (e.g., U [Utterance]: "She has the dowy" R [Reply]: "She has the dolly"). Exact imitations may also contain simple acknowledgments (e.g., U: "She jumps" R: "Yes, she jumps") and simple denials that do not change the direction of the conversation (e.g., U: "He won't" R: "No, he won't"). Exact imitations NEVER include required changes.

1a. Complete Imitations

A complete imitation includes all of the words of the imitated utterance in exactly the same order.

Examples:

U3: In the hole.
R3: In the hole?

U4: An apple.
R4: Yes, an apple.

1b. Reduced Imitations

A reduced imitation retains the order of the words but may not include them all. Reduced imitations may include only a portion of the prior utterance.

Examples:

U7: That's mean it's too much.
R7: Too much.

U8: And it's itchy.
R8: Itchy?

A broad definition of a *recast:*

A reply to an utterance is classified as a recast when the prior utterance is redisplayed in a changed sentence structure that still refers to the central events and relationships of the previous utterance. These structural differences usually refer to syntactic changes; however, semantic changes or corrections can also occur in a recast. Recasts are to be distinguished from an exact imitation of the prior utterance as previously defined. Expansions incorporate more morphemes and reductions fewer morphemes than the model. All recasts continue reference to some of the central events and central meanings of the prior model utterance.

2. Simple Recasts

These replies definitely continue reference to the central meanings in the preceding utterances but change the structure slightly. In a simple recast, by definition, such a change is limited to reordering of otherwise unchanged elements or to change in only ONE component of the previous utterance—a subject, a verb, an object, or a separate modifying phrase, such as a prepositional phrase, relative clause, or adverbial phrase.

2a. Simple Recasts–Expansions

Expansions are a subcategory of simple recasts. In our data, expansions involve change in just one major sentence component, and they expand on an incomplete sentence without reordering any elements of the utterance. For example, an expansion of the utterance "Broke" may be "The truck broke." A simple recast may also be given to a complete sentence (e.g., U: "The boy built that house" R: "Yeah, the boy did build that house"). A lengthening of the prior utterance should be evident. The addition of minimal acknowledgment, such as "yeah," "mm-hmm," or "well," or of minimal denials (e.g., "no") with no other changes does not count as a change in the sentence structure but does count in altering the number of morphemes.

Examples:

U11: Mom, turn off.
R11: Turn it off.

U12: Mommy awake?
R12: Mommy is awake.

2b. Simple Recasts–Reductions

Simple recast reductions comprise another subcategory of simple recasts. They contain many, but not all, of the words of the recasted utterance such that the reduction produces one structural change or correction. Often the replies fit the description of a reduced imitation; however, they differ in that they contain a single "required change." This is a change that is necessary because of the change in speaker (e.g., U: "I need it for *my* skin" R: "For *your* skin?") or a syntactic correction. In reduction recasts, a reduction in utterance length is evident.

Examples:

U19: She rolled it ball.
R19: She rolled that.

U20: She no like that.
R20: She doesn't?

NOTE: If the required change has not been made (e.g., U: "I need it for my skin" R: "For my skin"), the reply would be a reduced imitation.

2c. Simple Recasts–Other

A third major subcategory of simple recasts is referred to as other, indicating that these recasts neither expand nor reduce the recasted utterance but do include one structural change. Often such changes are "required changes." In such simple recasts, the absolute length of the recast is usually equal to that of the recasted utterance. Some of these simple recast–others will involve semantic changes in one or two words (e.g., U: "That's an orange" R: "That's an apple"). Another common example involves the reordering of exactly the same elements.

Examples:

U26: I want a pin.
R26: You want a pen?

U27: This is Art's.
R27: That is Art's.

3. Complex Recasts

If a recast keeps some explicit overlap in meaning but structurally changes two or more of the main components (e.g., subject, verb, object, article, prepositional or other modifying phrase) of the previous utterance, then it is coded as a complex recast. The changes involved could be supplying new subjects, verbs, or objects or could be revisions of what had been expressed in the prior utterance. When the prior utterance contains multiple clauses, any major component change in any clause counts as one change. Reordering of some elements also counts as one change.

3a. Complex Recasts–Expansions

These are defined as recast expansions with an increment in the recast complexity such that more than one structural change occurs. The utterance also increases in length.

Examples:

U30: Tim movie.
R30: Tim is watching the movie.

U31: Dis righ dere.
R31: This one goes right there?

3b. Complex Recasts–Reductions

These are recasts involving two or more structural changes that also result in a reduction of the recasted utterance (e.g., U: "Let's lock this one" R: "Lock it"; U: "I ate the cookie" R: "Yep, you did").

Examples:

U45: Sammy wore the green mittens.
R45: Yes, he wore them.

U46: Buy me a wittle car to put here.
R46: Buy you a little car?

3c. Complex Recasts–Other

This category includes recasts with two or more changes but without an increase or decrease in the number of morphemes. In addition, utterances are coded here that include both reductions and expansions.

Examples:

U51: Make britch.
R51: A bridge?

U52: I eat the pie.
R52: You ate the pie.

4. Assorted Continuations

These responses are comprised by all topic-continuing replies that do not meet the definitions for either recasts or imitations (which also continue topics). Continuations, as compared with recasts and imitations, maintain the topic without much explicit overlap in the words of the utterances. Structurally, they can have any degree of similarity or dissimilarity to the preceding utterance. Unlike recasts, assorted continuations do not combine clear reference to the same events of the prior utterance together with structural change in the continuation reply.

4a. Continuations–Default/Semantic Links

A number of utterance types are coded as continuations by default. These include short, interrupted or ambiguous utterances where no topic change is clearly indicated (e.g., U: "I want that block" R: "Look at this one").

In addition, scored here are those utterances that maintain a semantic link to the previous utterance but lack sufficient syntactic overlap to count as a recast or imitation. Semantic links are frequently maintained by pronouns (e.g., U:

"Here's a baby" R: "Let's put *her* over here") and by required changes (e.g., U: "Look at *this*" R: "*That's* an airplane"). Credit for semantic links should not be given when the link requires use of a superordinate category (e.g., U: "Here's a tyrannosaurus" R: "What other dinosaurs do you know?"). Utterances of this type are instead scored as topic changes.

Examples:

U63: This goes in there.   (Topic continued by this/that
R63: That's a tough one.   relationship)

U64: This car all wet.
R64: Well, dry it off.   ("It" continues topic of car)

4b.   Continuations–Minimal acknowledgments, denials, and placeholders

Minimal acknowledgments and denials are brief responses to the previous utterance but are neither imitations nor recasts of it (e.g., U: "This is a nice dog" R: "Yeah"; U: "I had an earache" R: "No"). They also include placeholders such as "very good," "that's nice," and "OK." If a minimal acknowledgment is also a reply to a question (e.g., U: "Does it go here?" R: "Yes"), it is *not* placed in this category but is scored below in the "Answers to questions" category.

Examples:

U72: He a mean cat.
R72: No.

U73: Me do it now.
R73: All right.

4c.   Continuations–Answers to questions

Coded here are answers to questions that do not contain enough explicit overlap to count as recasts but are more elaborate than minimal acknowledgments (e.g., U: "Does he have brown eyes?" R: "I think so"). Also included here are one-word minimal responses to questions.

Examples:

U77: When?
R77: I think she comes back tomorrow.

U78: Do you want this?
R78: No.

4d.   Continuations–Clarification requests

Clarification requests are utterances that arise from failure to hear correctly or from misunderstandings. The function of the utterance is to maintain the topic even though the partners do not completely understand each other (e.g., U:

"He's not the biggest one" R: "Excuse me?"; U: "Here's a green" R: "What?"). When a clarification request is combined with recast components in the same utterance, the utterance is categorized as a recast.

Examples:

U81:   He's not the biggest one.
R81:   What?

U82:   I wanna watch Batman.
R82:   Excuse me?

4e.   Continuations–Social greetings

Included here are utterances such as "Hi," and "Bye, Mom," which are either preceded by or followed by further discourse. This frequently occurs in the context of pretend play when partners assume the identity of toys or characters or carry on pretend telephone conversations.

Examples:

U85:   Hi, Mom.
R85:   Ili, Ryan.

U86:   Say bye-bye.
R86:   Bye, Grandma.

5.   Topic Changes

5a.   TC–1

Semantically, these replies provide a clear, abrupt change from the topic of the prior utterance and can be expressed in any syntactic form.

Examples:

U86:   See the kitten?
R86:   We're looking at the dog now.

U87:   Put the baby in the carriage.
R87:   Don't grind your teeth.

5b.   TC–2

Included here are utterances that depart less dramatically from the previous topic. The new topic is not an abrupt change but has some logical link to the previous utterance. The most common involves references to superordinate categories without mention of the exemplar in the original utterance (e.g., U: "There's the fork" R: "And there's the spoon"; U: "D is for dog" R: "And E is for elephant"). In these examples, dyads are talking about logically related items but have not explicitly linked them by focusing on the superordinate category (e.g., silverware, letters).

By contrast, when the superordinate category itself is the topic of conversation, lists of exemplars are not scored as topic changes but as default continuations; for example:

U: What animals did we see when we went to the zoo?
R: Bears.
U: And what else?
R: Tigers.
U: And we saw elephants.

Examples:

U88: I found a picture of triceratops.
R88: And here's a flying pteranodon.

(Semantic link here would require U88's use of superordinate categories, so R88 is not a continuation but a topic change.)

U91: I find a Q.
R91: Here's some other letters.

(Use of superordinate "letters" here establishes a new topic; if next utterance names a letter, it would be a continuation.)

As long as the follow-up utterance indicates clear departure from the previous topic, the presence of an acknowledgment (e.g., "Yeah," "Okay") does not affect the scoring.

Both types of topic changes can also be initiated by attention-getting statements such as "Hey" and "Lookit." If the subsequent utterances reveal that the topic does change, then the topic change is scored as initiating with these statements.

9

Linguistic Effects on Disfluency

John A. Tetnowski

LIKE MANY OTHER ASPECTS OF speech discussed in this text, fluency is an area that can be affected by higher levels of language formulation. Breakdowns in fluency can be studied to learn about the ways in which speech and language connections function. Some of these connections are obtained only for people who stutter (PWS), but many hold true for people who do not stutter and merely go through periods of nonfluency. The connections between the breakdowns in fluency and their relationship to speech and language variables are explored in this chapter, with an emphasis on factors related to fluency disruption.

This chapter specifically addresses how language variables influence speech production, both in children who stutter (CWS) and in those who do not. The chapter begins with a discussion of the distinction between stuttering and normal disfluency. Next, disfluency rates and types in children are described, and differences between stuttering and normal disfluency are defined. Linguistic and other variables that promote higher levels of disfluency are also discussed. Several models are presented that attempt to explain disfluencies in children and to show how various linguistic variables operate in these frameworks.

NONFLUENCY AND STUTTERING

Probably the most widely accepted definition of *stuttering* comes from Wingate, who described the primary symptoms of stuttering as the

> (a) Disruption in the fluency of verbal expression, which is (b) characterized by involuntary, audible or silent, repetitions or prolongations in the utterance of short speech elements, namely: sounds, syllables, and words of one syllable. These disruptions (c) usually occur frequently or are marked in character and (d) are not readily controllable. (1964, p. 488)

Not all disruptions in the fluency of speech are considered stuttering. Rather, only repetitions of short speech segments are so regarded (Wingate,

---

The term *normal disfluency* is used throughout the literature to distinguish between stuttering and nonstuttering disfluencies.

1964). Word, syllable, and sound repetitions; prolongations (i.e., dysrhythmic phonations); and stoppages (i.e., tense pauses) are the most typical types of disfluencies that are considered components of stuttering (Ham, 1989). Other disfluency types such as multisyllable word repetitions, phrase repetitions, interjections, and revision of incomplete phrases are not typically considered instances of stuttering.

These nonfluencies that are not stuttering are referred to as *disfluencies* or *normal disfluencies*. Ham defined *disfluency* as "the nonfluent speech of people who do not stutter; the nonstuttered, nonfluent speech of people who do stutter" (1990, p. 3). This definition indicates that individuals who stutter, as well as those who do not stutter, can be disfluent. Ham defined *dysfluency* as "the stuttered speech of stutterers; the stuttered speech of people who do not stutter usually" (1990, p. 3). By this definition, PWS can be dysfluent, but individuals who would not be considered PWS can also be dysfluent and use stuttering-like dysfluencies. The term *dysfluency* is used to refer to what the general population thinks of as stuttering.

Diagnostic difficulties arise in that both PWS and people not typically thought of as PWS exhibit all or most of the disfluency categories described. This is especially true in the case of children. Yairi (1981) showed that children between 2 and 3 years of age exhibit all of Johnson and Associates' (1959) disfluency categories. Differentiating CWS from children who are normally disfluent thus becomes very difficult. Even the task of identifying disfluencies themselves is challenging.

A considerable number of studies have used perceptual methods to examine the reliability of disfluency and stuttering identification tasks (Bar, 1969; Coyle & Mallard, 1979; Curlee, 1981; Ham, 1989; Ingham & Cordes, 1992; Kully & Boberg, 1988; MacDonald & Martin, 1973; Tuthill, 1946; Williams & Kent, 1958; Young, 1975). These studies show poor agreement among listeners as to where stuttering occurs. Poor agreement is also seen in the differentiation of stuttering and disfluency. Most of these studies indicate that the probability of highly reliable judgments of stuttering is no better than chance. Work by Ingham and colleagues (Cordes & Ingham, 1994a, 1994b; Ingham, Cordes, & Finn, 1993; Ingham, Cordes, & Gow, 1993) showed higher reliability using time analysis methods rather than through indicating exactly which word or syllable was stuttered. The technology necessary to complete this time analysis measure, though, has yet to reach the everyday consumer. Thus, it appears that perceptual judgments on the distinction between stuttering and disfluency are the only practical methods available.

DISFLUENCY RATES AND TYPES IN CHILDREN

The ages between 2 and 8 years are an important time for the development of language. Within this age span, children typically go through periods of disfluency. In general, disfluency rates decline substantially between preschool and high school ages (Yairi & Clifton, 1972). Disfluency rates averaged 7.65 per 100 words spoken for preschool children and declined to 3.83 per 100 words spoken for high school seniors.

Closer investigation of disfluency rates among young children show some interesting trends, however. Yairi (1982) investigated disfluency rates in two groups of 2-year-old nonstutterers: a younger group (24–26 months old at the beginning of testing) and an older group (29–33 months old at the beginning of testing). Speech samples were obtained on three or four occasions throughout an 8-month period for each child. Two distinct patterns emerged. The number of disfluencies increased for the younger children but decreased for the older children. This trend indicates that disfluencies typically increase through an age of about 30–32 months and then begin to decrease. Disfluency rates were also calculated for the entire 2-year-old group (Yairi, 1981) and revealed a mean disfluency rate of 6.49 disfluencies per 100 words uttered.

DeJoy and Gregory (1985) studied disfluency rates for slightly older children. They found a decrease in disfluencies as children progressed from 3½ to 5 years of age. A similar study was completed for children at 3-, 5-, and 7-year-old levels (Gordon & Luper, 1989). Disfluencies were found to decrease for the older children. This trend was similar for both imitative and elicitation tasks, despite the imitative task showing far fewer disfluencies than the nonimitative task. Haynes and Hood (1977) examined the disfluency rates of 4-, 6-, and 8-year-old children but did not find significant differences in disfluency rates among the three groups. Results of these and other studies of rate of disfluency are summarized in Table 1.

The studies in Table 1 show a trend of gradual decline in disfluencies with age. The individuals studied by Haynes and Hood (1977) showed this overall trend, but the differences did not reach significance. The younger individuals studied by Yairi (1982) showed a gradual increase in disfluency, followed by a decline after 29 months of age. Thus, for young children, it appears that the number of disfluencies increases between 24 and 30 months of age and then declines steadily through the age of about 4 years. The declining trend appears to slow for children between 4 and 8 years old but continues until at least high school age.

Another line of research has shown that, within this continual decline of disfluencies with age for children who do not stutter, the type of disfluency changes as well. Haynes and Hood (1977) found significantly more interjections in the speech of 8-year-old children who did not stutter than in the speech of 4- and 6-year-olds who did not stutter. In addition, there was a nonsignificant trend for whole-word repetitions to decrease with age. Other developmental trends indicate that as children progress through a stage of increased disfluency, the number of revisions and phrase repetitions also increases (Yairi, 1982). As the total number of disfluencies decreases, the number of part-word repetitions and interjections also decreases (Yairi, 1982). DeJoy and

Table 1. Summary of disfluency rates among children who do not stutter

Age	Disfluency rate (per 100 words)	Reference
2 years	6.49	Yairi (1981)
2 and 3 years	6.18	Yairi and Lewis (1984)
25 months[a]	3.67	Yairi (1982)
29 months[a]	5.11	Yairi (1982)
33 months[a]	3.81	Yairi (1982)
37 months[a]	6.90	Yairi (1982)
32 months[b]	8.43	Yairi (1982)
36 months[b]	5.10	Yairi (1982)
40 months[b]	4.26	Yairi (1982)
3.5 years	11.40	DeJoy and Gregory (1985)
5 years	9.30	DeJoy and Gregory (1985)
Preschool	7.65	Yairi and Clifton (1972)
High school	3.83	Yairi and Clifton (1972)
2 years	14.60	Wexler and Mysak (1982)
4 years	9.10	Wexler and Mysak (1982)
6 years	9.10	Wexler and Mysak (1982)
4 years	7.04	Haynes and Hood (1977)
6 years	7.20	Haynes and Hood (1977)
8 years	6.80	Haynes and Hood (1977)

[a]"Younger" 2-year-old group
[b]"Older" 2-year-old group

Gregory (1985) also indicated that repetitions, incomplete phrases, and dys-rhythmic phonations decrease with age; but the use of interjections and pauses (without tension) remains stable across age levels. In most of these studies, disfluency types typically related to stuttering (particularly dysrhythmic phonations and part-word repetitions) decrease as children develop. Disfluencies not typically related to stuttering remain present in children who do not stutter. The decrease in disfluency rates can partially be attributed to the remission of stuttering-like disfluencies after the age of 3.

FACTORS RELATED TO DISFLUENCY IN NONSTUTTERING CHILDREN

Disfluency patterns in children have been linked to several factors. Many of these factors came from studies of CWS, which were followed up by studies of children who did not stutter but were still disfluent. Early studies by Brown (1945) indicated that stuttering in adults tended to occur during the first few words of a sentence, on longer rather than shorter words, on the initial phoneme of a word, and on the production of content words. Later, these findings were tested on CWS, rather than the adult groups used by Brown (1945), as well as on those not judged to be CWS. The results indicated that for children who did not stutter, who ranged in age from 5 years to 12 years, disfluencies tended to occur on longer words and words that were in the grammatical categories described by Brown (i.e., nouns, verbs, adjectives, adverbs) (Williams, Silverman, & Kools, 1969). These findings are in agreement with data obtained from adults who do not stutter (Silverman & Williams, 1967). Silverman (1975) also studied word variables related to initial phoneme (consonant or vowel) and length of word, according to number of syllables, in 4-year-old children. The results indicated that neither of these factors were related to amount of disfluency used by preschool children who did not stutter. From this group of studies, word factors relating to disfluency in children who do not stutter are centered around word function and word length. These factors were found to be significant in children between the ages of 5 and 12 years but did not hold true for children younger than age 5 years.

It has been hypothesized that length and complexity of utterance could have an impact on the amount of disfluency observed in children who do not stutter. Although it was originally thought that length of utterance had an effect on disfluency rates of these children, closer observation revealed that length and complexity interact to produce more disfluencies in 5-year-old children who do not stutter (McLaughlin & Cullinan, 1989; Ratner & Sih, 1987). Longer sentences and more complex utterances, as judged by levels assigned with the Developmental Sentence Score (Lee, 1974), produced higher levels of disfluency. Longer and more complex sentences produced higher levels of disfluency in 5-year-old children (McLaughlin & Cullinan, 1989), as well as in children between the ages of 3 years, 11 months, and 6 years, 4 months (Ratner & Sih, 1987). The factors of length and complexity were also found to influence disfluency levels in CWS (Logan & Conture, 1995).

These results were obtained in structured imitation tasks (McLaughlin & Cullinan, 1989). They did not hold true in spontaneous speech samples. There was not a relationship between length and/or complexity and disfluency levels in 5-year-old children who do not stutter during spontaneous speech tasks. It is hypothesized that the pressure to use longer and more complex utterances that are generated in a modeled imitation task would result in an increase in disfluency behavior. Furthermore, the children with tendencies to be disfluent may restrict their speech to utterances within their linguistic ability level to avoid problems.

For children who do not stutter, the results are fairly consistent. Disfluencies increase as linguistic complexity increases (Colburn & Mysak, 1982; Gordon & Luper, 1989; Gordon, Luper, & Peterson, 1986; Haynes & Hood, 1977; McLaughlin & Cullinan, 1989; Pearl & Bernthal, 1980; Ratner & Sih, 1987). Complexity of utterances in all of these studies was assigned by using a syntactic system. For example, simple declaratives were considered less complex than future tense or passive utterances. Complexity was also construed as a result of demand, that is, whether an utterance was imitated or generated from a modeling task. In these studies, it was shown that the presumedly less demanding imitation task elicited fewer disfluencies than a more demanding modeled or spontaneous production task (Gordon & Luper, 1989; Gordon et al., 1986). The findings are consistent that increased demand (i.e., task complexity as well as linguistic capacity) increases the probability and rate of disfluency in children who do not stutter.

Colburn and Mysak (1982) also examined the complexity issue over time but did not use age as previous studies had. Instead, language level was used. They observed the disfluency patterns of four children as they progressed from Brown's (1973) Stage I through Stage IV of syntactic complexity. They found that the children studied had a significant number of disfluent utterances at each level of linguistic complexity, without any clear pattern of disfluencies emerging. Analysis of each disfluency type showed no apparent trends other than the category "revisions of incomplete phrases" increasing for all subjects as they progressed developmentally. It appears that linguistically advanced children have increased awareness of their own speech and an increased ability to repair potentially disfluent utterances.

In summary, the following trends appear for disfluent behaviors in children who do not stutter:

- All types of disfluency are seen in young children, including those disfluency types that are associated with stuttering.
- Disfluency rates increase with higher levels of linguistic complexity.
- Type of disfluency changes with age. As children develop, they tend to use fewer stuttering-like disfluencies but use more interjections and revisions of incomplete phrases.
- Disfluency increases as task complexity increases.
- Disfluency rates increase with word length and word functionality. This trend does not hold true for children under the age of 5.

Based on the available data, it can be hypothesized that the effects of word length and function, language complexity, and task difficulty stress the operating language system. It is also possible that task difficulty can operate independently of linguistic complexity. Increased demand on any of these variables can cause disfluency. There are linguistic variables that affect motor speech patterns. In other words, stressing the linguistic capabilities of a child can cause speech to break down in the form of disfluencies. Length of utterance does not appear to be sufficient to cause fluency interruptions; however, length, in conjunction with other factors, can contribute to disfluency. This relationship is still unclear for typically disfluent children. Experimental designs that can manipulate complexity while sentence length is left constant address this issue. It also appears that certain types of disfluencies decrease with age; specifically, the types most closely related to stuttering rather than to typical disfluency decrease. In other words, even though stuttering-like disfluencies appear in the speech of very young children, their frequency decreases by the time a child is 3 or 4 years old. The remaining normal disfluencies continue to be present in the speech of children through high school. Finally, at least one type of disfluency increases during certain developmental periods. The increase in revisions of incomplete phrases observed by Colburn and Mysak (1982) may actually be a sign of increased linguistic awareness. The revisions of incomplete phrases could be the child's means of repairing incorrect utterances as his or her language system is maturing. The next section examines whether these trends also hold true for children who stutter.

DISFLUENCY IN CHILDREN WHO STUTTER

Several studies have explored developmental changes in disfluency among CWS. Although disfluencies decrease with age in children who do not stutter, the same trends do not appear for CWS (Yairi & Lewis, 1984). The most common disfluency types found in children who stutter are part-word repetitions, dysrhythmic phonations, and single-syllable–word repetitions. The most common types of disfluency for children who do not stutter are interjections, part-word repetitions, and revision of incomplete phrases. These typically occurring disfluencies decrease in frequency with age among children who do not stutter. The absence of a significant overall reduction in disfluency rates in CWS can be attributed to stuttering-like disfluencies not declining in frequency as they do for children who do not stutter. These patterns are apparent between the ages of 2 and 3 years.

Another group of studies explored whether the same linguistic factors that have an impact on disfluencies in children who do not stutter operate similarly in children who do stutter. The main areas explored were length and complexity of utterance. Ratner and Sih (1987) found that length of utterance is not related to number of disfluencies produced by CWS. However, a later group of studies did show that length of utterance has an effect on frequency of disfluencies among CWS (Gaines, Runyan, & Meyers, 1991; Logan & Conture, 1995; Weiss & Zebrowski, 1992). In addition, it has been shown that linguistic complexity of utterance is related to frequency of disfluency for CWS (Gaines et al., 1991; Kadi-Hanifi & Howell, 1992; Logan & Conture, 1995; Weiss & Zebrowski, 1992). The interaction effects of both length and complexity were studied explicitly by Logan and Conture (1995). They concluded that both length and complexity of utterance interact with each other to influence frequency of disfluency in CWS. Longer and more complex utterances elicit higher levels of disfluent behavior among children who stutter. In other words, as linguistic demands increase, disfluencies also increase.

In summary, at very early ages, the speech of CWS is difficult to distinguish from the speech of children who do not stutter. Frequency of disfluency does not appear to separate the two groups exclusively at early ages but is a more important factor after the age of about 3½. The types of disfluencies that remain after the age of 3 years are also important cues in differentiating normally disfluent children from CWS. CWS tend to produce more dysrhythmic phonations and single-syllable–word repetitions than normally disfluent children. Although part-word repetitions occur quite frequently in 2- and 3-year-old CWS, these disfluencies also occur in children of the same ages who do not stutter. Part-word repetitions cannot be used as the sole factor in differentiating the two groups until after the age of 3½. It appears that many of the linguistic factors that affect the speech of nonstutterers also affect the speech patterns of CWS. Length of utterance is one additional factor that increases disfluent behavior in CWS, although length does not affect fluency patterns in children who do not stutter.

DIFFERENTIATING NORMALLY DISFLUENT CHILDREN FROM CHILDREN WHO STUTTER

Although it is clearly important to differentiate CWS from normally disfluent children, the task of doing so is quite difficult. A large study conducted by Andrews and Harris (1964) indicated that more than 70% of individuals who stuttered as children spontaneously recovered before the age of 16. Based on this study, the common advice given to parents of young CWS was to leave them alone because there was a significant chance that the child would outgrow stuttering behaviors. Ramig (1993) criticized the methodology used in Andrews and Harris's study, however. He stated that the survey procedures used were flawed in that they involved only parent report and not direct assessment. Ramig argued that many of the children used in the Andrews and Harris study were actually going through periods of normal disfluency and were misdiagnosed as CWS. In his own study, Ramig (1993) found that more than 90% of the children who were originally diagnosed as CWS between the ages of 3 and 8 by a speech-language pathologist still stuttered when evaluated 5–8 years later. These children had not received therapy, for which the following reasons were given: Parents could not afford treatment, and another speech-language pathologist or physician had informed them that the child would outgrow the disorder. This finding is quite troublesome because the author's personal experiences suggest that the latter advice is commonly given, despite data that demonstrate the clinical ability to differentiate stuttering from normal disfluency by the time a child is about 3½ years of age.

Adams (1977) compiled a list (see Table 2) that can be used as a quick screening guide to determine whether disfluent children require further evaluation. If children exhibit several of the behaviors on Adams's list, they are generally regarded as being at risk for stuttering because confirmed stutterers also show the behaviors listed. The appearance of fewer than two of the behaviors listed by Adams (1977) is thought to be more indicative of normal disfluency.

Table 2. Differentiating the normally nonfluent child from the incipient stutterer

Children who stutter tend to exhibit the following behaviors:
1. Disfluency rates of at least 10%
2. Part-word repetitions and prolongations (both silent and audible are the predominant types of disfluencies)
3. Three or more repetitions per unit during part-word repetitions
4. Difficulty in initiating, or abrupt cessation of voice or airflow
5. During part-word repetitions, the schwa vowel is often substituted for the target vowel

Adapted from Adams (1977).

Other tools that seek to differentiate stuttering from disfluencies were reviewed by Gordon and Luper (1992).

The guidelines and tools proposed by Adams (1977) are very useful in a clinical sense, but much progress in the differential diagnosis of stuttering from normal nonfluency has been accomplished since 1977. A considerable amount of this progress comes from an ongoing series of research projects conducted by Yairi and associates. This research has explored the speaking behaviors of children near the point at which they first began to stutter. The children in these studies were all under the age of 6. They were followed longitudinally to determine which speaking patterns were typical of children who showed typical disfluencies but were not diagnosed as CWS and to distinguish these from the speaking patterns of children who were diagnosed as CWS (Yairi & Ambrose, 1992b). The results indicated that CWS under the age of 6 showed the following disfluent behaviors (in rank order): part-word repetitions, dysrhythmic phonations (usually within-word prolongations), and single-syllable–word repetitions. The control group of children who did not stutter showed the following disfluent patterns (in rank order): interjections, part-word repetitions, and revisions or incomplete phrases. The mean number of disfluencies per 100 words was 21.54 for the CWS group and 6.16 for the group of children who did not stutter. These results indicate that CWS show a significantly higher number of disfluencies of all types than do nonstutterers by the time they are 3½ years old. It was also noted that all stuttering behaviors observed in CWS were also observed in children who do not stutter. Further works by Yairi and others have indicated that CWS show significantly more repetitions per unit than children who do not stutter (Ambrose & Yairi, 1995; Yairi & Lewis, 1984). CWS show a high number of stuttering clusters (i.e., two or more disfluencies on the same or adjacent words) (Hubbard & Yairi, 1988). Findings indicated that stuttering had its onset at a mean age of 32 months (Yairi & Ambrose, 1992b), and stuttering-like disfluencies decreased in both typically disfluent children and CWS over the 12-month period of the study (Yairi & Ambrose, 1992a; Yairi, Ambrose, & Niermann, 1993). Children who continued to be diagnosed as CWS after almost 2 years of follow-up continued to show a higher frequency of stuttering-like disfluencies (i.e., part-word repetitions and prolongations).

THEORIES OF STUTTERING

There have been many theories that attempt to explain the existence and development of stuttering. Among the more popular theories of stuttering are Johnson and Associates' (1959) semantogenic theory, Sheehan's (1953) conflict theory of stuttering, and Travis's (1931) cerebral dominance theory. Although these theories had their place in the history of this disorder, they have been replaced by several more contemporary views of stuttering. Shames and Rubin (1986) provided a review of these theories.

Although many theories look specifically at stuttering, several can explain the occurrence of disfluencies as well. Some can additionally explain the link between the occurrence of disfluency and linguistic variables. One of these theories that has received interest and support is the demands and capacities model of stuttering (Adams, 1990; Starkweather & Gottwald, 1990). This theory states that all individuals have a certain capacity to speak fluently based on their genetic disposition. Some individuals have a greater capacity to be fluent speakers, whereas others have less capacity to speak fluently. The second factor of this theory has to do with demands, specifically the demands of speaking. These demands can include pressure to talk quickly, pressure to speak in front of a large group, and linguistic pressures for longer and more complex utterances. According to this theory, whenever the demands of speaking exceed the speaker's capacity, stuttering can occur. The high demand can be motor, social, emotional, or linguistic. In this model, children who have linguistic delays or disorders can stutter, but children who have typical or even advanced linguistic ability can also stutter. The demands and capacities model has empirical support in that stuttering has been shown to occur more frequently when linguistic demands are increased (Gaines et al., 1991; Logan & Conture, 1995; Ratner & Sih, 1987; Weiss & Zebrowski, 1992).

A potential weakness of the demands and capacities model is that it does not separate stuttering from disfluency. Another theory partially addresses this problem. The neuropsycholinguistic theory (Perkins, Kent, & Curlee, 1991) states that speech requires a coordination of motor, linguistic, and paralinguistic components (see Figure 1). When these elements of speaking are not in synchrony, the person exhibits either stuttering or a disfluency. The determination of whether stuttering or disfluency will occur is dependent on the speaker's loss of control. If the speaker loses control, stuttering will occur; if not, a disfluency will occur. The factors responsible for the loss of control are related to time pressures, which are defined as the ability to initiate or continue speaking. Again, a genetic predisposition to stutter, influenced by the speaking environment, can be responsible for stuttering. This theory accounts for both stuttering and disfluencies.

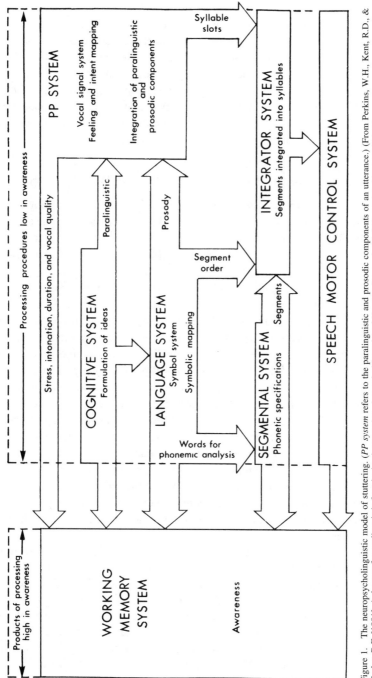

Figure 1. The neuropsycholinguistic model of stuttering. (*PP system* refers to the paralinguistic and prosodic components of an utterance.) (From Perkins, W.H., Kent, R.D., & Curlee, R.F. [1991]. A theory of neurolinguistic functioning in stuttering. *Journal of Speech and Hearing Research, 34,* 740; reprinted by permission.)

One final theory that has gained some popularity is referred to as the *covert repair hypothesis* (Kolk, 1991). In this theory, stuttering is thought to be a result of the speaker's trying to repair the errors made while speaking. These repairs are made on the typical repetitions and hesitations that exist in speech. In other words, stuttering is a result of an adaptation to an impairment rather than an impairment in itself. Careful evaluation of linguistic context can be useful in indicating where these adaptations take place and determining whether they are related to linguistic or other variables.

STUTTERING AND CENTRAL NERVOUS SYSTEM DYSFUNCTION

The theories mentioned in the previous section indicate that stuttering and/or disfluency have a basis in a decreased potential or a decreased ability to speak fluently. This lack of potential is theorized to be innate; thus, the central nervous system (CNS) is viewed as a possible source of this lack of innate potential.

There are a few studies that have explored the role of the CNS in connection with stuttering. A study by Pool, Devous, Freeman, Watson, and Finitzo (1991) examined these differences through regional blood flow studies (rCBF) in 20 adults who stutter and a matched group of adults who did not stutter. The rCBF measures were lower for PWS than in an age- and gender-matched group of people who did not stutter. Specifically, significant relative flow asymmetries were found for the anterior cingulate, superior temporal gyri, middle temporal gyri, and the inferior frontal gyrus. The implication of this study is that PWS differ neurologically from a matched group of people who do not stutter, specifically in the function of frontal and temporal lobes. These areas are associated with both motor initiation and motor programming for speech, as well as language processing. However, the differences have been shown only in adults who stutter. These differences in rCBF could be a factor in the reduced capacity models mentioned previously. They also show the connection between the linguistic processing and the motor production areas of the brain.

A follow-up study explored regional blood flow differences in three groups: 1) PWS who also show linguistic impairments (as measured by discourse analysis and complex story comprehension tasks), 2) PWS who do not show linguistic impairments, and 3) a matched control group of people who do not stutter without linguistic impairments (Watson et al., 1994). The results indicated left–right asymmetry differences in rCBF in the motor and linguistic areas of the brain between typical controls and PWS with typical linguistic abilities. Furthermore, PWS with linguistic impairments showed a different pattern in the middle temporal and inferior frontal areas. Thus, it appears that not only does stuttering relate to left–right asymmetry in language and motor areas of the brain, but, when linguistic impairments are also considered, the rCBF studies show a distinct pattern of asymmetries. These kinds of studies may eventually help to discriminate disfluent individuals who demonstrate both stuttering and linguistic disorders from those with stuttering alone. The relationship of stuttering, disfluency, and language proficiency is still unclear from a neurological standpoint; but rCBF studies seem to indicate subtle differences between PWS and people who do not stutter, as well as differences between those with language impairments and those without. Future research in this area can help clarify the link between language processing in the brain and the motor processes involved in speech. Using children who are disfluent in rCBF studies could also indicate whether stuttering and typical disfluency affect the same areas of the brain. These findings could potentially offer more support for the neuropsycholinguistic theory (Perkins et al., 1991) or the demands and capacities model (Adams, 1990; Starkweather & Gottwald, 1990) and establish a link between linguistic competence and motor production of speech.

FLUENCY AND A LINGUISTIC SUBTYPE OF STUTTERING

If the results of the rCBF studies previously mentioned can be substantiated, they will provide support for a subtyping taxonomy within the disorder of stuttering. Among the subtypes would be normal disfluency, stuttering with linguistic impairment, and stuttering with motor impairment. This subtyping scheme could help determine whether typically disfluent children are substantially different from beginning stutterers. However, such a scheme is a matter of debate. There continues to be a call for longitudinal studies to substantiate whether different subtypes of stuttering do exist (Borden, 1990; Yairi, 1990). That is, there may be a number of different causes, a number of different developmental patterns, and a number of different behaviors and severities, and thus several possible schemes, for subtyping stuttering and disfluency. Borden (1990) reviewed the literature and found that stuttering has been subclassified according to etiology, reactive behaviors, phonetic context of the stuttering, locus of the moment of stuttering, manifestation of stuttering, and the severity of stuttering.

Van Riper (1971) was one of the first to suggest subtyping stuttering. He described four distinct subtypes based on the factors of onset, attitudes and awareness, developmental trends, and associated language behaviors. Van Riper's (1971) subclassification scheme held that about 50% of the children experienced the onset of stuttering between the ages of 2 and 3 following typical speech and language development. Another 25% of the children experienced the onset of stuttering in close approximation with the appearance of their first sentences. In addition, these children experienced language and articulation delays.

Culatta and Goldberg (1995) also provided a subclassification system for disfluency types. Their classification system included the separation of fluency failures into two categories: normal disfluencies and abnormal disfluencies. The abnormal disfluencies are then subcategorized into stuttering, neurogenic dysfunction, psychogenic dysfunction, language delay, and mixed fluency failure. Although these categories are not perfectly defined, many researchers and practitioners support their usage (Borden, 1990; Culatta & Goldberg, 1995; Helm-Estabrooks, 1993). If these subcategories do exist, they might explain some of the inconsistencies noted throughout the stuttering literature and could potentially aid in the understanding of normal disfluency.

FACTORS INFLUENCING STUTTERING

CWS can potentially have other speech, language, and/or learning disorders. Most studies reveal a higher incidence of articulation deficits in children who stutter than in the population that does not stutter. This section addresses the other speech, language, or learning problems in children who stutter.

Phonology and Articulation

A survey completed by Blood and Seider (1981) indicated that 68% of CWS possess other speech, language, or learning problems. Of this group, 16% had an articulation disorder or delay. St. Louis and Hinzman (1988) found similar results. Ryan (1992), however, found that there were no significant differences in articulation skills between CWS and preschool children who do not stutter in his study. Ragsdale and Sisterhern (1984) found more disfluencies in the spontaneous speech of children with articulation disorders than in the spontaneous speech of children with typical articulation skills. Although the relationship between stuttering and articulation ability is somewhat unclear, it does appear that a number of the children who stutter possess articulatory deficiencies.

Wolk, Edwards, and Conture (1993) looked at the phonological skills of children with both stuttering and phonological disorders. They compared this group with a matched group of children who also stuttered but did not have a phonological disorder. The results of their study indicated that there was a greater number of prolongations, but a lower number of iterations per repetition for the stuttering group that also had signs of disordered phonology. From these data, the authors assumed that there are several different types of fluency disorders, including a type accompanied by impaired phonological systems.

Another study looked at effects of phonological complexity in children who stutter (Throneburg, Yairi, & Paden, 1994). The results of this study indicated that stuttering is not affected by the phonological difficulty of the word that was stuttered, nor is it affected by the phonological difficulty of the word following an instance of stuttering. Loci of stuttering were not related to phonological category.

In summary, the studies relating stuttering to articulation and phonological disorders reveal that a significant number of children who stutter also possess articulation and/or phonological disorders. This is not true of all CWS. The results of these studies indicated that there may be a subtype of fluency disorders that includes significant articulation and/or phonological disorders. In addition, these findings may indicate that difficulty in phonological or motor processes involved in speech could throw the entire central language system out of balance and cause disfluency. This would support the neuropsycholinguistic model proposed by Perkins et al. (1991).

Language Onset

Many clinicians have believed that children who stutter are slower to say their first word and slower to develop language than their peers who do not stutter. The results of a study by Andrews and Harris (1964) indicated that CWS are delayed in attaining certain language milestones. A closer examination of these results indicated that differences may be as small as 6 months. Furthermore, these differences could also be a result of other concomitant disorders, such as mental retardation or learning disabilities. Blood and Seider (1981) found that 7% of the CWS in their study were also being treated for a learning disability, and 5% of the CWS were also labeled as having some degree of mental retardation. These percentages could account for the difference in group means and could erroneously lead to the belief that children who stutter have later language acquisition times.

A more controlled study was completed by Seider, Gladstein, and Kidd (1982). They eliminated specific groups of other disorders, such as mental retardation and cerebral palsy, to eliminate confounding variables. They also collected data on siblings of each CWS and, to rule out gender differences, compared only males with males and females with females. With these variables controlled for, this study indicated no differences in language onset between children who stutter and those who do not.

Semantics and Syntax

Evaluating and diagnosing semantic skills in individuals who stutter can be a difficult task, primarily because many stutterers avoid feared words or sounds. Some researchers have attempted to work around this problem by measuring the receptive semantic skills of individuals who stutter. Studies by Westby (1979) and Williams, Melrose, and Woods (1969) indicated that a group of children who stuttered scored lower on measures of semantics than a matched group of children who did not stutter. Although the children in the stuttering group did score lower, the subjects in Westby's (1979) study were still within the normal range. It has been suggested that this does not indicate that stutterers have lower semantic abilities than children who do not stutter, but rather that there is a wide range of semantic abilities in children who stutter. This finding can be taken as further support of the possibility of subgroups among CWS. In addition, children with semantic disabilities could be disfluent because of the imbalance of one part of the language system with other production systems, as described by Perkins et al. (1991).

One hypothesis described in the neuropsycholinguistic model states that when language, segmental, or paralinguistic inputs become dyssynchronous, disfluency can occur. The dyssynchrony mentioned is a result of one area of skill (i.e., semantic, phonological, syntactic) below the level of the other language components. The production of language is then thrown out of balance as different components arrive at a central language integrator at different times and thus have a mistimed impact on the motor production of speech. This motor speech imbalance can result in either disfluency or stuttering, depending on other internal pressures and genetic predisposition (see Figure 1).

The syntactic abilities of PWS also have been evaluated and compared with their peers who do not stutter. These studies typically assess syntactic ability and complexity through measures such as mean length of utterance (MLU) or developmental sentence scoring (DSS) (Lee, 1974). As a group, children who stutter do not differ, or differ only slightly, from their peers in terms of syntactic production (St. Louis, Hinzman, & Hull, 1985; Wall, 1980; Westby, 1979). Blood and Seider (1981) found that 10% of school-age CWS also possess a language disorder. Statistics for the population that does not stutter estimate the prevalence of language disorders in school-age children to be between 3.9% and 5.8% (Van Hattum, 1982). This increased prevalence of language problems in CWS suggests the need for screening for syntactic abilities during evaluation.

Maske-Cash and Curlee (1995) examined this relationship in more detail by measuring vocal reaction times as they relate to syntactic complexity. For a group of kindergartners through fifth graders, they found that vocal reaction times were slower for CWS than for children who did not stutter across all levels of tasks. In addition, they found that the reaction times for CWS were slower than for the group who did not stutter as length and meaningfulness of an utterance increased. They also found that vocal reaction times were greater for CWS who possessed another speech or language disorder than for those who stuttered and had otherwise typical speech and language. These reaction times increased as length and meaningfulness of utterances increased. Although these findings are consistent with previous reaction time studies, the language component had not been studied previously in this context. The findings could lend more support to theories that emphasize the role of demands on the speaker in the genesis of stuttering (Adams, 1990; Starkweather & Gottwald, 1990).

Logan and Conture (1995) also found significant relationships between length and complexity of utterances and the occurrence of stuttering. They examined this relationship with the articulatory rate (as calculated from a sample of utterances between the child and the mother in free conversation) for children between 36 and 66 months of age. They determined that the articulatory rate, when considered with length and complexity of an utterance, was not responsible for the occurrence of stuttering. It would appear that the increased probability of stuttering results primarily from the length and complexity variables but is not associated with differences in articulatory rate.

The interaction of speaking rate and linguistic complexity was also studied by evaluating how several linguistic variables affect motor processes. Van Lieshout, Starkweather, Hulstijn, and Peters (1995) found that speakers use shorter vowel durations at sentence initial position, sentence final position, and in longer words. This shorter vowel duration decreases motor reaction time and thus increases stress on the motor system. The reaction to pushing the motor system to its limits could be a potential cause of stuttering. However, this study was conducted on speakers who did not stutter and the results are hypothesized only for what would happen for PWS. It does, though, further document the influence of linguistic complexity on speaking demand.

Pragmatics and Parent Interaction

Weiss and Zebrowski (1992) studied the context of stuttering loci from a pragmatic viewpoint. Their study found that more stuttering was observed for CWS on assertive utterances as opposed to responsive utterances. When these assertive utterances were later analyzed by MLU and DSS (Lee, 1974), they were found to be longer and more complex in nature. Although this study suggested an increase in stuttering as a function of pragmatic factors, the increase could have been due to the effects of length and complexity.

In another study, Weiss and Zebrowski (1991) analyzed discourse abilities of CWS and a matched group of children who did not stutter in a classroom setting. The results of this study indicated that almost twice as many children who did not stutter as those who did used all of the discourse features noted by Bedrosian (1985). These results could be an effect of delayed or disordered pragmatic language skills. They could also be related, however, to the avoidance behaviors often exhibited by PWS.

Nippold, Schwarz, and Jescheniak (1991) analyzed the narrative abilities of CWS and compared them with a group of children who do not stutter. Their results showed no significant differences between the groups on story reproduction, story length and syntactic complexity, story comprehension, and story grammar components. The mean scores of the CWS were lower on many tasks, but differences never reached statistical significance. There were no differences on measures of language as measured by the Clinical Evaluation of Language Fundamentals–Revised (Semel, Wiig, & Secord, 1987) or on nonverbal intelligence as measured by the Test of Nonverbal Intelligence (Brown, Sherbenou, & Dollar, 1982). Again, these results may be questionable because of subtyping issues. Although narrative analyses and evaluation of pragmatic abilities may eventually help in the accurate assessment and differential diagnosis of stuttering subtypes, significant differences between PWS and non-stutterers have yet to be consistently documented in these areas.

Parent Interactions

It has been hypothesized that stuttering onset is related to speaking variables of the parents of children who stutter. One variable that has been examined is the speaking rate of parents. Many stuttering treatment programs attempt to modify the speaking characteristics of parents of CWS. Meyers and Freeman (1985b) found that parents of CWS used a more rapid speaking rate than did parents of children who do not stutter. Kelly and Conture (1992) completed a similar study but did not find significant differences in the speaking rate of parents. The relationship of parents' speaking rates to stuttering is still unclear.

Turn-taking behaviors of parents of CWS have also been studied through the measurement of response time latencies and the use of interruptions. Parental response time latency did affect speaking rate but did not affect frequency or duration of stuttering (Kelly & Conture, 1992). The effects of interruptions by parents on the speech of their children were studied by two groups of researchers (Kelly & Conture, 1992; Meyers & Freeman, 1985a). These studies provided opposing results. Kelly (1994) indicated that the differences may be a result of stuttering severity. Participants in the Meyers and Freeman (1985a, 1985b) study had higher ratings of stuttering severity, which may have accounted for the observed differences, with parents of children with more severe stuttering altering their rate and interrupting more often. (For a thorough review of parent interactions with children who stutter, see Nippold & Rudzinski, 1995.)

Kelly (1994) and Kelly and Conture (1992) assessed the role of both fathers and mothers as conversational partners with CWS. They did not find significant differences in the speaking patterns of parents of CWS in terms of interruptions, delay time, and speaking rates. Nippold and Rudzinski (1995) thoroughly reviewed the literature and concluded that there is not enough empirical evidence to support the modification of parents' speech as the sole component of treatment.

There is some evidence, however, to support the observation that the modification of speaking behaviors by a conversational partner can decrease disfluencies (Winslow & Guitar, 1994). Caution must be taken when interpreting this finding, primarily because it is based on case study information from a single subject. Further research in this area should be undertaken, but there is definitely not enough support for indirect therapy as the sole means of treating young children who stutter.

This summary of the relationship of language to stuttering suggests that group differences in the language skills of PWS versus people who do not stutter can be documented, but this does not mean that PWS have delayed language skills. The most consistent findings indicate that both stuttering and typical disfluencies tend to occur more often as linguistic complexity increases. Nippold (1990), in a very thorough review, criticized some of the techniques used when comparing the language behaviors of PWS and people who do not stutter. Many studies are based on small samples, survey research, or procedures with other methodological flaws. Although validity and reliability of many of these studies are questionable, the one point they have in common is that there is a wide range of language skills within the population that stutters. An impairment in only one area of language formulation can cause an imbalance in the entire language system and cause disfluencies to occur. These findings could lend further support for the neuropsycholinguistic model (Perkins et al., 1991).

Effects of Language Therapy on Stuttering

There is some evidence to indicate that language intervention can have an influence on fluency. A study by Flack, Phelps-Terasaki, and Sartin-Lawler (1979) indicated that language therapy can actually have a positive effect on fluency, whereas a study by Hall (1977) indicated that language therapy can have a negative effect on fluency. Concurrent treatment of phonological and fluency disorders is also debatable. Conture, Louko, and Edwards (1993) reported positive gains in fluency by children who were in phonological process therapy programs. However, Merits-Patterson and Reed (1981) reported that some children actually began to stutter following phonological intervention. These inconsistent results indicate that language and/or phonological intervention can affect fluency patterns in both directions. Some individuals improve during language or phonological intervention, whereas others decline. Again, differential diagnosis and the possible subtyping of PWS could influence more informed therapy decisions.

CONCLUSIONS

It appears that a complex interaction takes place among disfluency, stuttering-like disfluency, linguistic difficulty, maturation, and motor demands. For speech to occur in a relatively fluent manner, several factors must be present. The speaker must be capable of formulating a thought and expressing it within current linguistic and motor capabilities. If a speaker's capabilities are exceeded, fluency breakdowns can occur. These breakdowns occur frequently as children master their language system and mature. The breakdowns in fluency can occur when exceeding capacity in any one area (e.g., length, complexity, task difficulty, interruption, syntax, grammar, phonology, motor demand) or in a combination of several areas. All children go through these growth periods, as evidenced by the higher levels of disfluency in younger children and the decline in disfluency rate with increases in age or linguistic ability.

Two different models help explain this phenomenon. The demands and capacities model (Adams, 1990; Starkweather & Gottwald, 1990) is helpful in its simplicity. Although it was not the original intention of the authors to do so, this theory does help explain the disfluencies in typical children as well as the stuttering in PWS. Whenever demands (e.g., linguistic, motor) exceed a person's internal capacity to speak fluently, disfluencies occur. The weakness of this model is in its inability to distinguish between stuttering and other disfluencies. Despite this deficiency, this model highlights the link between linguistic capacity and motor performance. For both CWS and children who do not stutter, increased linguistic complexity affects motor speech performance, exhibited as increased disfluency levels.

The distinction between stuttering and normal disfluency is shown more clearly in the neuropsycholinguistic model (Perkins et al., 1991). This model accounts for the occurrence of disfluencies when demands for fluent speech exceed internal capacity and when only one part of the central language component is stressed. This throws the entire central language component out of synchrony, and thus disfluencies can occur. Increased stress on any part of the language-processing system can affect motor speech. The determination of disfluency or stuttering depends on internal time pressure to begin or continue talking. However, to speak fluently, a person's cognitive system, language system, phonetic system, and motor system for speech must all be in synchrony. Whenever one area is delayed or disordered, the potential for throwing the entire language production system out of balance exists. In this model, a clear link exists between language and speech processes.

In some ways, the neuropsycholinguistic model places stuttering and normal disfluency patterns on a continuum. Disfluencies occur, but the distinction between typical disfluency and stuttering is determined on a continuum of control or time pressure. The continuum concept also makes theoretical sense in that the same linguistic factors that affect fluency in people who do not stutter also affect fluency in PWS. This does not indicate that PWS and individuals with disfluency possess the same capabilities and qualities. Rather, it indicates that although the two groups may have very different capabilities, both groups are affected by the same linguistic variables. Thus, the same links between language and speech are present for both children with disfluency and CWS. Future research should indicate which variables affect fluency in the same ways for both individuals who stutter and those who do not stutter.

The data reviewed here highlight the connection of language and speech because so many linguistic variables affect speech production. Increased linguistic demand has the effect of fluency breakdowns in both normally disfluent and stuttering populations. The connection is even more apparent when looking at the effects of disfluency on rCBF studies. Both the frontal and temporal areas of the brain are affected. These areas have traditionally been regarded as controlling motor planning and execution for speech, as well as language formulation and comprehension. Thus, the evidence from a variety of sources in the disfluency literature supports one integrated view of speech and language in both theoretical and clinical studies of communication and its disorders.

REFERENCES

Adams, M.R. (1977). A clinical strategy for differentiating the normally nonfluent child from the incipient stutterer. *Journal of Fluency Disorders, 2,* 141–148.

Adams, M.R. (1990). The demands and capacities model I: Theoretical elaborations. *Journal of Fluency Disorders, 15,* 135–141.

Ambrose, N.G., & Yairi, E. (1995). The role of repetition units in the differential diagnosis of early childhood incipient stuttering. *American Journal of Speech-Language Pathology, 4,* 82–88.

Andrews, G., & Harris, M. (1964). *The syndrome of stuttering.* London: Heinemann.

Bar, A. (1969). Effects of types of listeners and listening instructions on the attention to manner and content of a severe stutterer's speech. *Journal of Communication Disorders, 2,* 344–349.

Bedrosian, J. (1985). An approach to developing conversational competence. In D. Ripich & F. Spinelli (Eds.), *School discourse problems* (pp. 231–255). San Diego: College-Hill Press.

Blood, G.W., & Seider, R. (1981). The concomitant problems of young stutterers. *Journal of Speech and Hearing Disorders, 46,* 31–33.

Borden, G.J. (1990). Subtyping adult stutterers for research purposes. *ASHA Reports: Research Needs in Stuttering: Roadblocks and Future Directions, 18,* 58–62.

Brown, L., Sherbenou, R.J., & Dollar, S.J. (1982). *Test of Nonverbal Intelligence.* Austin, TX: PRO-ED.

Brown, R. (1973). *A first language: The early stages.* Cambridge, MA: Harvard University Press.

Brown, S.F. (1945). The loci of stutterings in the speech sequence. *Journal of Speech Disorders, 10,* 181–192.

Colburn, N., & Mysak, E.D. (1982). Developmental disfluency and emerging grammar: I. Disfluency characteristics in early syntactic utterances. *Journal of Speech and Hearing Research, 25,* 414–420.

Conture, E.G., Louko, L.J., & Edwards, M.L. (1993). Simultaneously treating stuttering and disordered phonology in children: Experimental treatment, preliminary findings. *American Journal of Speech-Language Pathology, 2,* 72–81.

Cordes, A.K., & Ingham, R.J. (1994a). Time interval measurement of stuttering: Effects of interval duration. *Journal of Speech and Hearing Research, 37,* 779–788.

Cordes, A.K., & Ingham, R.J. (1994b). Time interval measurement of stuttering: Effects of training with highly agreed or poorly agreed exemplars. *Journal of Speech and Hearing Research, 37,* 1295–1307.

Coyle, M.M., & Mallard, A.R. (1979). Word-by-word analysis of observer agreement utilizing audio and audiovisual techniques. *Journal of Fluency Disorders, 4,* 23–28.

Culatta, R., & Goldberg, S.A. (1995). *Stuttering therapy: An integrated approach to theory and practice.* Needham Heights, MA: Allyn & Bacon.

Curlee, R.F. (1981). Observer disagreement on disfluency and stuttering. *Journal of Speech and Hearing Research, 24,* 596–600.

DeJoy, D.A., & Gregory, H.H. (1985). The relationship between age and frequency of disfluency in preschool children. *Journal of Fluency Disorders, 10,* 107–122.

Flack, F., Phelps-Terasaki, D., & Sartin-Lawler, P. (1979). Relationships between language usage and fluency: A case study. *Journal of Childhood Communication Disorders, 3,* 128–138.

Gaines, N.D., Runyan, C.M., & Meyers, S.C. (1991). A comparison of young stutterers' fluent versus stuttering utterances on measures of length and complexity. *Journal of Speech and Hearing Research, 34,* 37–42.

Gordon, P.A., & Luper, H.L. (1989). Speech disfluencies in nonstutterers: Syntactic complexity and production task effects. *Journal of Fluency Disorders, 14,* 429–445.

Gordon, P.A., & Luper, H.L. (1992). The early identification of beginning stuttering: I. Protocols. *American Journal of Speech-Language Pathology, 1,* 43–53.

Gordon, P.A., Luper, H.L., & Peterson, H.A. (1986). The effects of syntactic complexity on the occurrence of disfluencies in five-year-old nonstutterers. *Journal of Fluency Disorders, 11,* 151–164.

Hall, P. (1977). The occurrence of disfluencies in language disordered school-aged children. *Journal of Speech and Hearing Disorders, 42,* 364–369.

Ham, R.E. (1989). What are we measuring? *Journal of Fluency Disorders, 14,* 231–243.

Ham, R.E. (1990). *Therapy of stuttering: Preschool through adolescence.* Englewood Cliffs, NJ: Prentice-Hall.

Haynes, W.O., & Hood, S.E. (1977). Language and disfluency variables in normal speaking children from discrete chronological age groups. *Journal of Fluency Disorders, 2,* 57–74.

Helm-Estabrooks, N. (1993). Stuttering associated with acquired neurological disorders. In R.C. Curlee (Ed.), *Stuttering and related disorders of fluency* (pp. 205–219). New York: Thieme.

Hubbard, C.P., & Yairi, E. (1988). Clustering of disfluencies in the speech of stuttering and nonstuttering preschool children. *Journal of Speech and Hearing Research, 31,* 228–233.

Ingham, R.J., & Cordes, A.K. (1992). Interclinic differences in stuttering-event counts. *Journal of Fluency Disorders, 17,* 171–176.

Ingham, R.J., & Cordes, A.K., & Finn, P. (1993). Time interval measurement of stuttering: Systematic replication of Ingham, Cordes, and Gow. *Journal of Speech and Hearing Research, 36,* 1168–1176.

Ingham, R.J., Cordes, A.K., & Gow, M.L. (1993). Time interval measurement of stuttering: Modifying interjudge agreement. *Journal of Speech and Hearing Research, 36,* 503–515.

Johnson, W., & Associates. (1959). *The onset of stuttering.* Minneapolis: University of Minnesota Press.

Kadi-Hanifi, K., & Howell, P. (1992). Syntactic analysis of the spontaneous speech of normally fluent and stuttering children. *Journal of Fluency Disorders, 17,* 151–170.

Kelly, E.M. (1994). Speech rates and turn-taking behaviors of children who stutter and their fathers. *Journal of Speech and Hearing Research, 37,* 1284–1294.

Kelly, E.M., & Conture, E.G. (1992). Speaking rates, response time latencies, and interrupting behaviors of young stutterers, nonstutterers, and their mothers. *Journal of Speech and Hearing Research, 35,* 1256–1267.

Kolk, H.H.J. (1991). Is stuttering a symptom of adaptation or of impairment? In H.F.M. Peters, W. Hulstijn, & C.W. Starkweather (Eds.), *Speech motor control and stuttering* (pp. 131–140). Amsterdam: Elsevier.

Kully, D., & Boberg, E. (1988). An investigation of interclinic agreement in the identification of fluent and stuttered syllables. *Journal of Fluency Disorders, 13,* 309–318.

Lee, L. (1974). *Developmental sentence analysis*. Evanston, IL: Northwestern University Press.

Logan, K.J., & Conture, E.G. (1995). Length, grammatical complexity, and rate differences in stuttered and fluent conversational utterances of children who stutter. *Journal of Fluency Disorders, 20*, 35–61.

MacDonald, J.D., & Martin, R.R. (1973). Stuttering and disfluency as two reliable and unambiguous response classes. *Journal of Speech and Hearing Research, 16*, 691–699.

Maske-Cash, W.S., & Curlee, R.F. (1995). Effect of utterance length and meaningfulness on the speech initiation times of children who stutter and children who do not stutter. *Journal of Speech and Hearing Research, 38*, 18–25.

McLaughlin, S.F., & Cullinan, W.L. (1989). Disfluencies, utterance length and linguistic complexity in nonstuttering children. *Journal of Fluency Disorders, 14*, 17–36.

Merits-Patterson, R., & Reed, C.G. (1981). Disfluencies in the speech of language delayed children. *Journal of Speech and Hearing Research, 46*, 55–58.

Meyers, S.C., & Freeman, F.J. (1985a). Interruptions as a variable in stuttering and disfluency. *Journal of Speech and Hearing Research, 28*, 428–435.

Meyers, S.C., & Freeman, F.J. (1985b). Mother and child speech rates as a variable in stuttering and disfluency. *Journal of Speech and Hearing Research, 28*, 436–444.

Nippold, M.A. (1990). Concomitant speech and language disorders in stuttering children: A critique of the literature. *Journal of Speech and Hearing Disorders, 55*, 51–60.

Nippold, M.A., & Rudzinski, M. (1995). Parents' speech and children's stuttering: A critique of the literature. *Journal of Speech and Hearing Research, 38*, 978–989.

Nippold, M.A., Schwarz, I.E., & Jescheniak, J. (1991). Narrative ability in school-age stuttering boys: A preliminary investigation. *Journal of Fluency Disorders, 16*, 209–308.

Pearl, S.Z., & Bernthal, J.E. (1980). The effect of grammatical complexity upon disfluency behavior of nonstuttering preschool children. *Journal of Fluency Disorders, 5*, 55–68.

Perkins, W.H., Kent, R.D., & Curlee, R.F. (1991). A theory of neurolinguistic functioning in stuttering. *Journal of Speech and Hearing Research, 34*, 734–752.

Pool, K.D., Devous, M.D., Freeman, F.J., Watson, B.C., & Finitzo, T. (1991). Regional cerebral blood flow in developmental stutterers. *Archives of Neurology, 48*, 509–512.

Ragsdale, J., & Sisterhern, D. (1984). Hesitation phenomena in the spontaneous speech of normal and articulatory-defective children. *Language and Speech, 27*, 235–244.

Ramig, P.R. (1993). High reported spontaneous stuttering recovery rates: Fact or fiction. *Language, Speech, and Hearing Services in the Schools, 24*, 156–160.

Ratner, N., & Sih, C. (1987). Effects of gradual increases in sentence length and complexity on children's dysfluency. *Journal of Speech and Hearing Research, 52*, 278–287.

Ryan, B.P. (1992). Articulation, language, rate and fluency characteristics of stuttering and nonstuttering preschool children. *Journal of Speech and Hearing Research, 35*, 333–342.

Seider, R.A., Gladstein, K.L., & Kidd, K.K. (1982). Language onset and concomitant speech and language problems in subgroups of stutterers and their siblings. *Journal of Speech and Language Research, 25*, 482–486.

Semel, E., Wiig, E.H., & Secord, W. (1987). *Clinical Evaluation of Language Fundamentals–Revised (CELF–R)*. San Antonio, TX: The Psychological Corporation.

Shames, G.H., & Rubin, H. (1986). *Stuttering then and now*. Columbus, OH: Charles E. Merrill.

Sheehan, J.G. (1953). Theory and treatment of stuttering as an approach-avoidance conflict. *Journal of Psychology, 36*, 27–49.

Silverman, E.M. (1975). Effect of certain word attributes on preschoolers' speech disfluency: Initial phoneme and length. *Journal of Speech and Hearing Research, 18*, 430–434.

Silverman, F.H., & Williams, D.E. (1967). Loci of disfluencies in the speech of nonstutterers during oral reading. *Journal of Speech and Hearing Research, 10*, 790–794.

Starkweather, C.W., & Gottwald, S.R. (1990). The demands and capacities model: II. Clinical applications. *Journal of Fluency Disorders, 15*, 143–157.

St. Louis, K.O., & Hinzman, A.R. (1988). A descriptive study of speech, language and hearing characteristics of school-aged stutterers. *Journal of Fluency Disorders, 13*, 331–355.

St. Louis, K.O., Hinzman, A.R., & Hull, F.M. (1985). Studies of cluttering: Disfluency and language measures in young possible clutterers and stutterers. *Journal of Fluency Disorders, 10*, 151–172.

Throneburg, R.N., Yairi, E., & Paden, E.P. (1994). Relation between phonologic difficulty and the occurrence of disfluencies in the early stage of stuttering. *Journal of Speech and Hearing Research, 37*, 504–509.

Travis, L.E. (1931). *Speech pathology*. Englewood Cliffs, NJ: Prentice-Hall.

Tuthill, C.E. (1946). A quantitative study of extensional meaning with special reference to stuttering. *Speech Monographs, 13*, 81–98.

Van Hattum, R.J. (1982). *Speech-language programming in the schools* (2nd ed.). Springfield, IL: Charles C Thomas.

Van Lieshout, P.H.H.M., Starkweather, C.W., Hulstijn, W., & Peters, H.F.M. (1995). Effects of linguistic correlates of stuttering on Emg activity in nonstuttering speakers. *Journal of Speech and Hearing Research, 38*, 360–372.

Van Riper, C. (1971). *The nature of stuttering*. Englewood Cliffs, NJ: Prentice-Hall.

Wall, M.J. (1980). A comparison of syntax in young stutterers and nonstutterers. *Journal of Fluency Disorders, 5*, 345–352.

Watson, B.C., Freeman, F.J., Devous, M.D., Chapman, S.B., Finitzo, T., & Pool, K.D. (1994). Linguistic performance and regional cerebral blood flow in persons who stutter. *Journal of Speech and Hearing Research, 37*, 1221–1228.

Weiss, A.L., & Zebrowski, P.M. (1991). Patterns of assertiveness and responsiveness in parental interactions with stuttering and fluent children. *Journal of Fluency Disorders, 16*, 125–142.

Weiss, A.L., & Zebrowski, P.M. (1992). Disfluencies in the conversations of young children who stutter: Some answers about questions. *Journal of Speech and Hearing Research, 35*, 1230–1238.

Westby, C.E. (1979). Language performance of stuttering and nonstuttering children. *Journal of Communication Disorders, 12*, 133–145.

Wexler, K.B., & Mysak, E.D. (1982). Disfluency characteristics of 2–4- and 6-year-old males. *Journal of Fluency Disorders, 7*, 37–46.

Williams, D.E., & Kent, L.R. (1958). Listener evaluations of speech perception. *Journal of Speech and Hearing Research, 1*, 124–131.

Williams, D.E., Melrose, B.M., & Woods, C.L. (1969). The relationship between stuttering and academic achievement in children. *Journal of Communication Disorders, 2*, 87–98.

Williams, D.E., Silverman, F.H., & Kools, J.A. (1969). Disfluency behavior of elementary-school stutterers and nonstutterers: The consistency effect. *Journal of Speech and Hearing Research, 12,* 301–307.

Wingate, M.E. (1964). A standard definition of stuttering. *Journal of Speech and Hearing Disorders, 29,* 484–489.

Winslow, M., & Guitar, B. (1994). The effects of structured turn-taking on disfluencies: A case study. *Language, Speech, and Hearing Services in the Schools, 25,* 251–257.

Wolk, L., Edwards, M.L., & Conture, E.G. (1993). Coexistence of stuttering and disordered phonology in young children. *Journal of Speech and Hearing Research, 36,* 906–917.

Yairi, E. (1981). Disfluencies of normal speaking two-year-old children. *Journal of Speech and Hearing Research, 24,* 490–495.

Yairi, E. (1982). Longitudinal studies of disfluencies in two-year-old children. *Journal of Speech and Hearing Research, 25,* 155–160.

Yairi, E. (1990). Subtyping child stutterers for research purposes. *ASHA Reports: Research Needs in Stuttering: Roadblocks and Future Directions, 18,* 50–57.

Yairi, E., & Ambrose, N.G. (1992a). A longitudinal study of stuttering in children: A preliminary report. *Journal of Speech and Hearing Research, 35,* 755–760.

Yairi, E., & Ambrose, N.G. (1992b). Onset of stuttering in preschool children: Selected factors. *Journal of Speech and Hearing Research, 35,* 782–788.

Yairi, E., Ambrose, N.G., & Niermann, R. (1993). The early months of stuttering: A developmental study. *Journal of Speech and Hearing Research, 36,* 521–528.

Yairi, E., & Clifton, N. (1972). Disfluent speech behavior of pre-school children, high school seniors and geriatric persons. *Journal of Speech and Hearing Research, 15,* 714–719.

Yairi, E., & Lewis, B. (1984). Disfluencies at the onset of stuttering. *Journal of Speech and Hearing Research, 27,* 154–159.

Young, M.A. (1975). Observer agreement for marking moments of stuttering. *Journal of Speech and Hearing Research, 18,* 530–540.

10

Phonology, Metaph
and the Development

Linda K. Swank and Linda S. Larrivee

THIS CHAPTER DISCUSSES THE ROLES of phonology and metaphonology in the processing and production of written language development. It emphasizes the importance of recognizing reading and writing in concert with oral language. To acquire written forms of language, especially alphabetic written language, facility with phonological aspects of oral language is essential.

The first section of this chapter defines and addresses factors influencing the emergence of phonology. Factors of influence include speech perception and speech production. Next, the theoretical construct of phonological processing is addressed. A discussion of the abstract character of a phoneme lays the foundation for the discussion in the second section, in which *metaphonology* is defined, factors that influence its emergence are examined, and speech experiences that have proved facilitative of the development of metaphonology are reviewed. In the third section, the relationship among literacy acquisition and phonology and metaphonology is addressed by considering issues concerning the written alphabetic language system. The relationship is further elucidated by a review of research on typical language and reading and on populations with language and reading disorders. In the fourth section, identification, assessment, and treatment of metaphonological disorders in children who exhibit phonological processing and/or phonological production impairments are discussed. Finally, connections among speech production and perception and the acquisition of written language are summarized.

PHONOLOGY

Phonology may be defined simply as the rule system that governs the speech sounds of a language. Phonology is part of the form of language (morphology and syntax are the other parts). Phonology, however, is anything but simple. Phonology traces its beginnings from infants' perceptual capacities, in the evolving repertoire of vocal resources or productive abilities of the first year nd in the emergence of a link between perception and production. unicative and cognitive development eventually permit the assembling system of interconnected sound patterns along with an emerging knowledge of the nature of naming and reference (Vihman, 1996).

Early models of phonological development emerged from generative linguistic models. The basic tenets of generative phonological theory include the following:

- Phonological descriptions can be formulated in terms of precise and explicit statements and notations.
- Segments are analyzable as a complex of features.
- There are two levels of representation, one corresponding to the underlying (abstract) level and the other to the (surface) phonetic level.
- Phonological rules mediate between the two levels.
- Phonological rules interact.

Stampe applied the generative rules to acquisition when he described his phonological processes, which relate the alternating forms of morphemes as they are reshaped or adjusted in different phonological contexts. Phonological processes reflect "natural responses to phonetic forces" (Donegan & Stampe, 1979, p. 130), based on the limitations of human speech perception and production. Stampe's Natural Phonology assumes that the processes are universal and innately available. Children need to learn to suppress, limit, and order these processes as required by the language. It is argued that the child's initial phonological system represents a language-innocent state. To produce the wider range of phonological oppositions found in the adult inventory, the child must learn to suppress those processes that do not make up a part of the phonology of the input language.

Models of nonlinear phonology have shifted the emphasis from rules to representations. These models offer important advantages in accounting for developmental data. Menn (1983) identified two properties of autosegmental formalism that aid in describing emerging phonological systems. The first is the possibility of specifying domains of application for phonetic features that extend beyond the segment, such as a syllable or word. The second involves the freedom from sequential ordering of features that results from placing them on separate tiers or levels of organization. Vihman (1996) suggested that the separate specifications of features that affect only consonants (i.e., glottalization, retroflexion) or only vowels (i.e., vowel harmony, advanced or retracted tongue root) in adult language provide a natural formal treatment for consonant harmony, which is notorious in child phonology but rare in adult production. The reordering of adult segments, or metathesis, is often observed in child production and disordered productions of children with specific language impairment and specific reading disabilities. The idea of specifying different features on different tiers provides a useful account for the reordering of heterogeneous segments. The first stage in phonological acquisition may involve autosegmental representation of certain features (i.e., placement of a feature on a separate tier) (e.g., a tier for nasals or velars only). This would explain the observed harmony processes in early speech production. Nonlinear models also include underspecification of features as an explanation of the relative lack of sophistication in the child's initial representations (see Vihman, 1996, for a review).

In principle, nonlinear models are equally compatible with nativist and functionalist developmental approaches to the acquisition of phonology. Bernhardt proposed a nativist interpretation:

> If a child comes to the language-learning situation with a representational framework and a set of universal principles, "templates" are then available to utilize for decoding and encoding. . . . Exposure to the input language(s) will both confirm the universally-determined representation (e.g., that, as expected, the language has CV units and stop consonants) and also result in "setting" of parameters where options are available (e.g., that the language has final consonants and that stress is syllable-initial in a given language). (1994, p. 161)

Vihman and Boysson-Bardies (1994) adopted an alternative functionalist interpretation of the establishment of the expectation of consonant–vowel (CV) syllables and stop consonants, which follows naturally from the character of vocal development in the first year. They go on to state, however, that

> whether these options are available to all children, specified by innate parameters, determined by some characteristics of the language to which the child is exposed, "chosen" by the child based on idiosyncratic perceptual, physiological, or cognitive biases, or some combination of the above is an open and widely debated question. In any case, the course of phonological development includes the addition of complexity to any or all of these aspects of the representation. (1994, p. 163)

Connectionist models have revived the role of both (input) frequency and (output) variability. These models depict a network of units interconnected by a set of input and output nodes. The connections are weighted to express the degree of relatedness or potential influence (positive or negative) between each pair of units. In addition, each unit filters the input it receives through its threshold or activation level, which may increase or decrease as a function of its recent activity. In other words, if the neural pathway is frequently stimulated, then the neural connections would be stronger and more easily activated. Conversely, with little or no use, the neural signal needed to accomplish a task would be weak and unable to perform the task. A "use it or lose it" proposition is postulated. Units may be arranged in multiple layers; within each layer, units compete to participate in a pattern of activity. Multiple influences may be expressed in parallel, as in the case of effects on word recognition (*top-down* lexical effects, from the syntactic or semantic context, and *bottom-up* phonetic effects from the auditory signal; McClelland & Elman, 1986).

Pinker and Mehler (1988) criticized the connectionist models as the new associationism discredited in the 1950s. Fodor and Pylyshyn (1988) argued, however, that the connectionist models are quite different from the associationism of the past; they viewed the connectionist models as "analog machines for computing [statistical] inferences" (p. 68), whereas learning is "basically a sort of statistical modeling" (p. 31). In the contrasting classical cognitive view, learning involves "theory construction, effected by framing hypotheses and evaluating them against evidence" (Fodor & Pylyshyn, 1988, p. 69).

Vihman (1996) argued that connectionist models offer several potential advantages in dealing with unruly aspects of developmental phonological data. Menn and Matthei argued that, in such models,

> we expect fuzzy boundaries, we expect forms to interact with each other, we expect frequency effects—and, crucially, we also expect both input and output forms to be stored in some linked way. We also have instance-based learning. . . . If we have storage of both input and output forms, we at least have the potential for modeling all of the good things that the two-lexicon model buys us, and we may be able to get rid of the aspects of the model that were getting oppressive. (1992, p. 228)

In his connectionist model, Stemberger (1992) supplemented frequency, described as one of two factors contributing to accessibility (or relative strength of a unit), with ease of articulation. Stemberger, however, dismissed the issue of perception by saying that he assumes the child's representations are identical to those of adults. He docs propose an adjustment of perceptuo-motor control functions for "a small number of learned mappings between perception and production, which can then be used to realize [adult] words" (1992, p. 173*n*, cited in Vihman, 1996). This tuning results in a few strong output states that tend to be overused, substituting for less common target patterns. Thus, it could be argued that consonant sequence reduction is overused, as is stopping for strident sounds, until the child is exposed to and attempts some of the less common target patterns.

The review of theoretical perspectives of developmental phonology underscores the lack of consensus among researchers in the field of child phonology. Each generation of knowledge builds on the previous generation's theories and research. Nonlinear theories and optimality theories are moving the field of child phonology forward toward resolution of many of the questions of how children acquire a mature phonology.

Factors that Influence the
Development of Phonology and Metaphonology

An examination of the development of phonology is incomplete without an examination of the parameters that influence speech perception and speech production. This review provides insight into how children eventually acquire, or do not acquire, metaphonology. Children must first be able to use the phonology of their language before they can consciously reflect on the phonological system. Perception and production are requisite abilities that lead to the eventual acquisition of metaphonology. Speech perception issues are addressed first.

Speech Perception Vihman's (1996) review of the literature in the area of categorical perception research provides a framework within which to consider why some children efficiently process and produce phonological units and thus acquire metaphonology and others exhibit limited phonological processing and production and thus exhibit limited metaphonology. To decode the speech signal, the typical child must process rapidly paced human speech flows; process speech productions that vary because of individual vocal tract sizes, rate of individual speakers, and a variety of other prosodic features; and process the results of the dynamic nature of speech production because articulatory gestures interact. In other words, coarticulation results in no two speech-sound productions being alike (e.g., no two phones are alike, just like snowflakes). So how does the infant discriminate between speech sounds or phoneme boundaries?

Research in infant perception (see Vihman, 1996, for review) arose from attempts to understand and model adult speech perception (Kuhl, 1987). It was research on adults' ability to discriminate between contrasting syllables using synthetic speech based on spectrographic representation of the acoustic signal that led to an appreciation of the extremely complex relationship between phonetic perception and the underlying acoustic events. Such tests revealed the striking phenomenon of categorical perception.

To investigate categorical perception, a continuum of syllables is synthesized so that the acoustic dimension of interest is altered in small, equal steps. The first acoustic dimension to be tested in this way was the cue to place of articulation differences between the stops /b/, /d/, and /g/. Place categories identification was found to be dependent on the relationship between the frequency of the stop release burst and that of the second formant in the following vowel (Cooper, Delattre, Liberman, Borst, & Gerstman, 1952). Liberman, Harris, Hoffman, and Griffith (1957) found that listeners shifted abruptly in their labeling of the utterance-initial consonant (e.g., from /b/ to /d/ and from /d/ to /g/), despite the stimuli presented being evenly graded along a continuum. Listeners showed very poor discrimination of sounds within each category but easily discriminated between categories. For the perception of consonants, absolute identification of specific phonemes proved to be generally almost as accurate as discrimination of differences. This type of discrimination accuracy is not seen in nonlinguistic contexts such as musical pitch (Vihman, 1996).

It was initially argued that categorical perception reflected the effects of long-term learning or experience in producing and perceiving the categories of the native language (*acquired distinctiveness*). "The possibility that the discrimination peaks are innately given," however, was not dismissed (Liberman, Harris, Eimas, Lisker, & Bastian, 1961, p. 178). Conversely, the relationship between perception and articulation seemed to be closer than the relationship between either articulation or perception and the acoustic stimulus itself (Cooper et al., 1952). This observation facilitated the development of the motor theory of speech perception (Studdert-Kennedy, Liberman, Harris, & Cooper, 1970). This theory postulated that the speech signal is a particularly efficient special code in which, because of the effects of coarticulation, an individual acoustic cue relays information simultaneously as the phonemic units are processed (Liberman, Cooper, Shankweiler, & Studdert-Kennedy, 1967).

If infants gave evidence of responding preferentially to the categorical voice onset time (VOT) contrasts characteristic of English (/ba/ versus /pa/) compared with the acoustically comparable distinctions represented by synthesized syllables selected from within one of these categories, then neither experience with the sounds of language (the learning theory account) nor reference to the articulatory patterns underlying speech sounds (the motor theory account) could reasonably be invoked as the source of the categorical nature of the adult response. In a study of 1- and 4-month-old infants, the results revealed infants' ability to discriminate the stimuli, or react to a change, only when the synthetic syllables (which differed by 20 milliseconds in all cases) cross the VOT category boundary characteristic of English and not when they are drawn from within either the short-lag (/b/) or the long-lag (/p/) category. Because 1- and 4-month-old infants have not begun to produce phonetic segments, the motor theory account did not provide the answer to how children discriminate change across phoneme boundaries. Likewise, because infants have limited experience with the speech sounds of the language, the learning theory account did not provide clear evidence of how children discriminate across phoneme boundaries. Thus, "the possibility that the discrimination peaks are innately given" could not be dismissed (Liberman et al., 1961, p. 178).

Building from these early foundational studies, Merzenich et al. (1996) and Tallal et al. (1996) applied the knowledge of speech perception to a population with specific language impairment (SLI). It has been documented that individuals with identified SLI exhibit a temporal-processing impairment expressed by limited abilities at identifying some brief phonetic elements presented in specific speech context (Tallal et al., 1996). Furthermore, these individuals exhibit poor performances at identifying or sequencing short-duration acoustic stimuli presented in rapid succession. It is argued that some individuals with SLI have difficulty with recognizing fast-element (usually consonant) phonetic segments because of an inappropriate integration with or masking by the following or preceding speech elements (usually vowels). However, there is a lack of parametric psychophysical studies. Thus, the proposed behavior may apply only within frequency channels because these children apparently have less difficulty identifying CV pairs with brief consonants in which consonant transitions and vowel formants are within largely nonoverlapping channels (Tallal et al., 1996).

It is hypothesized that the impairments underlying the phonetic reception limitations of some children with SLI might arise in early life as a consequence of atypical perceptual learning that then may contribute to atypical language learning (Merzenich et al., 1996), which may eventually lead to specific reading and academic problems. To test this hypothesis, the Merzenich and Tallal groups used a training paradigm with children who exhibited SLI between the ages of 5 and 10 years. The authors manipulated the speech signals by applying a two-stage processing algorithm. In the first processing stage, the duration of the speech signal was prolonged by 50% while preserving its spectral content and natural quality. In the second processing stage, fast (3–30 hertz) transitional elements of speech were differentially enhanced by as much as 20 decibels. This processed speech had a staccato quality in which fast (primarily consonants) elements were exaggerated relative to more slowly modulated elements (primarily vowels) in the ongoing speech stream. The authors reasoned that amplifying the fast elements should render those elements more salient and thus more reliably temporally integrated and less likely to be subject to forward or backward masking by neighboring, more slowly modulated speech elements. Following 1 month of daily training with acoustically modified speech, a repeated measures analysis of variance showed that posttraining test scores significantly improved by approximately 2 years in participants' speech discrimination and language comprehension. No measures of speech production were assessed.

Speech Production Speech perception studies provide one part of the story about how an individual is able to process and produce speech, develop a mature phonology, and become aware of the phonology of his or her language. However, perception is only one piece of the puzzle. Another piece of the puzzle is speech production ability. The relationship between perception and production has been examined to determine whether faulty perception is the source of some speech production errors. Eilers and Oller (1976) compared ease of perception of a contrast with frequency of production errors involving the contrast. The authors evaluated 14 children ages 22–26 months using paired real and nonsense words. Familiar objects such as fish were paired with nonsense toys given minimally contrasting names, such as "thish." The paired word forms included three types: 1) pairs in which the first element typically substitutes for the second element in child production (e.g., /f/ versus "th", /r/ versus /w/), 2) pairs of elements that do not typically substitute for one another (e.g., aspirated /p/ versus aspirated /t/), and 3) a nonminimal pair (e.g., /p/ versus aspirated /k/). Eilers and Oller postulated that if substitutions were influenced by perceptual confusions, then the first type of pairs should be more difficult for children to discriminate than the second or third types of pairs (Vihman, 1996).

Eilers and Oller (1976) were able to partially confirm their hypothesis. No child was able to discriminate the fricatives ("th" versus /f/; however, many adults have difficulty discriminating these phonemes), most infants could discriminate the glides, and all could discriminate the nonminimal pair. An unanticipated finding was that the pair that differed in aspiration (i.e., VOT) proved easily discriminable. A further analysis of the children's imitative production revealed that the first type of contrasts were not preserved in production. Conversely, some children produced a place contrast for the aspirated /p/ and /t/, although these same children did not exhibit discrimination on the perception task. Eilers and Oller concluded that no simplistic formula could capture the observed relationship between production and perception, even though evidence that perceptual difficulties played some role in production errors was observed. Vihman (1996) suggested that the results are in positive agreement with the general conclusions that some phonemic contrasts remain difficult to discriminate perceptually as late as 3 years of age and older (e.g., "th," /f/, /r/, /w/). Thus, it is presupposed that production errors involving these pairs may emanate from a lack of attention to the perceptual contrast.

The complexity of speech production may be better understood by a theory of tip-of-the-tongue (TOT) phenomenon, called the *node-structure theory* (NST). The NST is based on the information-processing model. NST posits that the memory system consists of a vast network of processing units called nodes. The nodes are organized hierarchically and have symmetrical connections. A bottom-up connection implies a corresponding top-down connection and vice versa. NST postulates that speech production uses three hierarchically related systems of nodes, including semantic, phonological, and motor (Burke, MacKay, Worthley, & Wade, 1991). Burke et al. hypothesized that TOT phenomena occur when the connections between lexical and phonological nodes become weakened as a result of infrequent use, nonrecent use, and aging, causing a reduction in the transmission of priming. They examined young, middle-age, and older-age adults' performance on TOT phenomenon tasks to find whether NST was supportable. They found that alternate (i.e., incorrect) words shared phonological and grammatical class with the TOT target words. In addition, they found that words that were less frequently used in the adults' vocabulary (e.g., names of friends not frequently called or seen) were more often the victim of the TOT phenomenon. The authors concluded that limited use of specific vocabulary appears to weaken nodes, with the result being reduced transmission of priming for the target words. The findings may have implications for language acquisition in children. If a child is not exposed to a typical linguistic environment and/or has limited opportunity to use newly acquired linguistic skills, then the connections among phonologic, semantic, and motoric nodes may not develop or may be weak. In addition, limited practice in saying a word (i.e., the motoric output) may result in a weakened kinesthetic image. NST may expand the understanding of the complexity of processing and producing phonological sequences. A breakdown may occur anywhere in the network of connections and affect processing and production of phonological sequences.

Interaction of Speech Perception and Speech Production   An important question in considering how children eventually become "meta" about the phonology of their language is "To what extent is the child's perceptual attention guided by his or her vocal (motoric) experience?" (Vihman, 1996, p. 162). Vihman noted that little research has been done to address this issue but identified Shvachkin (1973) as proposing that there is an intimate connection between the two processes, as did Studdert-Kennedy (1991). Straight (1980) is characterized as generally insisting on an autonomous relationship between the processes of perception and production. Straight, however, suggested that the child's own simplified or garbled production may, in some cases, result in an imprecise internal image that then underlies the child's ensuing spontaneous productions. Thus, a false or imprecise perceptual image leads to distorted speech production. Studdert-Kennedy (1993) emphasized that a priority function of perception is to guide production in the infant. In other words, by learning to listen, the child learns to speak. As the child explores the relationship between the sounds heard and the sounds produced, attention is focused on the phonetic (i.e., articulatory) properties of the native speech sounds. Walley (1993) stressed the need for studies of perceptual development beyond infancy. These studies could document the relationship between changes in perception and other areas of development, including cognitive or representational, lexical, and (expressive) phonological advances. Walley stated that "very little is known about how individual variation in perceptual abilities or proclivities contributes to developmental advances" (1993, p. 175).

The authors of this chapter strongly agree with Walley's statement. The theoretical construct of phonological processing, discussed later in this chapter, emanates from cognitive psychology. This research has not examined in depth speech perception and speech production and their relationship to various phonological processing abilities. There is a need to examine speech perception and speech production development from an interactive perspective of these two foundational abilities. Such examination would provide an enhanced understanding of how children develop mature receptive and expressive phonology, as well as how metaphonology emerges from receptive and expressive phonological abilities. This information would also provide insights into why some individuals have significant difficulties with metaphonological abilities that relate to reading and spelling skills.

Phoneme Abstractness: How Does One "Become Meta"? The previous review of the complexity of the development of the perception and production of speech in children leads to a discussion of how children eventually become aware of the phonemic unit. A brief review of what a phoneme is will highlight the difficulty an individual faces when required to "become meta" about phonemes. Phonemes are inherently abstract units responsible for distinguishing meaning (Bloomfield, 1933). Important as a unit at this tacit, representational level, however, the phoneme does not exist as a discrete element in articulation or in the rapidly paced human speech signal (Liberman, Cooper, Shankweiler, & Studdert-Kennedy, 1967). Rather, phonemes are realized in speech as part of coarticulated syllabic segments. Therefore, articulation or the resultant acoustic signal cannot simply be divided into precise phonemes. However, given the appropriate experience or training, it is possible to come to an appreciation of the existence of speech-sound units or articulatory gestures roughly equivalent to phonemes. For example, attention given to words beginning or ending in the same way provides assignment of a unit value (phoneme) to these beginnings and endings. However, such realization does not generally emerge from everyday use of speech. Rather, explicit awareness or sensitivity to phonemes appears to develop as a result of learning an alphabetic orthography (Stuart & Colthart, 1988).

Model of Phonological Processing Construct

The acquisition of a phonology system is complex, encompassing cognitive, linguistic, and motoric factors that influence the ability to obtain a mature phonology (Vihman, 1996). For the purpose of this chapter, a model of phonology that emphasizes the relationship among phonological processing, metaphonology, and reading acquisition is discussed. This model comprises four ability areas on a continuum from automatic to tacit to meta knowledge. Metaphonology is the fifth ability area but by its very definition is at a more conscious level of reflection. This model has been referred to in the literature as the *phonological processing construct* (Catts, 1991a; Wagner & Torgesen, 1987). Phonological processing is the ability to code (i.e., both encode and decode) abstract representations of the sound attributes of spoken and written words in the form of individual units of speech known as *phonemes*. Phonological processing ability also includes the implicit knowledge of rules for ordering phonemes (Vellutino & Denckla, 1991). The five components comprising the phonological processing construct are distinct yet interrelated in their characteristics and relationship to reading. The phonological processing construct assumes a basic impairment in the ability to generate, maintain, and operate on phonological representations in working memory. This supplies a unified account of the diverse verbal-processing–skill impairments observed in readers with disabilities (Shankweiler & Crain, 1986). Researchers theorize that language-coding impairments are the reflection of a more general underlying deficiency in the phonological processing component of working memory (Brady & Fowler, 1988; Liberman & Shankweiler, 1985, 1991; Liberman, Shankweiler, & Liberman, 1989; Mann, 1987; Mann, Cowin, & Schoenheimer, 1989; Stanovich, 1987, 1988a, 1988b, 1991a, 1991b). Each ability area of the phonological processing construct is addressed in the following discussion.

Phonological Encoding Phonological encoding is the ability to process rapidly paced human speech that requires the listener to impose a phonemic identity on incoming speech sounds. As the speech-sound sequences are identified, it is then possible to figure out which words are represented in the signal (Yeni-Komshian, 1993). This requires analyzing the speech signal perceptually, deriving the phonological structure of words, and storing the phonological representations or names of these words in long-term or semantic memory (Catts, 1991c; Swank, 1994). Phonological encoding ability includes phonetic and phonemic perception (e.g., speech perception).

Phonological Coding in the Context of Lexical Access Phonological coding in the context of lexical access refers to gaining access to the referent of a word in our lexicon or internal dictionary of words. There are two kinds of phonological coding in the context of lexical access. One type is the retrieval of phonological codes, and the second is the use of phonological codes to gain access to the lexicon. Retrieving phonological codes refers to retrieving the speech sounds associated with an object from long-term memory (Denckla & Rudel, 1976; Stanovich, 1991b; Wolf, 1982, 1984, 1989, 1991). This skill is needed for word-finding and naming tasks. The second type, using phonological codes to gain access to the lexicon, refers to coding written words into a speech-sound–based representational system as a means of gaining access to the word's lexical referent (i.e., decoding in reading; Catts, 1991b). This is the skill used in reading when the indirect or phonetic approach is used. For example, if a child sees the written word *dinosaur*, he or she needs to phonologically recode the print into a speech-sound–based code to read *dinosaur* (Swank, 1994).

Research shows that poor readers are slower on tasks that require rapid automatized naming of colors, letters, numbers, or objects (Denckla & Rudel, 1976). Wolf (1984) established a relationship between naming speed and later reading. Katz (1986) and Wolf (1991) both examined the issue of phonological versus semantic deficits in naming. Katz found that children's naming errors were often related to the target word phonologically (e.g., number of syllables, stress patterns, vowels) but not semantically. These findings suggest that the lexical retrieval deficits of poor readers may be due to phonological representations that are incomplete or deficient.

Phonological Coding in Working Memory Phonological coding in working memory is the ability to efficiently maintain phonological information on-line in working memory until a specified task is completed. For example, tasks such as decoding decontextualized words or repeating a string of digits, numbers, or letters do not require long-term storage. The phonological code is maintained temporarily in working memory until the task is completed (i.e., decoding a decontextualized word or dialing a telephone number). In addition, implicit rules for ordering phonemic units are required for phonological coding in working memory (Chomsky & Halle, 1968). Compared with good readers, poor readers have been found to have impairments in the short-term recall of digits (Cohen & Netley, 1981; Miles, 1974), letters (Shankweiler, Liberman, Mark, Fowler, & Fischer, 1979), words (Byrne &

Shea, 1979; Vellutino & Scanlon, 1991), and sentences (Mann, Liberman, & Shankweiler, 1980). This difficulty is observed whether the stimuli are presented in a visual or auditory mode (Shankweiler et al., 1979). Research findings indicate that phonological codes are the most efficient for storing verbal information (Baddeley & Hitch, 1974; Conrad, 1964). It is the use of the phonological code in working memory that is particularly problematic for children with reading disabilities (Catts, 1991a). Poor readers also are less sensitive to phonologically confusable items on recall tasks. These deficiencies are restricted to the linguistic domain because other types of materials, such as nonsense designs and faces, generally can be retained in working memory by poor readers (Holmes & McKeever, 1979; Katz, Shankweiler, & Liberman, 1981; Vellutino & Scanlon, 1991). The phonological processing impairment hypothesis proposes that a reduced ability to code serial speech-sound patterns in working memory is the culprit that results in individuals with reading disabilities having difficulty using phonological information efficiently (Cohen & Netley, 1981).

Expressive Phonological Coding   Expressive phonological coding involves producing complex speech-sound sequences and multisyllabic words (Catts, 1986, 1991b). Results of research indicate that adolescents with reading disorders have difficulty with tasks requiring production of phonologically complex words (e.g., ambulance, thermometer) and the repetition of phonologically complex phrases (e.g., "brown and blue plaid pants," "the priest blessed the bread"; Catts, 1986). Encoding difficulties may prevent subjects with reading disorders from representing the phonological detail needed to accurately produce some stimulus words. Catts (1986) argued that phonetic similarity in common monosyllabic words in phrases results in speech planning or articulation problems. Research results show that subjects with reading disorders do have significantly more problems than do good readers in producing phonologically complex words.

METAPHONOLOGY

The terms *phonological awareness* and *metaphonology* are used interchangeably in the literature by researchers. Metaphonology is the awareness or manipulation of the speech-sound units of language (Hakes, 1982; Stanovich, 1988a), and it is sensitivity to speech-sound units of the language. In other words, metaphonology is the ability to consciously think about and perform mental operations on speech-sound units, such as segmenting, blending, deleting, and changing the order of speech-sound sequences.

Metaphonology is generally considered to be a component of metalinguistic awareness. Metalinguistic awareness involves the ability to focus on linguistic form apart from the context or content of a message (Hakes, 1982; van Kleeck, 1990). Language form leads to message content. Individual sentences do not stand in isolation but are integrated into a meaningful message through text-level processing. This is generally an automatic process that is executed rapidly and requires little attention (Hakes, 1982). In contrast, metalinguistic ability has been described as opaque. This suggests that metalinguistic performance focuses on the language forms apart from context and content. Metalinguistic ability is exhibited when "the language system itself is treated as an object of thought, with control processes being employed to perform mental operations on the products of the mental mechanisms involved in normal language processing" (Hakes, 1982, p. 207). Thus, metaphonology is the ability to treat phonology as an object of thought, and it is the ability to perform mental operations on the phonology of a language.

Factors Influencing the Emergence of Metaphonology

What factors influence the emergence of metaphonology in the typical child? Researchers have focused on tasks measuring children's ability to manipulate speech units ranging from words, syllables, onsets, rhymes, and phonemes (Bryant, Maclean, Bradley, & Crossland, 1989; Stanovich, Cunningham, & Cramer, 1984; Yopp, 1988). Swank (1991) addressed the issue of identifying factors that influence the emergence of metaphonology in young prereaders. The author examined the theoretical construct of metaphonology from a two-level perspective in a group of typically developing kindergarten children. The study found support for a two-level construct of metaphonology. The two levels of metaphonology were identified as supraphonemic (i.e., speech-sound units larger than the phoneme) and phonemic awareness. Furthermore, the empirical findings supported the hypothesis that supraphonemic awareness was primarily dependent on oral language and general literacy knowledge. This finding has been supported by other studies that investigated the relationship between metaphonology and oral language ability (Bowey & Patel, 1988; Catts, 1991a; Smith & Tager-Flusberg, 1982) and knowledge of nursery rhymes (Bradley & Bryant, 1985; Bryant, Maclean, & Bradley, 1990; Bryant, Maclean, Bradley, & Crossland, 1989). Bowey and Patel (1988) and Smith and Tager-Flusberg (1982) also found significant correlations between measures of metaphonology at the supraphonemic level and oral language ability. Bryant, Bradley, et al. (1989) found that children's supraphonemic awareness (i.e., rhyme awareness) was significantly related to their oral language ability.

Studies that have examined the relationship between general literacy experience and metaphonology have focused on nursery rhyme knowledge (Bradley, 1980; Bradley & Bryant, 1983, 1985; Bryant, Bradley, et al. 1989; Goswami & Bryant, 1990). Swank (1991) also found a similar relationship between supraphonemic awareness and nursery rhyme knowledge. A relationship was also found, however, between supraphonemic awareness and a broader assessment of general literacy knowledge. The measure used to assess general literacy knowledge included assessment of print awareness and yielded a significant correlation with the supraphonemic measures (.51).

Swank also found that the phonemic level of metaphonology was primarily dependent on alphabetic knowledge, thus supporting previous empirical evidence suggesting that it is the formal training in an alphabetic written language system that is the major influence on the emergence of phonemic awareness (Bowey & Francis, 1991; Ehri & Wilce, 1980, 1985, 1987, 1989; Mann, 1986; Morais, 1991; Morais, Bertleson, Cary, & Alegria, 1986). In addition, Swank found a relationship among phonemic awareness and oral language and general literacy knowledge. She argued that perhaps the relationship among these is hierarchical in nature and mediated by way of supraphonemic awareness. The hierarchical model suggests that the foundational knowledge areas are oral language and emergent literacy knowledge. These knowledge areas are proposed as the foundation leading to the emergence of supraphonemic awareness. Supraphonemic awareness then influences acquisition of the alphabet, which in turn influences phonemic awareness. Initial support for the proposed hierarchical relationship was found.

Research has shown metaphonology to be a primary determinant of early reading success. Although general indices of intelligence, vocabulary, and listening comprehension also predict reading ability, metaphonology has been found to be highly related to reading (Bradley & Bryant, 1983, 1985; Juel, 1991, 1994; Lundberg, Olofsson, & Wall, 1980; Maclean, Bryant, & Bradley, 1987; Stanovich, Cunningham, et al., 1984; Tunmer & Nesdale, 1985; Vellutino & Scanlon, 1991; Wagner & Torgesen, 1987; Yopp, 1988). The nature of the relationship between metaphonology and reading has been a matter of debate. One view is the precursor–causal relationship view of metaphonology and reading. It is argued that metaphonology provides and is necessary for reading ability, specifically word recognition or written word decoding. Another view is the resultant view. Supporters of this view argue that it is metaphonology that is the result of acquiring reading skills via formal training in a written alphabetic language. Likewise, it has been argued that both groups are describing different sides of the same coin. This argument suggests that a reciprocal relationship exists between metaphonology and reading such that metaphonology is both a precursor of and a result of reading. This view is the reciprocal model.

The precursor studies examine how subjects perform on measures of metaphonology taken before formal reading instruction and on measures of reading ability administered after reading instruction and found support for the precursor–causal relationship between metaphonology and reading ability (Bradley & Bryant, 1983; Bryant, Bradley, et al., 1989; Juel, 1991; Lundberg et al., 1980; Maclean et al., 1987). Moreover, training studies provide compelling evidence of the precursor–causal link between metaphonology and reading. These studies have shown that improved metaphonology following specific training programs results in a significant enhancement of reading ability (Alexander, Anderson, Heilman, Voeller, & Torgesen, 1991; Ball & Blachman, 1988, 1991; Blachman, 1994; Hatcher, Hulme, & Ellis, 1994; Lundberg, Frost, & Peterson, 1988).

The resultant studies investigate the effects of formal training in a written alphabetic language system on metaphonology. Findings suggest that awareness of phoneme size units appears to be dependent on exposure to and experience with the written alphabetic system (Morais, 1991). Read, Zhang, Nie, and Ding (1986) compared readers of alphabetic and/or nonalphabetic written language systems and found that readers of an alphabetic written language system performed better on tasks of metaphonology than did readers of a nonalphabetic written language system. Another group of researchers (Bertelson & de Gelder, 1989; Bertelson, de Gelder, Tfouni, & Morais, 1989; Morais, Cary, Alegria, & Bertelson, 1979) compared performance of literate and illiterate adults on tasks of metaphonology and found that the performance of the literate group was superior to that of the illiterate group on all tasks of metaphonology.

A meta-analysis of studies that investigated the relationship between metaphonology and reading identified the relationship as reciprocal (Smith, Simmons, & Kameenui, 1995). The authors' review of empirical research determined that metaphonology facilitates and is influenced by reading acquisition. The existence of a reciprocal relationship means that metaphonology is important before and during reading acquisition. The practical importance of the reciprocal relationship between reading and metaphonology has been emphasized by several authors (e.g., Adams, 1990; Stanovich, 1988a; Vellutino & Scanlon, 1991; Wagner & Torgesen, 1987). From the review of the literature, we found consistent recommendations for early identification of children at risk for reading failure (e.g., limited metaphonology) and for early, explicit instruction in metaphonology before and in tandem with beginning reading instruction (e.g., Ball & Blachman, 1991; Cunningham, 1990; Slocum, O'Connor, & Jenkins, 1993).

In conclusion, metaphonology is a significant influence on the acquisition of early reading (written word decoding) and spelling skills. Thus, it is an ability that needs to be present before introducing formal reading instruction. If metaphonology is limited, then stimulation and explicit training need to be implemented.

Speech and Language Experiences Facilitative of Metaphonology

In a meta-analysis of metaphonology training studies, Smith et al. (1995) identified six speech and language strategies that are most facilitative of metaphonology. First, the child's ability to manipulate speech-sound units was made overt with concrete representation of speech-sound units (e.g., colored blocks, tokens). Second, phonemic units were orally modeled by the instructor and produced by the child (e.g., kinesthetic image developed). Third, explicit instruction was specifically recommended by researchers (e.g., as opposed to whole-language proponents, who argue that the form of language will be discovered implicitly). Fourth, a sound–symbol correspondence component was added to metaphonology interventions (e.g., mapping the phoneme to a written alphabetic symbol). Fifth, the dimension of segmenting or combinations of segmenting, blending, and detection of phonemic units received focus. Sixth, linguistic complexity was scaffolded (e.g., word length, size of phonological unit, relative difficulty of phoneme position in words, relative difficulty of phonological properties of words).

Speech and language behaviors that are most effective in facilitating the emergence of metaphonology include production of the phoneme being targeted. Elicitation of the phoneme is achieved by methods of modeling, tactile and kinesthetic stimulation and feedback, imitating a production provided by a more competent peer or teacher, and discriminating similar speech sounds and phonological patterns. In addition, pairing the phoneme production with a visually concrete stimuli (e.g., colored blocks, tokens, mouth shape cards, written alphabetic symbols) to track and sequence phonological strings provides the scaffolding needed to move toward written word decoding and spelling.

RELATIONSHIP BETWEEN LITERACY AND PHONOLOGY AND METAPHONOLOGY

To understand why phonology and metaphonology are so important to reading, what is meant by reading in an alphabetic written language must first be understood. This section defines the alphabetic written language and its components and discusses the relationship between reading and metaphonology.

The Alphabetic Written Language

More than 4,000 years ago, the first alphabetic written language was devised by the Greeks. Before that time, written languages were pictographic or logographic. These types of written languages had written symbols that represented concepts. Thus, thousands of symbols had to be learned to write in a pictographic or logographic written language. The idea of a written language based on speech sounds of the language was revolutionary and a quantum leap for eventually providing a written language system to the masses. No longer did a person have to spend years learning all the symbols that represent the thousands of concepts that an oral language conveys; rather, one could learn a few basic written symbols that represented the dozens of speech sounds in a spoken language and thus have an infinite reservoir of ideas to convey via writing. Alphabetic written languages provided an efficient way to communicate ideas. To emphasize this point, a basic review of what is known about our spoken language is helpful.

In English, there are 44 phonemes represented by 26 alphabetic symbols, with more than 250 orthographic correspondences used to convey communication via the written language system. Thus, it is apparent—though basics are sometimes easily overlooked—that knowledge of the speech-sound system (i.e., metaphonology) is a necessity when learning an alphabetic written language system. In preparing individuals to read, it should be remembered that, first and foremost, the English written language system is an alphabetic written language system. What does this mean for those who are interested in identifying, diagnosing, and implementing training to teach individuals to read? In educational practice, new methodologies of instruction are frequently implemented before empirical evidence validates such methods. One area with significant and irrefutable evidence of its relationship to reading outcome, however, is metaphonology.

A basic tenet of learning how to read in an alphabetic written language system is that metaphonology is a necessity. The novice reader has to consciously reflect on the phonemes of the language to be able to break the alphabetic code. In other words, if the novice reader is not able to "map" the speech sounds onto the written symbol system, then decoding or the ability to sound out printed words will be impeded.

How did such a basic building block of the written language system become an obscure and frequently ignored area when considering how to best prepare individuals for reading? Frequently forgotten in reading instruction is that an alphabetic written language system is based on the principle that graphemes (i.e., the written alphabetic symbol) in print represent phonemes (actually phonetic segments) in speech. Learning the grapheme–phoneme correspondences requires the individual to extract and attend to the phonemes and the graphemes that represent the phonemes. Thus, the purpose of graphemes is to serve as a medium by which recognition of phonemes occurs (Morais, 1991). Emergence of phonemic awareness, it is argued, is inhibited without the formal training in a written alphabetic system. Research has documented the difficulties prereaders (Lundberg & Hoien, 1991; Stahl & Murray, 1994), people who are illiterate (Morais et al., 1979), and readers of nonalphabetic orthography (Read et al., 1986) have with phonemic awareness.

Morais (1991) suggested that children who are creative spellers have been told the phonemic values of letters and frequently question parents with regard to letter-to-sound correspondences. In other words, creative spellers have considerable experience with preliteracy and early metaphonological activities (e.g., being read to, reciting nursery rhymes, inventing rhyming games to play with phonological units). Liberman and Liberman (1990) suggested that the goal in teaching reading is to transfer phonology from speech to script. They proposed that this transfer occurs only through training in the alphabetic principle. In other words, only through alphabetic knowledge does the child grasp that words are distinguished from each other by the phonological structure (i.e., phonemic awareness). Studies have supported this argument. Alphabetic knowledge has been found to be the primary influence on phonemic awareness.

In summary, alphabetic languages such as English create access to written-word meaning via a phonological representation or the phonetic approach. The phonetic approach requires the reader to recode the visually perceived letters into their corresponding phonemes. Individual phonemes are then blended to form a phonological sequence that is matched to a similar sequence in the lexicon. Research of Perfetti and Bell (1991) suggested that good readers are much more dependent on the indirect or phonetic approach than previously thought. Thus, a necessary component of reading instruction in an alphabetic language (e.g., English) requires explicit training in the phonological component of language. Therefore, formal instruction in phonological coding abilities, such as metaphonology, is crucial when providing reading instruction.

Blachman (1994) identified five conclusions about the relationship between metaphonology and reading from her review of the literature. First, there is a significant relationship between metaphonology and beginning reading achievement. Second, performance on metaphonology tasks by preschool, kindergarten, and first-grade children is a powerful predictor of later reading achievement. Third, explicit training in metaphonology has a positive and significant impact on reading and spelling skills. Fourth, metaphonology can be effectively trained before literacy instruction with subsequent positive effect on reading ability. Fifth, children trained in both metaphonology and letter names and sounds, especially when trained in separate activities and not simultaneously, do better in reading than children trained in metaphonology only.

Research on the Relationship Among
Phonology, Metaphonology, Reading, and Spelling

Research clearly establishes the importance of the relationship among phonology, metaphonology, reading, and spelling. The conclusions drawn from some of the studies suggest that metaphonology precedes and influences reading, whereas other research findings suggest that reading influences the development of metaphonology. Studies examining the relationship among phonology, metaphonology, and reading are referred to in the literature as *phonological processing*. As previously discussed, there are five interrelated areas considered part of the phonological processing construct: 1) phonological encoding, 2) phonological coding in the context of lexical access or retrieval of phonological information (i.e., word finding), 3) phonological coding in working memory, 4) expressive phonological coding, and 5) phonological awareness or metaphonology (for a review, see Catts, 1991b; Swank, 1994).

This section reviews studies that look at phonological coding in the context of lexical access, phonological coding in working memory, and expressive phonological coding. The purpose of the review is to provide insight on the relationship between speech perception and speech production abilities that lead to phonological processing abilities and acquisition of reading and spelling. Studies that examine phonological encoding and metaphonology are enfolded into other studies of the various areas of phonological processing.

Phonological Coding in the Context of Lexical Access Studies that investigate the relationship between speech production and phonological coding in the context of lexical access (e.g., word finding) provide insight into the relationship between phonological abilities and metaphonology. In these studies, children are asked to perform some tasks of metaphonology as well as tasks of naming (rapid or discrete) of verbal items to assess phonological coding in the context of lexical access.

Poor readers often exhibit word retrieval problems (Catts, 1986; Fried-Oken, 1984; German, 1979, 1982; Kamhi, Catts, Mauer, Apel, & Gentry, 1988; Katz, 1986; Wolf, 1982, 1991), which have been explained generally in terms of impairments in memory storage or retrieval processes (Kail & Leonard, 1986; Katz, 1986; Wolf, 1991). The storage impairment hypothesis proposes that both semantic and phonological factors play a role in storage limitations. The storage impairment hypothesis is supported by research showing that poor readers have particular difficulty in recalling low-frequency words (Denckla & Rudel, 1976; German, 1979; Wolf, 1991).

The retrieval impairment hypothesis was examined by Wolf (1991), who completed a series of longitudinal studies by developing an internal multiple-choice component and testing it at three different stages. Stage I was before reading acquisition (i.e., prereading stage). Stage II was during reading acquisition (i.e., reading decoding stage). Stage III was during later grades (i.e., reading comprehension stage). Wolf examined word retrieval processes with and without the influence of written language skills. The design of an internal multiple-choice component allowed for examination of retrieval of vocabulary distinctions within the same set of words. Wolf compiled more than 4,000 naming errors of children using the Boston Naming Test (BNT; Goodglass & Kaplan, 1983) from 115 primary school–age children. Classification of errors via computer permitted selection of the most common phonological, semantic, and visual errors for each item on the BNT (e.g., target: "helicopter"; phonological error: "hoptacopter"; semantic error: "airplane"; visual error: "wasp"). These three types of foils plus the target became the multiple-choice component for the children's version of the BNT. Following test completion, the booklet was again reopened; each picture was represented and the child was auditorily given the three foil words and target word. If the subject consistently selected the correct target, then a retrieval impairment in vocabulary knowledge was not indicated. If one type of foil (i.e., phonological, semantic, visual) was consistently chosen, then further testing in that area was recommended. If no pattern in target foil was revealed, vocabulary was indicated.

Through a series of analyses, Wolf drew several conclusions from her longitudinal studies. Results suggested that naming measures emphasizing speed appeared particularly powerful in both prediction and group differentiation (typical population versus population with reading disabilities). Also, no significant differences were identified in discrete naming ability (i.e., BNT) between individuals with specific reading disabilities (i.e., individuals who had documented phonological processing impairments) and garden-variety poor readers (e.g., individuals with delays related to limited environmental stimulation). The error analysis, however, revealed that children with specific reading disabilities frequently knew the word but could not name it, whereas the garden-variety poor reader did not know the concept (i.e., vocabulary impairment). Finally, the naming system proved capable of pinpointing, before reading is acquired, impediments in specific processes later used in reading development. Wolf concluded that naming impairments may be connected to corresponding occurrences of speed problems in name retrieval and in motoric domains. Given the strong demands for rapid rates of processing in naming and reading, these two systems and their individual subprocesses may be particularly vulnerable (especially phonology, and especially in acquisition stages) to temporal mechanism failure (see Merzenich et al., 1996; Tallal et al., 1996).

Research in the area of word-finding problems reveals that impairments in the storage of phonological and semantic information are the key to word-finding problems. If an individual does not have an accurate auditory and kinesthetic image for a word or series of speech sounds, then storing the code for later retrieval will result in word-finding problems. It appears that the impairment of phonological coding in the context of lexical access is related to both speech perception and speech production abilities.

Phonological Coding in Working Memory   Another component of the phonological processing construct is one of phonological coding in working memory. Few studies have examined speech production abilities and their relationship to other areas of language acquisition. One reason is that studies of skilled adult speakers failed to demonstrate any direct associations between short-term memory and language production (see Gathercole & Baddeley, 1993, for review). However, Adams and Gathercole (1995) argued that the absence of any apparent contribution of phonological coding in working memory to skilled language production in adults does not rule out its involvement in children learning to speak. Bock (1982) theorized that the development of speech production is such that a progression from controlled to automatic processing might be especially likely for lower-level processes, such as articulation and word production. Elber and Wijjnen (1992) demonstrated how attainment of this level of speech production abilities may depend on the development of grammatical and phonological encoding processes and the efficient application of these in sentence planning. The authors proposed that the formulation of these skills comes about through the effort of the child, specifically the effort involved in producing the forms in the child's own speech (Adams & Gathercole, 1995).

Adams and Gathercole (1995) investigated whether phonological working memory is associated with spoken language development by assessing speech corpora taken from 3-year-old children grouped in terms of their phonological memory abilities. Quantitative and qualitative indices of the children's spontaneous speech output were taken during structured play sessions. The authors found significant differences, with children of good phonological memory abilities producing language that was more grammatically complex, contained a richer array of words, and included longer utterances than children with poor phonological memory abilities. The authors found that the rate of articulation mediated the link between nonword repetition and syntactic complexity of the children's utterances. They also found that children with poorer phonological memory skills produced more phonological errors in speech production, although this difference did not reach statistical significance.

Adams and Gathercole (1995) reviewed evidence of a positive relationship between phonological memory skills and speech production abilities in children. Children with developmental disorders of language, who exhibit limited vocabulary knowledge and limited syntactic production (Scarborough, Rescorla, Tager-Flusberg, Fowler, & Sudhalter, 1991), also have limited phonological memory skills (Gathercole & Baddeley, 1990; Taylor, Lean, & Schwartz, 1989). Adams and Gathercole argued that the co-occurrence of impairments in both phonological memory and language production fits well with the view that the memory system plays an important role in supporting the developing speaking skills of the child.

Speidel (1989, 1993), in reviewing two cases of bilingual siblings, provided evidence for specific association between phonological memory abilities and a whole range of speaking skills. Both siblings had competent intellectual abilities and good comprehension skills in their two languages. One sibling, however, exhibited language production comparable to her language comprehension level. Conversely, the other sibling had exhibited limited language production ability since infancy. This sibling exhibited poor performance on conventional verbal short-term memory tests such as digit span and auditory serial recall.

Speidel (1993) argued that the poor phonological memory of this sibling is related to his undoubtedly weak articulatory skills during the early stages of language acquisition. Furthermore, the limited phonological memory abilities of this individual will lead to impairments of long-term memory of the words and phrases used to build syntactic patterns in spontaneous speech. These words and phrases are imitations of adult models. These patterns are retained in long-term memory and constitute the foundation for the acquisition of adult language forms. Phonological memory abilities are argued to affect both the efficiency with which the adult models can be incorporated into long-term memory and the inventory of syntactic forms (Adams & Gathercole, 1995).

Gathercole and Baddeley (1989) also investigated how the short-term phonological storage component of working memory relates to vocabulary acquisition of 4- and 5-year-old children. Short-term phonological memory at age 4 accounted for a significant amount of variance in vocabulary at age 5, above that accounted for by vocabulary scores the previous year. The authors concluded that phonological coding in working memory is involved in the acquisition of new vocabulary in children. This finding expands the view that it is world-experiential knowledge that leads to increases in the mental lexicon. The word-finding studies previously discussed indicated that many children comprehend concepts but cannot retrieve the phonological code necessary to either label an object or picture or read a word. Gathercole and Baddeley's (1989) findings suggested that phonological coding in working memory is a necessary building block for increases in a child's lexicon. Speidel (1989) extended this proposal to include long-term learning of phrases as well as individual words. According to these two accounts, phonological memory impairments disrupt and delay development of syntactic and productive vocabulary skills during childhood.

Finally, inefficient phonological coding in working memory may interfere with the development of phonological recoding (i.e., decoding) skills of reading in three ways. First, English orthography is not a one-to-one correspondence between graphemes and segments of the acoustic signal. Therefore, children must discover the correspondences by reflecting on the elements of written and spoken words. To do this, the child must map sounds onto print, which requires the child to maintain phonological segments in working memory. Second, beginning readers, who rely on sounding-out strategies to identify unfamiliar words, must perform blending operations that require serial processing of isolated sounds. Phonemes held in memory are then combined to form a candidate word, which is then compared with word candidates from the mental lexicon. Third, sentence context that is stored in working memory can be used to facilitate word identification. Impaired working memory ability may prevent the beginning reader from taking full advantage of sentence context as an aid to word identification.

Expressive Phonological Coding The final area to be discussed is that of expressive phonological coding. Poor readers have documented problems in the ability to produce complex phonological sequences (Blalock, 1982; Harris-Schmidt & Noell, 1983; Johnson & Myklebust, 1967; Miles, 1974). Catts (1986) examined the speech production impairments of a group of adolescent readers with disabilities compared with a group of typical readers on three production tasks: 1) naming of pictured objects with phonologically complex names (e.g., ambulance, thermometer), 2) the repetition of phonologically complex words (e.g., statistics, aluminum), and 3) the repetition of phonologically complex phrases (e.g., "brown and blue plaid pants," "the priest blessed the bread"). The poor readers produced significantly more speech articulation errors on each of the tasks compared with the group of typical readers. Analysis of the production errors revealed that the errors were generally word-specific substitutions or omissions of sound segments. The errors appeared not to be conditioned by the phonetic context in which they occurred. Catts proposed that such an error pattern may reflect difficulties in encoding phonological information in working memory (e.g., complex level of speech perception). It is argued that some poor readers have impairments in determining the nature and order of the phonemes in words and that this makes it difficult for them to accurately produce many less familiar multisyllabic words (see, e.g., Tallal et al., 1996).

Conversely, it has been argued that speech production errors of some poor readers are the result of a motor speech–planning deficit (e.g., speech production). Catts (1987) investigated the speech production abilities of college students with specific reading disabilities and with typical reading skills. Individuals rapidly repeated a series of phonologically complex and less complex phrases. The complex phrases were two and three syllables in length and contained similar phonetic segments or consonant clusters in similar syllabic positions (e.g., "she sews," "bright blue beam"). The less complex phrases had approximately the same number of segments as the complex items but contained less phonetic similarity across syllables (e.g., "he sews," "dark blue hat"). The group with specific reading disabilities repeated both the complex and less complex phrases at a significantly slower rate than did the typical group. These individuals also exhibited significantly more speech production errors on the repetition of complex phrases than did the group of typical readers. Neither group exhibited difficulty with the less complex phrases.

Catts's (1987) analysis of error patterns led him to conclude that the problems of speech production in the group with specific reading disabilities arose, at least in part, from difficulties during the motor speech–planning stage. The majority of the errors were "slips of the tongue" involving anticipation or perseveration (e.g., "blight blue beam" for "bright blue beam"). Catts explained that, in speech planning, abstract lexical units are converted into a serial order of phonological segments. It is during this conversion that errors may occur and result in phoneme segments being misordered or misproduced. Some individuals, who eventually have specific reading disabilities, apparently are slower and less accurate than typical individuals, who are able to efficiently convert lexical information into a sequential speech-sound–based code. Catts concluded that the production of complex phonological sequences appears to be the result of deficits in encoding phonological information (i.e., speech perception) as well as problems in planning and perhaps articulating (i.e., speech production) phonologically complex sound sequences.

In a subsequent study, Kamhi, Catts, and Mauer (1990) examined the motor speech and the encoding deficit hypotheses to compare and contrast the two. Poor readers and age-matched typical readers were evaluated in their abilities to produce four novel, multisyllabic nonsense words. The poor readers, even with more training opportunities, required significantly longer time than the typical readers to produce three of the four words. The recognition data from this study indicated that encoding limitations (e.g., complex level of speech perception) rather than speech production limitations were primarily responsible for the longer acquisition times. Speech production deficiencies seemed to account for only a small portion of the difficulty that the poor readers experienced learning the novel words. From these two studies (Catts, 1987; Kamhi et al., 1990), it appears that, depending on the words being produced, both hypotheses may be valid. In other words, production of common monosyllabic words in phonetically complex strings may be the result of a motor speech–planning problem, whereas production of multisyllabic low-frequency words may be the result of an encoding problem.

In a study that investigated long-term effects of speech production impairments, Clarke-Klein and Hodson (1995) investigated children who may have a predisposition for spelling problems because of histories of severe expressive phonological impairments. Associations among expressive phonological development, metaphonological skills, and spelling performance were found to be significantly related. The authors analyzed the written spelling errors of 61 third-grade children with and without histories of severe speech-sound disorders. A variety of phonological deviation patterns were evidenced in the misspellings of true-word and nonsense-syllable spelling items. Spelling errors were categorized broadly as errors of omission, class deficiency, phonemic substitution, context-related syllable structure alteration, voicing alteration, or assimilation. Results showed that, overall, children with histories of severe speech-sound disorders demonstrated significantly more types and numbers of phonological deviations in spelling errors than did phonologically typical children, and the individuals with phonological impairments also performed poorly on measures of metaphonology compared with the typical speech group.

Lewis and Freebairn (1992) also found that individuals with histories of preschool speech-sound disorders performed more poorly on assessments of metaphonology, reading, and spelling during the elementary, adolescent, and adult years than did people with typical phonological histories. Webster and Plante (1992), too, reported relationships between early speech-sound disorders and limitations of metaphonology. The authors concluded that speech intelligibility (i.e., speech production ability) may be a highly significant predictor of performance on tasks that require explicit awareness of phonemic segments (e.g., spelling).

ASSESSMENT AND TREATMENT OF
SPECIFIC PHONOLOGICAL IMPAIRMENTS

This chapter has focused on the relationships among phonology, metaphonology, and reading. It has discussed that phonology develops from children's speech perception and speech production experiences and that these experiences derive from an innate ability to acquire oral language. From acquiring the phonology of their language, children move toward procuring metaphonology. It is metaphonology that opens the door to reading acquisition. A key to opening the door to literacy is to have all of the component pieces necessary present for the acquisition of reading skills. This section addresses these issues. First, how does the speech-language pathologist differentially diagnose children who are in need of intervention because they lack the prerequisite skills to acquire reading? Second, once the differential diagnosis has been completed, how does the speech-language pathologist design appropriate and efficacious treatment?

Specific assessment techniques are described for children who exhibit specific phonological impairment (SPI). Students with SPI frequently are not identified until they are in intermediate, middle, or even secondary school. Poor performance on metaphonology measures and decreasing reading comprehension scores for individuals with average intelligence suggest an underlying SPI that has not been detected. Some students are able to rote-memorize many sight words and certain phoneme–grapheme correspondence rules, but their phonological processing abilities do not become automatic. Automaticity is a key to fluent, efficient reading decoding and comprehension. It is easy to identify students who are at risk for SPI in kindergarten or first grade by using measures of metaphonology (Swank, 1991; Swank & Catts, 1994; Swank, Meier, Invernizzi, & Joel, 1997).

Many referrals received by speech-language pathologists are for children who perform within the normal range on psychological and psychoeducational evaluations, yet they are not acquiring reading skills as expected. A subtle language disorder may be suspected. The subtle language disorder may be in the area of SPI. SPI generally has been overlooked because of the lack of information available to practitioners. Some general information is provided later in this section for assessment of each specific area of phonological processing.

Three subsets of children need to be considered for early identification. One subset is children who have expressive phonological impairments. Another subset is children who have receptive or phonological processing impairments. The third subset is a mixed group of children who exhibit both expressive and receptive phonological processing impairments.

The first subset traditionally has been easily identified by using measures that evaluate articulation and phonological processes. However, the term *phonological processes* (see Hodson & Paden, 1991) should not be confused with the term *phonological processing*. An assessment of speech production typically is given to most children during early childhood speech and language screening clinics. Therefore, children with moderate to severe expressive phonological impairments that result in moderate to high levels of unintelligible speech are easily identified.

The second subset is children who have an undetected impairment. These children are frequently given a cursory speech-language screening. They frequently pass because the appropriate measures have not been administered. To identify children who have phonological processing impairments, and consequently metaphonology limitations, specific tasks are needed to expose the impairments. For preschool children, measures of rhyme awareness and rhyme production provide insight into the child's early metaphonology development (Swank, 1993). At the kindergarten level, a task of syllable deletion can be given (Swank, 1991). In the first grade, a measure of syllable and phoneme deletion can be administered (Swank, 1991, 1996) as well as a sound–symbol association measure. Samples of these measures of metaphonology are provided in the appendix to this chapter.

The third group is the mixed group, which needs the same types of screening measures. Thus, all three subsets require assessments of productive phonology and metaphonology. For children at the second-grade level and above, a measure of expressive phonology should include a repeating multi-syllable word list (see Hodson and Paden, 1991, for such a list).

Screening is the first level of diagnosis. If children fail the screening phase, then a comprehensive language assessment needs to be conducted. Depending on what information is available on the child (e.g., review of past records, interviews with parents and teachers, observations, other testing), the assessment needs to measure all areas of language form, content, and function and to include an audiological examination. For the purpose of the discussion in this chapter, recommendations for an assessment that addresses SPI are limited.

A comprehensive phonological assessment includes assessing the five basic phonological processing areas. These may be assessed informally and/or formally. A conversational speech sample may eliminate the necessity of administering formal measures in each of these areas. However, this section provides suggestions for both formal and informal measures. First, a measure of intelligibility is needed. A standard articulation or phonological processes assessment may be used, as well as a speech sample that is analyzed for phonetic inventory, syllable structures, and existing phonological processes.

Assessing Phonological Encoding

Assuming that proficient hearing acuity has been documented, a note of caution is given when assessing phonological encoding. Although phonological encoding is the ability to perceive phonetic and phonemic information, many formal measures purporting to assess these areas may not be adequate in uncovering the problem. Many children who have SPI perform adequately on simple tasks of word discrimination. The phonological encoding problems often occur during conversational speech and/or when processing new phonological codes (i.e., new vocabulary) or complex phonological sequences. Phonological encoding may be assessed using formal measures such as the Goldman-Fristoe-Woodcock Auditory Test Battery (Goldman, Fristoe, & Woodcock, 1974), subtests of sound mimicry and sound recognition. These measures can be used as a starting point with the understanding that impairments in any ability area are on a continuum from mild to severe. Thus, some formal and/or informal measures may identify some phonological encoding problems, whereas more subtle impairments may require further observation and assessment in perhaps a natural linguistic environment. This caution is true for all areas of phonological processing. Reports of behaviors such as having difficulty listening in noisy environments or of miscues with phonologically complex sequences may indicate a problem with phonological encoding.

Assessment of Metaphonology

Again, a note of caution is given. Many prereading and reading curriculums used in public education assume that metaphonological abilities are present as a child enters formal schooling (i.e., kindergarten). A review of the prereading curriculum provided in many kindergarten classes reveals limited or no focus on metaphonological activities. This is an unfortunate finding because research has shown since the 1980s that ability in metaphonology predicts reading outcome. Thus, screening for these abilities is important (see Swank & Catts, 1994). Formal measures of metaphonology include the Test of Awareness of Language Segments (Sawyer, 1987), Screening Test for Phonological Awareness (Torgesen & Bryant, 1993), Lindamood Auditory Conceptualization Test (Lindamood & Lindamood, 1971), and the Phonological Awareness Literacy Screening (PALS) (Swank et al., 1997). Informal measures include syllabic and phonemic deletion, blending, segmentation, and word categorization by sound units for recommendations on how to establish local norms (see Catts, 1991c; Swank & Catts, 1994).

Assessment of Phonological Coding in the Context of Lexical Access

To assess phonological coding in the context of lexical access, two specific types of naming ability may be sampled. First, discrete naming measures evaluate the ability to name various types of vocabulary (i.e., nouns, verbs, adjectives, categorical classes). Second, rapid automatized naming (RAN) measures evaluate the ability to rapidly name common objects in a repeated series. Discrete naming may be assessed by the Test of Word Finding (German, 1986) and the BNT. Wolf (1989) developed a descriptive analysis procedure to accompany the BNT for the identification of the word-finding difficulties as related to phonological, semantic, or visual confusion. Informal measures of RAN include measures developed by Denckla and Rudel (1976) or use of the Clinical Evaluation of Language Fundamentals (CELF; Wiig & Semel, 1981) Confrontation Naming (Subtest 8). The RAN measures usually have colored shapes or pictured common objects. Wolf (1991) found that using rapid alternating stimulus measures (i.e., shapes, letters, numbers alternately displayed in a series) is particularly powerful in discriminating between good and poor readers. The poor readers have significantly more difficulty in naming this type of alternating sets stimuli (e.g., limited cognitive flexibility, shifting categories).

Assessing Phonological Coding in Working Memory

Phonological coding in working memory may be assessed by using formal measures such as Clinical Evaluation of Language Functions–Revised (CELF–R) (Semel, Wiig, & Secord, 1987), Oral Directions subtest, or Token Test for Children (DiSimoni, 1983). Sentence repetition tasks should highlight a pattern of either primacy or recency recall problems. If the individual recalls only the first part of the sentence or recalls only the last part of the sentence, he or she may be exhibiting an impairment in phonological coding in working memory. The errors are more likely to be syntactic and/or morphological if the gist of the sentence is recalled but grammatical information is reduced. Informal measures include recalling a series of letters, numbers, words, and sentences. Although phonological coding in working memory may be assessed by using serial recall, it does not follow that this would be appropriate intervention (e.g., drill on recalling numbers, letters, words). Whereas identifying the problem may use a specific task, using similar tasks to intervene with the problem is not necessarily efficacious practice.

Assessment of Expressive Phonological Coding

Expressive phonological coding in older children may be assessed using a multisyllabic screening instrument (Hodson, 1986). Informal measures include lists of multisyllabic words and phrases (see Catts, 1986, 1987; Kamhi et al., 1990). In addition, language samples of conversational speech can yield useful insights into a child's expressive phonology abilities. Does the child transpose phonemes? Is weak syllable deletion a consistent pattern? Is conversational speech muffled and less intelligible than one-word productions? This type of pattern may indicate expressive phonological coding problems. People with this impairment sometimes appear almost disfluent at times as they stumble over a difficult-to-produce word.

 The goal of the preceding discussion on assessment was to inform, educate, and challenge speech-language pathologists to identify children who may have SPI. The focus was to highlight specific skills that relate the phonology of language to reading outcome. The SPI construct provides a framework of assessment for the language specialist. Beginning readers probably can read as well as they can listen if inadequate recoding or phonological decoding is not holding them back (Tunmer & Hoover, 1993). Assessment of phonological abilities can provide the educational team with invaluable information for planning effective academic intervention. Speech-language pathologists have information and training in assessment techniques, phonology and articulation, and phonetics. Thus, they possess the requisite knowledge to assess children who have language-based reading disorders that are related to SPI. Theory, research results, and practices demand that speech-language pathologists provide differential diagnosis of phonologically based reading disorders. Research results have established that phonological abilities are a key component in acquiring reading skills. Thus, assessment of phonological abilities is imperative when evaluating reading failure.

Treatment of Specific Phonological Impairments

Treatment for articulatory or expressive phonological impairments has been addressed in a variety of texts and articles. Information on the treatment of receptive phonology or phonological processing is limited. Thus, this section focuses on those treatment issues. An overview of the six strategies identified as facilitating metaphonology begins this section. The following are the six strategies:

1. The child's ability to manipulate speech-sound units is made overt with concrete representation of speech-sound units (e.g., colored blocks, tokens).
2. Phonemic units are orally modeled by the instructor and produced by the child (i.e., kinesthetic image developed).
3. Explicit instruction about speech sounds and how they are made, how they are classified, and how they are different and similar is specifically recommended by researchers.
4. A sound–symbol correspondence component is added to metaphonology interventions (e.g., mapping the phoneme to a written alphabetic symbol).
5. The dimension of segmenting or combinations of segmenting, blending, and detection of phonemic units receive focus.
6. Linguistic complexity is scaffolded (e.g., word length, size of phonological unit, relative difficulty of phoneme position in words, relative difficulty of phonological properties of words).

A formal treatment regime that includes these six strategies is the Auditory Discrimination in Depth program (Lindamood & Lindamood, 1975). This program may be used as a resource for stimulation programs in kindergarten and primary grades. It may also be used as therapy for individuals who exhibit moderate to severe specific phonological impairments (e.g., receptive/phonological processing). Another resource for preschool and kindergarten levels is Sounds Abound (Catts & Verstatinen, 1994).

Important to a discussion about how phonology and metaphonology relate to reading acquisition and how to best treat individuals who exhibit a specific phonological impairment that affects reading acquisition is to remind the reader to have a balanced view of reading acquisition. Thus, Adams's (1990) and van Kleeck's (1995) model of metaphonology and reading outcome serves as an organizing framework for the domains of preliteracy knowledge. There are four major components of the model: 1) the orthographic processor that needs experience with print conventions and letter naming and recognition skills; 2) phonological processing that requires experience with rhyming and playing with speech-sound units; 3) a meaning processor that requires oral language experiences that lead to semantic, syntactic, and morphosyntactic knowledge; and 4) a context processor that requires experience with book conventions, narratives, expanded syntactic knowledge, and world experience. Two broad stages of preliteracy development are proposed. One stage is proposed as the *meaning* stage, and the other stage is proposed as the *form* stage. The model offers a novel resolution to the whole language (meaning emphasis) versus phonics (form emphasis) controversy regarding beginning reading pedagogy. For the purpose of this chapter, the focus is on the importance of the second stage, or phonics, phonology, and metaphonology abilities.

Van Kleeck (1990) identified the rudiments of metaphonology as deemphasizing meaning and focusing on speech-sound segments, as is done with rhyming books. A perusal of Mother Goose rhymes or the Dr. Seuss books demonstrates that meaning is not the main emphasis; rather, the focus is on speech-sound segments. Often, silly and nonsensical utterances are used for the purpose of creating a rhyme. Thus, as Bradley and Bryant (1983, 1985) have argued, rhyming is a way of focusing the child's attention on speech-sound segments (i.e., form of language) rather than strictly on meaning. Using such books and activities would be appropriate in teaching children to attend to speech-sound units.

CLINICAL IMPLICATIONS

Some children enter kindergarten with competent metaphonology, having broken the alphabetic code. Other typically developing children appear to have no phonemic awareness or alphabetic knowledge. Findings from studies indicate the need to identify who is at risk for reading problems and who is advanced in reading acquisition. Both populations need specific stimulation to allow for maximum academic progress. Thus, a quick screening using metaphonology deletion and segmentation tasks can identify which children need what type of instruction. This type of procedure can help identify and target specific treatment goals for children (Swank & Catts, 1994).

CONCLUSIONS

This chapter has addressed how speech perception and speech production interact with the development of phonological processing abilities, including metaphonology and development of expressive phonology. How these abilities influence the emergence of reading skills was reviewed. To emphasize the importance and complexity of developing phonology, metaphonology, and reading acquisition, some key points of this chapter are summarized.

First, studies that investigate the relationship between speech production and phonological coding in the context of lexical access (e.g., word finding) provide insight into the relationship among phonological abilities, metaphonology, and reading outcome. These studies clearly document that children who are poor readers often exhibit word retrieval problems. These problems have been explained generally in terms of impairments in memory storage or retrieval processes related to phonological processing, which is directly related to speech perception. This view is supported by research showing that poor readers have particular difficulty in recalling low-frequency words (Denckla & Rudel, 1976; German, 1979; Wolf, 1991).

Second, poor phonological memory may be related to weak articulatory skills during the early stages of language acquisition. Furthermore, limited phonological memory abilities lead to impairments of long-term memory of the words and phrases used to build syntactic patterns in spontaneous speech. These words and phrases are imitations of adult models. These patterns are retained in long-term memory and constitute the foundation for the acquisition of adult language forms. Some argue that phonological memory abilities affect both the efficiency with which the adult models can be incorporated into long-term memory and the inventory of syntactic forms. This impairment in phonological memory abilities is also related to vocabulary acquisition. The word-finding studies indicate that many children comprehend concepts but cannot retrieve the phonological code necessary to either label an object or picture or read a word. Thus, phonological coding in working memory is a necessary building block for increases in a child's lexicon. In addition, this proposal is extended to include long-term learning of phrases as well as individual words. According to these two accounts, phonological memory impairments disrupt and delay development of syntactic and productive vocabulary skills during childhood. Finally, inefficient phonological coding in working memory may interfere with the development of phonological recoding (e.g., decoding) skills of reading. Impaired working memory ability may prevent the beginning reader from taking full advantage of sentence context as an aid to word identification.

Third, productive phonological abilities also relate to reading outcome. Poor readers have documented problems in the ability to produce complex phonological sequences. Production errors are generally word-specific substitutions or omissions of sound segments. The errors appear not to be conditioned by the phonetic context in which they occurred. Thus, such an error pattern may reflect difficulties in encoding phonological information in working memory (e.g., speech perception). It is argued that some poor readers have impairments in determining the nature and order of the phonemes in words and that this makes it difficult for them to accurately produce many less familiar multisyllabic words (e.g., speech perception).

Fourth, meta-analysis of studies that investigated the relationship between metaphonology and reading identified the relationship as reciprocal. Metaphonology facilitates and is influenced by reading acquisition. The existence of a reciprocal relationship means that metaphonology is important before and during reading acquisition. The practical importance of the reciprocal relationship between reading and metaphonology has been claimed by several authors (e.g., Adams, 1990; Stanovich, 1988a, 1988b; Vellutino & Scanlon, 1991; Wagner & Torgesen, 1987). It is important to provide early identification of children at risk for reading failure (e.g., limited metaphonology) and to provide early, explicit instruction in metaphonology before and in tandem with beginning reading instruction. Metaphonology is a significant influence on the acquisition of early reading (i.e., written word decoding) and spelling skills. Thus, it is an ability that needs to be present before introducing formal reading instruction. If metaphonology is limited, then stimulation and explicit training need to be implemented.

In conclusion, this chapter has elucidated the significant and important relationships among speech perception, speech production, receptive and expressive phonology, metaphonology, and reading in an alphabetic written language system. This information is applicable to differential diagnosis of children and treatment planning for children who exhibit written language problems.

REFERENCES

Adams, A.M., & Gathercole, S.E. (1995). Phonological working memory and speech production in preschool children. *Journal of Speech and Hearing Research, 38,* 403–414.

Adams, M.J. (1990). *Beginning to read: Thinking and learning about print.* Cambridge, MA: MIT Press.

Alexander, A., Anderson, H., Heilman, P., Voeller, K., & Torgesen, J. (1991). Phonological awareness training and remediation of analytic decoding deficits in a group of severe dyslexics. *Annals of Dyslexia, 41,* 193–206.

Baddeley, A., & Hitch, G.J. (1974). Working memory. In G. Bower (Ed.), *The psychology of learning and motivation* (pp. 47–90). New York: Academic Press.

Ball, E., & Blachman, B. (1988). Phoneme segmentation training: Effect on reading readiness. *Annals of Dyslexia, 38,* 208–225.

Ball, E., & Blachman, B. (1991). Does phoneme awareness training in kindergarten make a difference in early word recognition and developmental spelling? *Reading Research Quarterly, 26,* 49–66.

Bernhardt, B. (1994). The prosodic tier and phonological disorders. In M. Yavas (Ed.), *First and second language phonology* (pp. 149–172). San Diego: Singular Publishing Group.

Bertelson, P., & de Gelder, B. (1989). Learning about reading from illiterates. In A.M. Galaburda (Ed.), *From neurons to reading* (pp. 1–23). Cambridge, MA: MIT Press.

Bertelson, P., de Gelder, B., Tfouni, L.V., & Morais, J. (1989). Metaphonological abilities of adult illiterates: New evidence of heterogeneity. *European Journal of Cognitive Psychology, 1,* 239–250.

Blachman, B. (1994). What we have learned from longitudinal studies of phonological processing and reading, and some unanswered questions: A response to Torgesen, Wagner, and Rashotte. *Journal of Learning Disabilities, 27,* 287–291.

Blalock, J. (1982). Persistent auditory language deficits in adults with learning disabilities. *Journal of Learning Disabilities, 15,* 604–609.

Bloomfield, L. (1933). *Language.* New York: Holt, Rinehart & Winston.

Bock, J.K. (1982). Toward a cognitive psychology of syntax: Information processing contributions to sentence formulation. *Psychological Review, 89,* 1–47.

Bowey, J.A., & Francis, J. (1991). Phonological analysis as a function of age and exposure to reading instruction. *Applied Psycholinguistics, 12,* 91–121.

Bowey, J.A., & Patel, R.U. (1988). Metalinguistic ability and early reading achievement. *Applied Psycholinguistics, 9,* 367–383.

Bradley, L. (1980). *Assessing reading difficulties: A diagnostic and remedial approach.* New York: Macmillan.

Bradley, L., & Bryant, P. (1983). Categorizing sounds and learning to read: A causal connection. *Nature, 30,* 419–421.

Bradley, L., & Bryant, P. (1985). Rhyme and reason in reading and spelling. *International Academy for Research in Learning Disabilities Monograph Series* (No. 1). Ann Arbor: University of Michigan Press.

Brady, S.A., & Fowler, A.E. (1988). Phonological precursors to reading acquisition. In R. Masland & M. Masland (Eds.), *Preschool prevention of reading failure* (pp. 204–215). Timonium, MD: York Press.

Bryant, P., Maclean, M., & Bradley, L. (1990). Rhyme, language, and children's reading. *Applied Psycholinguistics, 11,* 237–252.

Bryant, P., Maclean, M., Bradley, L., & Crossland, J. (1989). Nursery rhymes, phonological skills, and reading. *Journal of Child Language, 16,* 407–428.

Burke, D.M., MacKay, D.G., Worthley, J.S., & Wade, E. (1991). On the tip of the tongue: What causes word finding failures in young and older adults? *Journal of Memory and Language, 30,* 542–579.

Byrne, B., & Shea, P. (1979). Semantic and phonetic memory codes in beginning readers. *Memory and Cognition, 7,* 333–338.

Catts, H.W. (1986). Speech production/phonological deficits in reading disordered children. *Journal of Learning Disabilities, 19,* 504–508.

Catts, H.W. (1987, November). *Can't read, can't spell, can't talk so good either.* Paper presented at the Annual Conference of the American Speech-Language-Hearing Association, New Orleans, LA.

Catts, H.W. (1991a). Early identification of dyslexia: Evidence from a follow-up study of speech-language impaired children. *Annals of Dyslexia, 41,* 163–177.

Catts, H.W. (1991b). Early identification of reading disabilities. *Topics in Language Disorders, 12,* 1–16.

Catts, H.W. (1991c). Phonological processing deficits and reading disabilities. In A.G. Kamhi & H.W. Catts (Eds.), *Reading disabilities: A developmental language perspective* (pp. 101–132). Needham Heights, MA: Allyn & Bacon.

Catts, H., & Verstatinen, T. (1994). *Sounds abound.* East Moline, IL: LinguiSystems.

Chomsky, N., & Halle, M. (1968). *The sound pattern of English.* New York: Harper & Row.

Clarke-Klein, S., & Hodson, B.W. (1995). A phonologically based analysis of misspellings by third graders with disordered-phonology histories. *Journal of Speech and Hearing Research, 38,* 839–849.

Cohen, R., & Netley, C. (1981). Short-term memory deficits in reading disabled children, in the absence of opportunity for rehearsal strategies. *Intelligence, 5,* 69–76.

Conrad, R. (1964). Acoustic confusions in immediate memory. *British Journal of Psychology, 55,* 75–84.

Cooper, F.S., Delattre, P.C., Liberman, A.M., Borst, J.M., & Gerstman, L.J. (1952). Some experiments on the perception of synthetic speech sounds. *Journal of the Acoustical Society of America, 24,* 597–606.

Cunningham, A. (1990). Explicit vs. implicit instruction in phonological awareness. *Journal of Experimental Child Psychology, 50,* 429–444.

Denckla, M.B., & Rudel, R. (1976). Naming of pictured objects by children who exhibit dyslexia and other language-learning disabilities. *Brain and Language, 39,* 1–15.

DiSimoni, F. (1983). *Token Test for Children.* Hingham, MA: Teaching Resources.

Donegan, P.J., & Stampe, D. (1979). The study of natural phonology. In D.A. Dinnsen (Ed.), *Current approaches to phonological theory* (pp. 126–173). Bloomington: Indiana University Press.

Ehri, L.C., & Wilce, L.S. (1980). The influence of orthography on readers' conceptualization of the phonemic structure of words. *Applied Psycholinguistics, 1,* 371–385.

Ehri, L.C., & Wilce, L.S. (1985, Winter). Movement into reading: Is the first stage of printed word learning visual or phonetic? *Reading Research Quarterly, 20,* 163–179.

Ehri, L.C., & Wilce, L.S. (1987). Cipher versus cue reading: An experiment in decoding acquisition. *Journal of Educational Psychology, 79,* 3–13.

Ehri, L.C., & Wilce, L.S. (1989). The development of spelling knowledge and its role in reading acquisition and reading disability. *Journal of Learning Disabilities, 22,* 356–365.

Eilers, R.E., & Oller, D.K. (1976). The role of speech discrimination in the development of sound substitutions. *Journal of Child Language, 3,* 319–320.

Elber, L., & Wijjnen, F. (1992). Effort production skill and language learning. In C.A. Ferguson, L. Menn, & C. Stoel-Gammon (Eds.), *Phonological development: Models, research, and implications* (pp. 337–368). Timonium, MD: York Press.

Fodor, J.A., & Pylyshyn, Z.W. (1988). Connectionism and cognitive architecture: A critical analysis. *Cognition, 28,* 3–71.

Fried-Oken, M. (1984). *The development of naming skills in normal and language deficit children.* Unpublished doctoral dissertation, Boston University.

Gathercole, S., & Baddeley, A. (1989). Evaluation of the role of STM in the development of vocabulary in children: A longitudinal study. *Journal of Memory and Language, 28,* 200–213.

Gathercole, S., & Baddeley, A. (1990). Phonological memory deficits in language disordered children: Is there a causal connection? *Journal of Memory and Language, 29,* 336–360.

Gathercole, S.E., & Baddeley, A.D. (1993). *Working memory and language.* Hillsdale, NJ: Lawrence Erlbaum Associates.

German, D. (1979). Word-finding skills in children with learning disabilities. *Journal of Learning Disabilities, 12,* 176–181.

German, D. (1982). Word-finding substitutions in children with learning disabilities. *Language, Speech, and Hearing Services in the Schools, 13,* 223–230.

German, D. (1986). *Test of Word Finding.* Allen, TX: DLM Teaching Resources.

Goldman, R., Fristoe, M., & Woodcock, R.W. (1974). *Goldman-Fristoe-Woodcock Auditory Test Battery.* Circle Pines, MN: American Guidance Service.

Goodglass, H., & Kaplan, E. (1983). *Boston Naming Test (BNT).* Philadelphia: Lea & Febiger.

Goswami, U., & Bryant, P. (1990). *Phonological skills and learning to read.* Hillsdale, NJ: Lawrence Erlbaum Associates.

Hakes, D. (1982). The development of metalinguistic abilities: What develops? In S. Kuczaj (Ed.), *Language, cognition, and culture* (pp. 163–210). Hillsdale, NJ: Lawrence Erlbaum Associates.

Harris-Schmidt, G., & Noell, E. (1983). Phonology. In C. Wren (Ed.), *Language learning disabilities: Diagnosis and remediation* (pp. 39–71). Rockville, MD: Aspen Publishers.

Hatcher, P.J., Hulme, C., & Ellis, A.W. (1994). Ameliorating early reading failure by integrating the teaching of reading and phonological skills: The phonological linkage hypothesis. *Child Development, 64,* 41–57.

Hodson, B.W. (1986). *Assessment of Phonological Processes–Revised.* Austin, TX: PRO-ED.

Hodson, B., & Paden, E. (1991). *Targeting intelligible speech: A phonological approach to remediation.* San Diego: College-Hill.

Holmes, D., & McKeever, W. (1979). Material-specific serial memory deficit in adolescent dyslexics. *Cortex, 15,* 51–62.

Johnson, D., & Myklebust, H. (1967). *Learning disabilities: Educational principles and practices.* New York: Grune & Stratton.

Juel, C. (1991). Learning to read and write: A longitudinal study of 54 children from first through fourth grade. *Journal of Educational Psychology, 80,* 437–447.

Juel, C. (1994). *Learning to read and write in one elementary school.* New York: Springer-Verlag.

Kail, R.V., & Leonard, L.B. (1986). *Word-finding abilities in language-impaired children.* Rockville, MD: American Speech-Language-Hearing Association.

Kamhi, A., Catts, H., & Mauer, D. (1990). Explaining speech production errors in poor readers. *Journal of Learning Disabilities, 23,* 632–636.

Kamhi, A., Catts, H., Mauer, D., Apel, K., & Gentry, B. (1988). Phonological and spatial processing abilities in language and reading impaired children. *Journal of Speech and Hearing Disorders, 53,* 316–327.

Katz, R. (1986). Phonological deficiencies in children with reading disability: Evidence from an object-naming task. *Cognition, 22,* 225–257.

Katz, R., Shankweiler, D., & Liberman, I. (1981). Memory for item order and phonetic recoding in the beginning reader. *Journal of Experimental Psychology, 32,* 474–484.

Kuhl, P.K. (1987). Perception of speech and sound in early infancy. In P. Salapatek & L. Cohen (Eds.), *Handbook of infant perception 2* (pp. 275–382). New York: Academic Press.

Lewis, B.A., & Freebairn, L. (1992). Residual effects of preschool phonology disorders in grade school, adolescence, and adulthood. *Journal of Speech and Hearing Research, 35,* 819–831.

Liberman, A.M., Cooper, F.S., Shankweiler, D.P., & Studdert-Kennedy, M. (1967). Perception of the speech code. *Psychological Review, 74,* 431–461.

Liberman, A.M., Harris, K.S., Eimas, P.D., Lisker, L., & Bastian, J. (1961). An effect of learning on speech perception: The discrimination of the duration of silence with and without phonemic significance. *Language and Speech, 4,* 175–195.

Liberman, A.M., Harris, K.S., Hoffman, H.S., & Griffith, B.C. (1957). The discrimination of speech sounds within and across phoneme boundaries. *Journal of Experimental Psychology, 54,* 358–368.

Liberman, I.Y., & Liberman, A.M. (1990). Whole language vs. code emphasis: Underlying assumptions and their implications for reading instructions. *Annals of Dyslexia, 40,* 51–76.

Liberman, I., & Shankweiler, D. (1985). Phonology and the problem of learning to read and write. *Remedial and Special Education, 6,* 8–17.

Liberman, I., & Shankweiler, D. (1991). Phonology and beginning reading: A tutorial. In L. Reiben & C. Perfetti (Eds.), *Learning to read: Basic research and its implications* (pp. 3–17). Hillsdale, NJ: Lawrence Erlbaum Associates.

Liberman, I., Shankweiler, D., & Liberman, A. (1989). The alphabetic principle and learning to read. In D. Shankweiler & I. Liberman (Eds.), *Phonology and reading disability: Solving the reading puzzle* (pp. 1–33). Ann Arbor: University of Michigan Press.

Lindamood, C., & Lindamood, L. (1971). *Lindamood Auditory Conceptualization Test (LAC).* Chicago: Riverside.

Lindamood, C., & Lindamood, L. (1975). *Auditory Discrimination in Depth.* Chicago: Riverside.

Lundberg, I., Frost, J., & Peterson, O. (1988). Effects of an extensive program of stimulating phonological awareness in preschool children. *Reading Research Quarterly, 23,* 263–284.

Lundberg, I., & Hoien, T. (1991). Initial enabling knowledge and skills in reading acquisition: Print awareness and phonological segmentation. In D. Sawyer & B. Fox (Eds.), *Phonological awareness in reading: The evolution of current perspectives* (pp. 73–96). New York: Springer-Verlag.

Lundberg, I., Olofsson, A., & Wall, S. (1980). Reading and spelling skills in the first school years predicted from phonemic awareness skills in kindergarten. *Scandinavian Journal of Psychology, 21,* 159–173.

Maclean, M., Bryant, P., & Bradley, L. (1987). Rhymes, nursery rhymes, and reading in early childhood. *Merrill-Palmer Quarterly, 33,* 255–281.

Mann, V. (1987). Phonological awareness and alphabetic literacy. *Cahiers de Psychologie Cognitive, 7,* 476–481.

Mann, V., Cowin, E., & Schoenheimer, J. (1989). Phonological processing, language comprehension and reading ability. *Journal of Learning Disabilities, 22,* 76–89.

Mann, V.A. (1986). Phonological awareness: The role of reading experience. *Cognition, 24,* 65–92.

Mann, V.A., Liberman, A.M., & Shankweiler, D.P. (1980). Children's memory for sentences and word strings in relation to reading ability. *Memory and Cognition, 8,* 329–335.

McClelland, J.L., & Elman, J.L. (1986). Interactive processes in speech perception: The TRACE model. In D.E. Rumelhart, J.L. McClelland, & the PDP Research Group (Eds.), *Parallel distributed processing: Exploration in the microstructure of cognition* (pp. 58–121). Cambridge, MA: MIT Press.

Menn, L. (1983). Development of articulatory, phonetic, and phonological capabilities. In B. Butterworth (Ed.), *Language production 2: Development, writing, and other language processes* (pp. 3–50). New York: Academic Press.

Menn, L., & Matthei, E. (1992). The "two-lexicon" account of child phonology: Looking back, looking ahead. In C.A. Ferguson, L. Menn, & C. Stoel-Gammon (Eds.), *Phonological development: Models, research, and implications* (pp. 211–247). Timonium, MD: York Press.

Merzenich, M.M., Jenkins, W.M., Johnston, P., Schreiner, C., Miller, S.L., & Tallal, P. (1996). Temporal processing deficits of language-impaired children ameliorated by training. *Science, 271,* 77–81.

Miles, T. (1974). *Understanding dyslexia.* London: Priory Press.

Morais, J. (1991). Phonological awareness: A bridge between language and literacy. In D.J. Sawyer & B.J. Fox (Eds.), *Phonological awareness and reading: The evolution of current perspectives* (pp. 31–72). New York: Springer-Verlag.

Morais, J., Bertelson, P., Cary, L., & Alegria, J. (1986). Literacy training and speech segmentation. *Cognition, 24,* 45–64.

Morais, J., Cary, L., Alegria, J., & Bertelson, P. (1979). Does awareness of speech as a sequence of phones arise spontaneously? *Cognition, 7,* 323–331.

Perfetti, C.A., & Bell, L. (1991). Phonemic activation during the first 40 ms of word identification: Evidence from backward masking and priming. *Journal of Memory and Language, 30,* 473–485.

Pinker, S., & Mehler, J. (Eds.). (1988). *Connections and symbols.* Cambridge, MA: MIT Press.

Read, C., Zhang, Y., Nie, H., & Ding, B. (1986). The ability to manipulate speech sounds depends on knowing alphabetic writing. *Cognition, 24,* 31–44.

Rubin, H., & Liberman, I. (1983). Exploring the oral and written language errors made by language disabled children. *Annals of Dyslexia, 33,* 111–120.

Sawyer, D.J. (1987). *Test of Awareness of Language Segments.* Austin, TX: PRO-ED.

Scarborough, H.S., Rescorla, L., Tager-Flusberg, H., Fowler, A.E., & Sudhalter, V. (1991). The relation of utterance length to grammatical complexity in normal and language disordered groups. *Applied Psycholinguistics, 12,* 23–46.

Semel, E., Wiig, E.H., & Secord, W. (1987). *Clinical Evaluation of Language Fundamentals–Revised (CELF–R).* San Antonio, TX: The Psychological Corporation.

Shankweiler, D., & Crain, S. (1986). Language mechanisms and reading disorder: A modular approach. *Cognition, 24,* 139–168.

Shankweiler, D.P., Liberman, I., Mark, L., Fowler, C., & Fischer, F. (1979). The speech code and learning to read. *Journal of Experimental Psychology: Human Learning and Memory, 5,* 531–545.

Shvachkin, N.K.H. (1973). The development of phonemic speech perception in early childhood. In C.A. Ferguson & D.I. Slobin (Eds.), *Studies of child language development* (pp. 91–127). New York: Holt, Rinehart & Winston.

Slocum, T.A., O'Connor, R.E., & Jenkins, J.R. (1993). Transfer among phonological manipulation skills. *Journal of Educational Psychology, 85,* 618–630.

Smith, C.L., & Tager-Flusberg, H. (1982). Metalinguistic awareness and language development. *Journal of Experimental Childhood Psychology, 34,* 449–468.

Smith, S.B., Simmons, D.C., & Kameenui, E.J. (1995). *Synthesis of research on phonological awareness: Principles and implications for reading acquisition* (Tech. Rep. No. 21). Eugene: University of Oregon, National Center to Improve the Tools of Educators.

Speidel, G.E. (1989). Imitation: A bootstrap for learning to speak? In G.E. Speidel & K.E. Nelson (Eds.), *The many faces of language learning* (pp. 151–179). New York: Springer-Verlag.

Speidel, G.E. (1993). Phonological short-term memory and individual differences in learning to speak: A bilingual case study. *First Language, 13,* 69–91.

Stahl, S., & Murray, B. (1994). Defining phonological awareness and its relationship to early reading. *Journal of Educational Psychology, 86,* 221–234.

Stanovich, K. (1987). Perspectives on segmental analysis and alphabetic literacy. *Cahiers de Psychologie Cognitive, 7,* 514–519.

Stanovich, K. (1988a). Explaining the difference between the dyslexic and garden-variety poor readers: The phonological-core variable-difference model. *Journal of Learning Disabilities, 21,* 590–604.

Stanovich, K. (1988b). Science and learning disabilities. *Journal of Learning Disabilities, 22,* 366–369.

Stanovich, K. (1991a). Discrepancy definitions of reading disability: Has intelligence led us astray? *Reading Research Quarterly, 26,* 7–29.

Stanovich, K.E. (1991b). Word recognition: Changing perspectives. In R. Barr, M.L. Kamil, P. Mosenthal, & P.D. Pearson (Eds.), *Handbook of reading research* (Vol. 2, pp. 418–452). New York: Longman.

Stanovich, K.E., Cunningham, A.E., & Cramer, B.B. (1984). Assessing phonological awareness in kindergarten children: Issues of task comparability. *Journal of Experimental Child Psychology, 38,* 175–180.

Stemberger, J.P. (1992). A connectionist view of child phonology: Phonological processing without phonological processes. In C.A. Ferguson, L. Menn, & C. Stoel-Gammon (Eds.), *Phonological development: Models, research, implications* (pp. 165–189). Timonium, MD: York Press.

Straight, H. (1980). Auditory versus articulatory phonological processes and their development in children. In G.II. Yeni-Komshian, J.F. Kavanagh, & C.A. Ferguson (Eds.), *Child phonology: Vol. 1. Production* (pp. 43–67). New York: Academic Press.

Stuart, M., & Colthart, M. (1988). Does reading develop in sequence of stages? *Cognition, 30,* 139–181.

Studdert-Kennedy, M. (1991). Comment: The emergent gesture. In I.G. Mattingly & M. Studdert-Kennedy (Eds.), *Modularity and the motor theory of speech perception: Proceedings of a conference to honor Alvin M. Liberman* (pp. 29–39). Hillsdale, NJ: Lawrence Erlbaum Associates.

Studdert-Kennedy, M. (1993). Discovering phonetic function. *Journal of Phonetics, 21,* 147–155.

Studdert-Kennedy, M., Liberman, A.M., Harris, K.S., & Cooper, V.S. (1970). Motor theory of speech perception: A reply to Lane's critical review. *Psychological Review, 77,* 234–249.

Swank, L.K. (1991). *Phonological awareness: A two level hypothesis.* Unpublished dissertation, University of Kansas, Lawrence.

Swank, L.K. (1993, November). *Identifying preschoolers at risk for developing language-based reading problems.* Paper presented at the annual American Speech-Language-Hearing Association convention, Anaheim, CA.

Swank, L.K. (1994). Phonological coding abilities: Identification of impairments related to phonologically based reading problems. *Topics in Language Disorders, 14,* 56–71.

Swank, L.K. (1996, June). *Phonology, metaphonology, and prereading skills: The identification and intervention process in kindergarten.* Poster presented at the 17th Annual Symposium on Research in Child Language Disorders, Madison, WI.

Swank, L.K., & Catts, H.W. (1994). Phonological awareness and written word decoding. *Language, Speech, and Hearing Services in the Schools, 25,* 9–14.

Swank, L.K., Meier, J., Invernizzi, M., & Joel, C. (1997). *Phonological Awareness and Literacy Screening (PALS)*. Charlottesville: University of Virginia.

Tallal, P., Miller, S.L., Bedi, G., Byma, G., Wang, X., Nagarajan, S.S., Schreiner, C., Jenkins, W.M., & Merzenich, M.M. (1996). Language comprehension in language-learning impaired children improved with acoustically modified speech. *Science, 271,* 81–84.

Taylor, H.G., Lean, D., & Schwartz, S. (1989). Pseudoword repetition ability in learning disabled children. *Applied Psycholinguistics, 10,* 203–219.

Torgesen, J., & Bryant, P. (1993). *Screening Test for Phonological Awareness*. Austin, TX: PRO-ED.

Tunmer, W.E., & Hoover, W.A. (1993). Phonological recoding skill and beginning reading. *Reading and Writing, 5,* 161–179.

Tunmer, W.E., & Nesdale, A.R. (1985). Phonemic segmentation skill and beginning reading. *Journal of Educational Psychology, 77,* 417–427.

van Kleeck, A. (1990). Emergent literacy: Learning about print before learning to read. *Topics in Language Disorders, 10,* 25–45.

van Kleeck, A. (1995). Emphasizing form and meaning separately in prereading and early reading instruction. *Topics in Language Disorders, 16,* 27–49.

Vellutino, F.R., & Denckla, M.B. (1991). Cognitive and neuropsychological foundations of word identification in poor and normally developing readers. In R.T. O'Connell (Ed.), *Handbook of reading research* (Vol. II, pp. 571–608). New York: Longman.

Vellutino, F., & Scanlon, D. (1991). The preeminence of phonologically based skills in learning to read. In S. Brady & D. Shankweiler (Eds.), *Phonological processes in literacy* (pp. 237–252). Hillsdale, NJ: Lawrence Erlbaum Associates.

Vihman, M. (1996). *Phonological development: The origins of language in the child.* Oxford, England: Blackwell Publishers.

Vihman, M., & Boysson-Bardies, B. (1994). The nature and origins of ambient language influence on infant vocal production and early words. *Phonetica, 51,* 159–169.

Wagner, R.K., & Torgesen, J.K. (1987). The nature of phonological processing and its causal role in the acquisition of reading skills. *Psychological Bulletin, 101,* 192–212.

Walley, A.C. (1993). More developmental research needed. *Journal of Phonetics, 21,* 171–176.

Webster, P., & Plante, E. (1992). Effects of phonological impairments on word, syllable, and phoneme segmentation and reading. *Language, Speech, and Hearing Services in the Schools, 23,* 176–182.

Wiig, E., & Semel, E. (1981). *Clinical Evaluation of Language Fundamentals (CELF)* (1st ed.). San Antonio, TX: The Psychological Corporation.

Wolf, M. (1982). The word-retrieval process and reading in children and aphasics. In K. Nelson (Ed.), *Children's language* (Vol. 3, pp. 437–493). New York: Gardner Press.

Wolf, M. (1984). Naming reading and the dyslexias: A longitudinal overview. *Annals of Dyslexia, 34,* 87–115.

Wolf, M. (1989, March). *Boston Naming Test–Children's Version, Multiple-Choice Component.* Paper presented to the Biennial Conference of the Society for Research of Child Development, Kansas City, MO.

Wolf, M. (1991). Naming speed and reading: The contribution of the cognitive neurosciences. *Reading Research Quarterly, 26*(2), 123–141.

Yeni-Komshian, G. (1993). Speech perception. In F. Vellutino (Ed.), *Psycholinguistics* (pp. 90–133). New York: Harcourt Brace Jovanovich.

Yopp, H. (1988). The validity and reliability of phonemic awareness tests. *Reading Research Quarterly, 23,* 159–177.

Appendix A
Experimental Preschool Tasks
(chronological age = 42–60 months)

RHYME PRODUCTION

(Mean for children who do not speak standard English = .76 [.23 standard deviations])
(Mean for children who speak standard English = 3.11 [4.0 standard deviations])

Say: "We are going to play a game. Some words sound alike; they rhyme. If I say *hat, cat, sat,* they all sound alike. I am going to say some words, and I want you to say another word that sounds like the word I say. Let's try the game. If I say *hat,* what word sounds like *hat?*" If the child responds correctly, give positive feedback. If the child responds incorrectly, give corrective feedback and give another example using *toe, hoe.*

Carrier phrase: "Say a word that sounds like ____."

1.	me	knee	6.	moo	sue
2.	my	sky	7.	map	sap
3.	may	bay	8.	bed	led
4.	so	bow	9.	sit	mitt
5.	mop	top	10.	mutt	putt

RHYME MATCHING

(Mean for children who do not speak standard English = 2.76 [2.1 standard deviations])
(Mean for children who speak standard English = 4.76 [3.6 standard deviations])

Part A

Procedures are similar to those used by Swank (1991). The examiner says, "Listen carefully, I am going to show you four pictures and say the four words that go with each picture. One of the words sounds the same as the picture in

Source: Swank (1993).

the box. Here is an example: If I say *bag*, *nine*, *tag*, *bike*, the word that sounds the same as *bag* is *tag*."

Part B

Say: "Here are four pictures. I will name each picture; then I will say another word. You choose the picture of the word that sounds like the word I said. For example, if I say *boy*, then you will find the picture of a toy because *boy* and *toy* sound alike."

Part A   Test Stimuli

1.	man	car	marble	can
2.	pail	whale	pencil	wagon
3.	goat	carrot	coat	glass
4.	bear	ball	box	chair
5.	dog	cat	frog	duck

Part B   Test Stimuli

6.	hair	bear	rabbit	pig	doll
7.	hat	pencil	cat	horse	ball
8.	rock	can	duck	marbles	sock
9.	mail	house	dog	pail	man
10.	ball	frog	box	cow	doll

RHYME ODD WORD OUT

(Mean for children who do not speak standard English = 1.85 [1.7, 2 times standard deviations])
(Mean for children who speak standard English = 4.23 [3.4 standard deviations])

This task is similar to Bradley and Bryant (1985). *Say,* "I want you to tell me the word that does not belong with the other words. It does not sound like the other words. For example, if I say *map*, *cap*, and *boy*, then *boy* does not belong, because it does not sound like *map* and *cap*."

1.	swim	hop	top	6.	pill	bill	sing
2.	tap	go	cap	7.	rake	hen	men
3.	rake	take	home	8.	too	moo	fat
4.	toe	feet	seat	9.	book	cook	like
5.	kite	rat	bite	10.	go	toy	boy

SYLLABLE DELETION

(Mean for children who do not speak standard English = 3.71 [3.5, 2 times standard deviations])

(Mean for children who speak standard English = 6.06 [3.8 standard deviations])

"Now we are going to play a game where we say just a little bit of the word."

Example 1: "Cowboy." Show a picture of a "cow" and say the word "boy." "Say 'Cowboy.' Now I will say 'cowboy' without the 'cow' [covering picture of cow]. 'Cowboy' without 'cow' is 'boy.'" Remember, just say a little bit of the word." *Corrective feedback:* "'Cowboy' without 'cow' is 'boy.'" *Reinforcement:* "Yes, 'cowboy' without 'cow' is 'boy.'"

Example 2: "Say 'cupcake.' Now say 'cupcake' without 'cup.'" (same procedure as above).

Example 3: "Say 'toothbrush.' Now say 'toothbrush' without 'tooth'" (same procedure as above). No pictures are used for test stimuli.

Test Stimuli

1. seesaw
2. hallway
3. anthill
4. daytime
5. birthday
6. airplane
7. forget
8. Sunday
9. sometime
10. baby

Appendix B
Experimental Kindergarten Level
(chronological age = 62–78 months)

COMBINED SYLLABIC AND PHONEMIC DELETION (*N* = 815)

(Mean for syllabic level = 3.1 [2.5 standard deviations])
(Mean for phonemic level 1 = 1.3 [2.1 standard deviations])
(Mean for phonemic level 2 = .8 [1.8 standard deviations])

"Now we are going to play a game where we say just a little bit of the word."

Example 1: "Cowboy." Show a picture of a "cow" and say the word "boy." "Say 'Cowboy.' Now I will say 'cowboy' without the 'cow' [covering picture of cow]. 'Cowboy' without 'cow' is 'boy.' Remember, just say a little bit of the word." *Corrective feedback:* "'Cowboy' without 'cow' is 'boy.'" *Reinforcement:* "Yes, 'cowboy' without 'cow' is 'boy.'"

Example 2: "Say 'cupcake.' Now say 'cupcake' without 'cup.'" (same procedure as above).

Example 3: "Say 'toothbrush.' Now say 'toothbrush' without 'tooth.'" (same procedure as above). No pictures are used for test stimuli.

Syllabic level	Phonemic level 1	Phonemic level 2
1. Sunday	8. fat	14. snow
2. something	9. seat	15. scream
3. baseball	10. shout	16. thread
4. return	11. jar	17. cloud
5. baby	12. tall	18. twin
6. monkey	13. door	19. /fjew/
7. person		20. spring
		21. /skware/
Total 7	Total 6	Total 8

Source: Swank (1996).

SOUND–SYMBOL ASSOCIATION (*N* = 815)

(Mean = 4.0 [3.7 standard deviations])

Child is shown lower-case consonant letters and asked to "say the sound that the letter says." *Example:* Show "k" and ask child to make the sound the "k" says. Give corrective feedback or positive reinforcement. *Example:* Show "n," using same procedure.

Test Items:

Letter	*Sound*		*Letter*	*Sound*
1. b	/b/	6.	m	/m/
2. d	/d/	7.	p	/p/
3. f	/f/	8.	s	/s/
4. h	/h/	9.	z	/z/
5. l	/l/	10.	v	/v/

11

Connecting Speech and Language
Clinical Applications

Stephen M. Camarata

THE SPEECH–LANGUAGE CONNECTION HAS profound implications for clinical practice. The previous chapters in this volume discuss subtle speech–language interactions across developmental language levels. The ontogeny of such interactions is evident from early vocalizations (see Chapters 1 and 5), suggesting a speech–language connection that is thoroughly integrated into the overall linguistic system at multiple levels (see also Folkins & Bleile, 1990). Thus, it is no surprise that this integration of speech and language is evident in the diverse ways described in previous chapters. The most obvious clinical manifestation of this is in the comorbidity of speech and language disorders in clinical populations (see Chapter 4). Clinicians often have to target multiple speech and language goals during intervention and routinely are required to consider, either directly or indirectly, the developmental ramifications of integrating speech and language for the cases displaying this type of comorbidity. Most clinicians are perhaps familiar with this form of overt implication for speech–language interaction effects. However, the more subtle integration effects also often have a profound impact on clinical case management. This chapter provides a general framework for examining the speech–language connection in clinical practice and also discusses the clinical ramifications of the types of subtle and overt connection effects described in this volume.

This chapter is organized into three sections: 1) a brief review of four models of language, ranging from cognitive-linguistic to information processing, and a description of how the speech–language connection is implicitly and/or explicitly a part of each of these models; 2) a description of how the speech–language connection can be incorporated into different intervention approaches; and 3) a description of reported speech–language integration effects that demonstrate the importance of the speech–language connection in assessment and intervention.

THEORETICAL FRAMEWORKS FOR
CONSIDERING THE SPEECH–LANGUAGE CONNECTION

There are a number of theoretical frameworks that speech-language patholo-gists, linguists, and psychologists have used to examine language, and each of these frameworks has strengths and weaknesses for evaluating the speech–language connection (cf. Crystal, 1987). Even such diverse frameworks as op-erant psychology, which examines language strictly within a larger behavioral model (Skinner, 1957), and transformational grammar (Chomsky, 1957), which posits multiple native cognitive rules for syntax, can include important elements of a speech–language connection. For example, an operant analysis of language development could include speech prerequisites for acquisition of certain interrelated language structures (e.g., a child must at least approximate accurate production of /s/, /z/, and /ðz/ to use the plural morpheme; see Cama-rata, 1990; Camarata & Erwin, 1988; Camarata & Gandour, 1985). Con-versely, the surface structure for grammatical rules must include a phonologi-cal level to account for the actual production of syntax (e.g., the surface realization of the plural marker as /s/, /z/, or /ðz/ in the words *cats*, *dogs*, and *horses* requires systematic analysis of the phonetic context in which these al-ternating morphological forms appear; see Chomsky & Halle, 1968). These examples demonstrate the importance of considering the speech–language connection in any theory of language acquisition and, more important from a clinical viewpoint, in any model of language disorders and with intervention approaches ranging from traditional didactic (incorporating imitation and modeling; see section on clinician-oriented approaches in Fey, 1986; and the review in Paul, 1995) to play-based interventions (see Camarata, Nelson, & Camarata, 1994; and the section on child-oriented approaches in Fey, 1986; Paul, 1995). As discussed in this chapter, the speech–language connection is an important consideration within any intervention plan.

Despite this importance, there has been a long-standing tendency to view language acquisition and language disorders in terms of mastering a discrete set of modules, behaviors, or levels (Camarata, 1991; Crystal, 1987). For ex-ample, information-processing models of language (Bock, 1982; Kirk & Kirk, 1971; Osgood, 1971) include levels of input and output processes believed to be required for language use. These processes can include auditory discrimi-nation, auditory sequencing, verbal association, verbal sequencing, and other skills thought to relate to language. These models often focus on the mechan-ics of language processing rather than on the content (for an iteration of this model for language disorders, see Merzenich et al., 1996). Other models focus on the various parts of language rather than on language processing. Bloom and Lahey (1978) proposed a language model consisting of content, form, and speech and use. Content includes meaning, form includes rules for sentence construction and word endings (i.e., grammar), and *speech* and *use* are the social aspects of language. Crystal (1987) proposed a model that includes two levels of speech and three language domains: morphology, which includes prefixes and suffixes but is particularly focused on the 14 grammatical morphemes studied by Brown (1973); phonetics, pertaining to speech output; phonology, which pertains to the internal or cognitive aspects of speech; semantics, which includes meaning, with a focus on word meaning; and syntax, which describes the rules for constructing sentences out of words. Finally, a number of psychologists and linguists have adopted a model of language that includes morphology, phonology, pragmatics, semantics, and syntax (see Camarata, in press). In this latter model, morphology, semantics, and syntax are defined in the same way that Crystal defines them. *Phonology* is more broadly defined as the rules of speech (including Crystal's phonetic level), and *pragmatics* is considered to be the social use of language (as in "use" for Bloom and Lahey, 1978).

Content, Form, and Use: The Bloom and Lahey Model

Although the following review relies most heavily on the latter model, a description and review of the speech–language connection as it relates to clinical applications requires at least a brief description of these models. In addition to the orientation to the speech–language connection issues inherent in each model, this review also allows clinicians from diverse theoretical perspectives to apply this potential speech–language connection in their own work. Perhaps the most straightforward model is that presented by Bloom and Lahey (1978; see also Lahey, 1988). In this model, *language* is defined as the integration of content, form, and use (see Figure 1). As noted previously, the language level

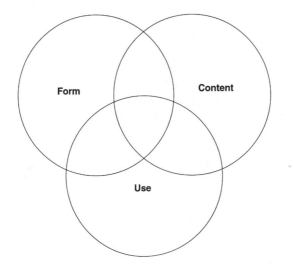

Figure 1. The integration of content, form, and use. (Adapted from Bloom and Lahey [1978].)

form includes speech in addition to morphology and syntax (and thus includes an implicit integration of these levels). Form is in turn integrated into the larger language context via interactions with content and use. An example of this implicit integration of levels was reported by Bloom, Lifter, and Hafitz (1980). They reported that children learning French (in typical acquisition) were more likely to acquire progressive morphemes (e.g., as in the present progressive) with verbs that displayed ongoing activities (and no clear conclusion; i.e., *play*), whereas past tense forms were more likely to emerge with verb forms that had a clear conclusion (i.e., *jump*). This example demonstrates how one aspect of the form level (i.e., morphology) can be connected to the content level (i.e., semantics) during acquisition, and it is clear that the Bloom and Lahey framework implicitly allows for speech–language interactions. However, details of specific potential integrations between speech and the other aspects of form and/or the other levels of language (i.e., content and use) are not provided. Despite this lack of details, those clinicians using this model for intervention can easily adapt the information presented in this section to the interactions among content, form, and use (i.e., the connection between phonology and syntax reported by Panagos and Prelock, 1982, can be translated into an interaction among components within the form level in the Bloom and Lahey model).

Information-Processing Models of Language

Those clinicians using an information-processing approach to language intervention may find the model presented by Bock (1982) to be useful for examining the speech–language connection. In this model, language is viewed as a distributed application of cognitive resources. The speech–language connection is included extensively in the model: Explicit phonological interfaces are described in lexical (i.e., word) selection, in syntactic processing (i.e., sentence formulation), and in the eventual end-point output (i.e., articulation). In this model, all of these processes require resource allocation in the form of working memory (see Figure 2). From a clinical perspective, the speech–language connection has important ramifications for any children with processing limitations: Increased complexity in one processing level results in increased allocation of working memory resources. This is precisely the effect described by Panagos and Prelock (1982) and by Panagos, Quine, and Klich (1979): Increased sentence length was associated with a decrease in phonological accuracy in children with language disorders. From a broader perspective, Bock's model predicts that any processing limitations in language acquisition (and language disorders) with a resulting impact on either overall working memory or poor input and/or output processing of semantic, syntactic, and/or phonological information when working memory demands are increased will result in limitations in the output. Thus, speech and language are directly connected within this model, and interaction effects are explicitly predicted.

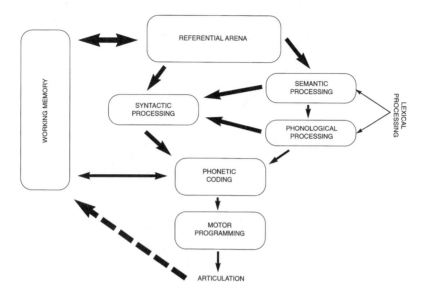

Figure 2. Processing levels involved in working memory. (From Bock, J.K. [1982]. Toward a cognitive psychology of syntax: Information processing contributions to sentence formulation. *Psychological Review, 89*, 24; reprinted by permission.)

Descriptive/Linguistic Model

A widely used model of speech and language in speech-language pathology, in linguistics, and in developmental psychology incorporates a descriptive rather than an explanatory view (as in the Bloom & Lahey, 1978, model). This model includes five levels of language: phonology, semantics, morphology, syntax, and pragmatics. *Language* is generally defined as a code for conveying ideas (i.e., thoughts), and this code is believed to consist of speech sounds, words, word endings (i.e., grammatical markers), sentence structures, and social context (Camarata, 1991). This model has a long and venerable history (e.g., Bloomfield, 1933) and was designed to "pursue the study of language without reference to any one psychological doctrine" (Bloomfield, 1933, p. vii). Thus, the model has been designed to be descriptive rather than explanatory in terms of psychological processes. Perhaps because of this descriptive orientation, applications of this model have largely been in each level (i.e., phonology, semantics, morphology, syntax, pragmatics) as an autonomous unit of study (see Figure 3).

These levels are integrated when actually communicating, and there is an implicit assumption that these parts of speech and language must be simultaneously (and appropriately) managed. However, the primary focus has been on the isolation and detailed description of key features of each part rather than on how the levels are integrated. This orientation in linguistics and psychology

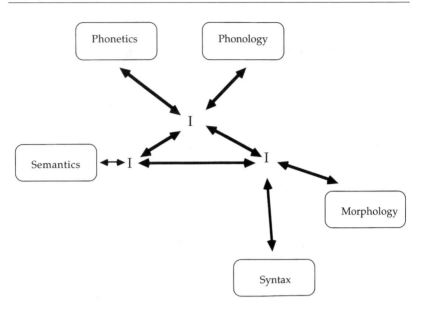

Figure 3.   Five levels of language as an autonomous unit of study in a descriptive model. (Adapted from Crystal [1987].)

is often replicated in speech-language pathology. Clinical diagnostic sessions are often designed to provide samples of the child's comprehension and production within each of the language levels. For example, the Test of Auditory Comprehension of Language–Revised (TACL–R; Carrow-Woolfolk, 1985) includes subtests for assessing word classes (i.e., semantics), grammatical morphemes (i.e., morphology), and elaborated sentences (i.e., syntax). Similarly, most speech assessment instruments (e.g., the Arizona Test of Articulation Competence, the articulation subtest on the Test of Language Development–2 Primary [Hammill & Newcomer, 1988]) include sound production only in single word contexts. The focus of assessment and treatment is often on performance within each of the language levels rather than on the integrated use of these levels and, more important, on whether integrating levels results in important changes in the child's language behavior.

An Integrated Descriptive Model: Crystal

Unlike the models presented previously, Crystal (1987) directly addressed the speech–language connection in children with language disorders. His model is designed to incorporate interactions among language levels, including levels of speech and levels of language in children with speech and language disorders. Adopting a descriptive framework rather than a processing model (although information processing and elements of models such as that of Bock,

1982, are implicit in the descriptive framework), Crystal viewed language and language disorders in the context of interactions among what he calls *levels*. These levels include morphology, phonetics, phonology, semantics, and syntax, which Crystal hypothesized may be integrated in a number of potential ways. As might be guessed from the explicit incorporation of two levels involving speech (i.e., phonetics and phonology), this model includes multiple interactions between speech and language. Crystal provided four models of integration, including one with the levels that are central to learning and use and interaction effects that are more marginal; one with the levels essentially coalescing and all language essentially being the product of integration effects; one with integration effects that are central and autonomous levels that are marginal; and one in which clusters of levels are associated with interaction effects. However, not all levels are necessarily associated with integration effects (see Figure 4).

Crystal provided evidence relating to all of these models; but perhaps the most important from a clinical viewpoint is the fourth model, in which one or more clusters of levels result in interaction effects. For example, in this view, the integration of phonology, phonetics, semantics, and morphology may result in an interaction effect. Clinically, this would imply that increased phonological complexity coupled with morphology may result in trade-off effects. Consider the plural morpheme: At the semantic level, this is a relatively straightforward concept (i.e., number) that involves a relatively concrete word class (i.e., nouns). At the morphological level, English uses an open form (i.e., no marker) for singular and a bound morpheme to denote two or more. There are some irregular forms (e.g., goose/geese, mouse/mice), but the use of the bound morpheme is relatively consistent. At the phonological level, the English plural in regular forms is derived from one phoneme, /s/; but, at the phonetic level, the phoneme /s/ appears as [s], [z], or [ðz] based on phonetic context. That is, [s] appears when the final consonant of the stem is voiceless and is not an alveolar (or palatal) fricative or affricate (e.g., *cats, books, lamps*); [z] appears when the stem includes a final vowel or voiced consonant that is not an alveolar or palatal fricative or affricate (e.g., *dogs, boas, lads, rings*); and [ðz] is used when the final consonant in the stem is an alveolar or palatal fricative or affricate (e.g., *matches, glasses, buses, judges*). Looking across levels, it appears that the semantic and morphological levels are straightforward, and the consistent underlying phonological form /s/ is used for plural. However, the phonetic form is relatively complex, having three distinct forms conditioned by phonetic context. Also, the addition of the marker results in a final cluster (e.g., *cats, dogs*) that is relatively difficult to produce, and the production of one phonetic form [z] is contrary to general patterns of word-final devoicing in child language acquisition (Ingram, 1976). It is clear that the integration of the phonetic level into the others indicates that plural may be difficult to master for children with speech and language disorders.

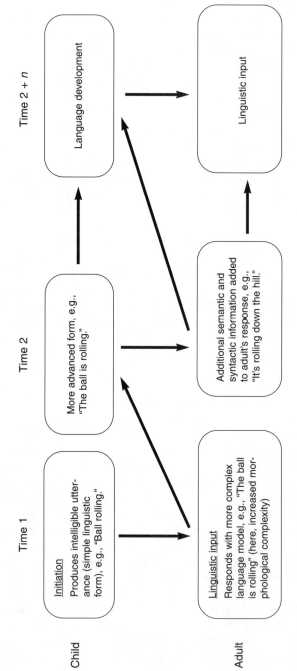

Figure 4. The transactional model of language acquisition.

306

This kind of speech–language connection can also be seen in cross-linguistic comparisons of morphological acquisition. According to Brown (1973) and Miller (1981), the plural morpheme is mastered at approximately age 2 years in most children. However, in languages that use marking that is less difficult in terms of the phonetic level (e.g., Italian uses a vowel alternation; Leonard, 1992), the plural morpheme is acquired at an earlier age. A parallel finding was reported in Camarata (1990) in an English-speaking child who mastered the final /s/ at a young age and also used the appropriate plural marker much earlier than age 2. Finally, Camarata and Gandour (1985) reported a child with speech and language disorders who used suprasegmental form to mark the plural, presumably because the typical segmental form was beyond his capability. To summarize, the speech–language connection can be an integral part of acquisition (Crystal, 1987) for typically functioning children and children with speech and language disorders. The previous example describing the acquisition of the plural in English in children with speech and language disorders and in comparisons of plural acquisition across languages illustrates how different speech and language levels (in the case of plural, phonology, phonetics, semantics, and morphology) can coalesce to produce integration effects.

INCORPORATING THE
SPEECH–LANGUAGE CONNECTION INTO INTERVENTION

This section presents various ways that the speech–language connection can be integrated into treatment of children with speech and language impairments. This section includes a discussion of the implications of integrating speech into language, a rationale for simultaneous monitoring of speech and language during remediation, and the potential applications of the integration effects during various types of speech and language interventions.

Speech as an Integrated Part of Language: Implications
for the Speech–Language Connection During Intervention

Researchers and clinicians have traditionally subdivided the study of language (and language disorders) into autonomous parts (cf. Bloomfield, 1933; Camarata, in press; Crystal, 1987). Historically, language researchers have attempted to isolate and study in detail these individual components of language. Clinicians also have often treated speech and language skills as autonomous behaviors. Without minimizing the importance of conducting research and treatment in such a manner, there are crucial advantages to studying and treating speech and language levels simultaneously, regardless of the particular theoretical orientation adopted regarding assessment and remediation. Jakobson captures the importance of a clinical balance between autonomous levels and integration of levels:

> Too often, attempts to treat the linguistic aspect of aphasia [or language disorders] suffer from inadequate delineation of the linguistic levels. One could even say that today the most important task in linguistics is to learn how to delimit the levels. The various levels of language are autonomous. [But] autonomy doesn't mean isolationism; *all levels are interrelated.* Autonomy does not exclude integration, and even more, autonomy and integration are closely linked phenomena. . . But in all linguistic questions and especially in the case of aphasia, it is important to approach language and its disruption in the framework of a given level, while remembering at the same time that any level is what the Germans call *das Teilganze* and that the totality and the interrelation between the different parts of the totality have to be taken into account. (1980, pp. 94–95; emphasis added)

Intervention has all too often been conducted primarily with each level in isolation from the other aspects of language (see the review and arguments in Crystal, 1987).

Preliminary attempts to examine the interrelationships among language dimensions have revealed important integration effects between phonology and the other dimensions of language. Such studies have indicated that each of the other language dimensions can be interrelated with speech in children with language and phonological impairments. Perhaps the most consistent finding among these studies is the relationship between phonology and syntax. For example, Panagos and his colleagues (Panagos, 1974; Panagos & Prelock, 1982; Panagos et al., 1979); Paul and Shriberg (1982); and Schwartz, Leonard, Folger, and Wilcox (1980) reported that increases in syntactic complexity are associated with changes in speech-sound production accuracy. That is, increased syntactic complexity is often associated with an increase in the number of phonological errors. This effect is often attributed to processing limitations, such as those described in Bock (1982), and a direct interface between phonological and syntactic processing. Some have argued that the effect is more basic, noting that increased syntactic complexity is often directly related to an increased number of phonetic units (i.e., complex sentences tend to include more words and more syllables) (see Panagos & Prelock, 1982).

From a clinical perspective, regardless of the source of the integration effect between speech and syntax (i.e., processing limitations or production constraints on the number of syllables), the key issue is that children are likely to make more speech errors when attempting syntactically more complex sentences. This issue has several important practical ramifications. First, traditional single-word articulation assessments are likely to represent the child's highest level of speech competence, and these children may make more errors in syntactic contexts and in running speech. There have been numerous cases of children referred with regard to a concern about speech intelligibility who performed within the normal range on traditional articulation tests, but who scored dramatically lower in multiword utterances (e.g., using the revised Percentage Consonants Correct Index for spontaneous speech; see Shriberg, 1993). Second, single words are likely to be a less complex, easier context for production from a speech–language integration perspective. This issue should be examined directly within intervention studies to determine whether the conventional wisdom regarding treating speech disorders is in fact true (see Camarata, 1993, 1995, for a discussion of context in the treatment of speech disorders). A reverse effect for phonology and syntax has also been reported. Panagos and Prelock (1982) noted that children attempting more difficult (i.e., more developmentally advanced) phonemes tended to use shorter, syntactically simpler sentences. From a clinical perspective, this would suggest that teaching more complex syntactic forms is likely to be more successful when introduced with words containing easier speech sounds (perhaps selected from an inventory of existing sounds that the child uses correctly). Again, this issue should be evaluated directly within intervention studies. Clearly, the speech–syntax connection has the potential for a direct impact on speech and language intervention.

A similar integration effect for the semantic level and the speech level was reported by Camarata and his colleagues (Camarata & Leonard, 1986; Camarata & Schwartz, 1985), who conducted a series of studies that revealed the interrelation between semantics and phonology. In this case, greater semantic complexity (object words compared with action words) was associated with a decrease in phonological accuracy (i.e., lower percentage of consonants produced correctly). These latter studies included a high degree of control of confounding factors (e.g., diversity of morphological markers, frequency of presentation, phonological structure of the lexemes within each class), suggesting again that processing limitations may result in trade-offs among language domains. Clinically, this would appear to suggest that production of nouns (as on articulation tests) is likely to be more accurate than other word classes (e.g., verb forms). Taken with the findings for syntax and speech integration, it appears likely that traditional articulation tests overestimate speech production skills when integrated into other language contexts. Also, the findings appear to suggest that new speech sounds introduced during treatment are more likely to be used correctly in noun contexts.

A similar reverse semantic and speech effect has also been reported. The findings of Leonard et al. (1982) indicated that new words containing old (i.e., already mastered) speech sounds are more likely to be learned than identical words containing new (i.e., more difficult) sounds (see also Schwartz & Leonard, 1982). This finding was replicated in typical children and in children with language impairments, suggesting, from a clinical point of view, that new vocabulary should be selected that minimizes phonological challenges for the child: New words should be selected that include sounds already mastered by the child.

Campbell and Shriberg (1982) reported a speech–pragmatics integration effect, indicating that phonology and pragmatics are interrelated during language acquisition. They observed that children with phonological impairments make fewer errors when producing words that are new topics in the conversational context compared with words produced as comments in the discourse (i.e., those that reflect an already established shared reference were produced with more errors). In this case, increased phonological accuracy was used only when listener uncertainty was likely to be high, whereas lower levels of accuracy may suffice when the conversational partner is already aware of the topic (see also Gallagher, 1977). This finding suggests that children attempt to manage processing load by cutting accuracy of speech production when the context allows. One question is whether this processing resource conservation in speech was associated with allocation of working memory or other processing resources to other language levels (i.e., increased semantic, syntactic, or morphological accuracy and/or complexity).

The clinical implications of this finding are as follows. During evaluation, speech production is more likely to be accurate in topic contexts compared with comments. Speech samples should be examined in terms of pragmatic context to determine variability on this dimension. In samples including predominantly comments (a likely category in many clinical samples), the child's capability for speech may have been underestimated. This capability would be a particularly important consideration when selecting speech targets for intervention that are ostensibly absent from the child's inventory (i.e., the sound may be in the inventory if a topic context is sampled). An extrapolation of the results of Campbell and Shriberg (1982) suggests that new sounds should be introduced in contexts that are most likely to facilitate accurate production (i.e., inducing the child to use new sounds in topic contexts). Again, this potential implication should be examined in more detail using intervention studies.

Finally, as noted previously, work by Camarata (1990), Camarata and Erwin (1988), and Camarata and Gandour (1985) suggested an integration effect between morphology and speech. These authors reported that difficulty in producing grammatical markers (e.g., plural) can lead to shifts in the phonological patterns used to signal the grammatical change (e.g., use of variations in duration, intensity, and/or F_0) and, more important, that phonological complexity is likely to have an impact on grammatical morpheme acquisition. From a clinical viewpoint, this integration effect appears to indicate that grammatical morphemes should be introduced in words with the least phonological complexity (i.e., in stems that include sounds that are already produced correctly by the child).

Rationale for Monitoring Speech and
Language Levels Simultaneously During Treatment

Perhaps the most important implication of the studies discussed in the previous sections of this chapter for the speech–language connection is the simultaneous monitoring of speech and language acquisition during treatment. As described previously, the analysis and treatment of speech and language disorders historically have been viewed as being rather autonomous endeavors. For example, leading texts often examine speech disorders to the exclusion of other kinds of language disorders (e.g., Bernthal & Bankson, 1988; Stoel-Gammon & Dunn, 1986). Researchers examining the treatment of speech disorders also do not include attempts to monitor simultaneous acquisition of morphological, phonological, syntactic, and semantic milestones. However, several other chapters in this volume suggest that phonological and language acquisition are integrated from the earliest stages of development and that monitoring these language domains simultaneously can provide important information (see, e.g., Chapters 1, 3, and 5).

In a broader sense, Slobin (1973) noted that acquisition of new structures is often coordinated with existing (i.e., old) language structures. He observed that any new form first appears with an already established function. This appears to have important clinical implications: Acquisition of new targets may be facilitated if already established elements are included. As described previously, acquisition of new lexical items may be facilitated when the words selected include already acquired speech sounds (see Leonard et al., 1982). Conversely, Schwartz and Leonard (1982) reported that children avoid producing words containing phonemes not present in their phonological systems. Perhaps the most familiar example of phonological and lexical integration is the progressive idiom (Ingram, 1976; Leonard, Newhoff, & Mesalam, 1981; Leopold, 1947), in which there is an apparent regression in phonological competence as the child's lexical inventory increases. For example, Leopold reported that his daughter Hildegard initially used correct speech production for the word *pretty* but subsequently produced this word with misarticulations. He theorized that the rapid expansion of Hildegard's vocabulary resulted in a decay in her phonological skills. This type of speech–language connection also appears to have important clinical ramifications: Advances in vocabulary size may be associated with decreased phonological accuracy. Clinicians electing to simultaneously teach speech sounds and lexical items may observe this kind of integration effect. However, the decay in speech performance is inexplicable unless it is viewed within the framework of a speech–language connection.

There is clearly the potential for these types of integration in speech and language levels within the population with language disorders. Crystal stated his view rather directly, "that levels of interactions between levels are of considerable clinical import. Indeed, a good case can be made to say that the traditional preoccupation with levels has led us to ignore what may well be a central issue in the investigation of language disabilities" (1987, p. 8). Consider the treatment implications of progressive idioms as previously presented: A regression in phonological performance may actually be associated with advances in the lexical domain. However, traditional treatment paradigms that examine speech as an autonomous construct fail to account for this regression and lead the clinician to conclude that the treatment is not effective. Thus, the literature provides a strong rationale for monitoring language domains simultaneously during treatment and indicates that the treatment of speech disorders should not be conducted in isolation (Crystal, 1987).

The preceding literature review reveals that speech can interact with other aspects of language to produce interesting and important covariance. In addition, there is direct evidence to suggest that speech competence plays a more fundamental role in language acquisition and in the remediation of language disorders. For example, Miller and Leddy (Chapter 7) report that speech capability was the most predictive factor in the remediation of language disorders in children with Down syndrome. In this view, speech can serve as a choke point or flow restrictor for the other aspects of language; that is, children with language impairments must be at least minimally proficient in speech production in order to be successful in overall language production (see Camarata, 1996). In a very fundamental way, speech and language are directly interrelated: The use of language requires at least minimal intelligibility. Consider the implications for morphology when a child cannot produce the final /s/ (and the allophonic variations of /s/: [s], [z], and [∂z]). Such a child has difficulty in producing plural (*books*), contracted copula and auxiliary (e.g., *she's nice, she's walking*), possessive (e.g., *Janet's*), and regular third-person singular (e.g., *she walks*). Realization of the language forms is predicated directly upon speech.

THE SPEECH–LANGUAGE CONNECTION TRANSCENDS
DEVELOPMENTAL LEVELS AND DISABILITY TYPOLOGIES

At first glance, the chapters in this volume appear to be quite diverse in terms of developmental context and disability typology, ranging from typically developing infants (see Chapters 1 and 3) to infants with tracheostomies (see Chapter 5) to preschool children with speech and language-learning disabilities (see Chapters 3 and 4), children with hearing impairments (see Chapter 8), children with Down syndrome (see Chapter 7), children (and, in some studies discussed, adults) who stutter (see Chapter 9), augmentative system users (see Chapter 6), and children with reading difficulties (see Chapter 10). However, this diversity also serves to validate the clinical importance and pervasive nature of the speech–language connection. Although all chapters include detailed information on the specific aspects of the speech–language connection within the developmental levels and within the disability typology described therein, this section examines some of this information in the general framework of speech–language integration discussed above.

Locke (see Chapter 3) provides a discussion of the potential grammatical origins of developmental language disorders and presents a model founded on the evolutionary roots of language and language acquisition as the potential basis for language disorders. He points to an important paradox in the literature on language-learning disorders when viewed from an exclusively grammatical perspective: Such children often display aspects of language-learning disorders before the onset of grammatical use. Although grammar acquisition is often problematic in children with developmental language disorders (see Fey, 1986; Leonard, in press; and Paul, 1995, for reviews), Locke has provided a convincing argument for an ontogeny for developmental language disorders beyond grammar, particularly within the social-cognitive domains. It could be added that strictly grammatical accounts are inconsistent with the types of speech–language interaction effects described previously. In addition to the co-occurrence of speech and language disorders (Aram & Kamhi, 1982; Chapter 4), there have been numerous reports of direct integration effects for speech and language in children with developmental language-learning disorders (as in Chapter 7).

From an evolutionary viewpoint and while viewing grammar as one aspect of a larger linguistic context, Chapter 7 describes the pivotal role of speech skills in later lexical and grammatical acquisition in children with Down syndrome. Miller and Leddy have found that level of speech competence is one of the strongest predictors of later success in language-teaching programs. In addition to illustrating the integrated nature of speech and language in development in this population, these findings perhaps provide a window into the evolutionary dependence of language (and grammar) on differentiated speech. The development of grammar and other language skills may have a foundation upon differentiated, articulate speech. As in Miller and Leddy, lack of differentiated, intelligible speech may dramatically alter development of language both in the individual (although language use without speech is possible; see Chapters 6 and 8) and perhaps within the species as well. It is clear that accounts of developmental language disorders should include the speech–language connection.

Chapter 2 provides further insight into this potential process. Stoel-Gammon has described the factors that may lead to rapid lexical acquisition in typically developing children. These factors overlap key aspects of the Locke model but also include a criterion of being easy to pronounce. Furthermore, Stoel-Gammon has traced the acquisition of words from potential origins in babbling (see Chapter 1) through first words. She has provided a detailed account of the interrelations between speech and language acquisition in typically functioning talkers and in late talkers (Thal, Oroz, & McCaw, 1995), noting that late talking is related to impoverished phoneme inventories. This analysis directly parallels what was seen in Miller and Leddy (and described in Camarata, 1995); that is, speech development can serve as a limiting factor in subsequent language acquisition. In a related model, Swank and Larrivee (Chapter 10) have provided evidence that reading skills are, in part, related to speech and language skills. In addition to the well-known increased risk of reading disabilities in children with preschool speech and/or language disorders, Swank and Larrivee describe the ways that speech perception; speech production; and, most important, metaphonology relate to the use (and comprehension) of abstract alphabetic symbols. In a broader sense, the acquisition of written language is directly related to facility with the speech domain, a speech–language connection that is similar to that presented for children with Down syndrome, in children who are late talkers, and in typical language acquisition.

Chapter 9 illustrates a kind of integration effect for the speech–language connection that is the reverse of what has been discussed previously in the present chapter. In the case of stuttering, language (including grammar, lexical characteristics, and morphology) is directly and/or indirectly related to speech skills. Stuttering has traditionally been viewed as predominantly, if not exclusively, a speech behavior. Because extensive tests of language skills have failed to reveal systematic abnormalities in any aspects of language, the role of linguistic aspects of stuttering was not examined in detail. Chapter 10 has provided evidence that, though language disorders per se are not directly associated with stuttering, linguistic variables are important conditioning factors for stuttering behavior. That is, linguistic characteristics such as clause structure, grammatical complexity, lexical selection, and morphological factors can have a dramatic influence on stuttering behavior. It appears that detailed understanding of stuttering requires insight into the linguistic factors that facilitate or inhibit fluent speech. Thus, the speech–language connection in stuttering involves linguistic variables as conditioning factors in speech production. The factors that decrease fluency are remarkably similar to the factors reported to decrease speech production accuracy in children who do not stutter but have phonological disorders (cf. Panagos & Prelock, 1982). Although at least a portion of this variability can potentially be attributed to the increased motor complexity of longer grammatical strings (i.e., linguistic complexity and motor complexity in terms of utterance length are often confounded), the effect has been observed in stutterers (see Chapter 9) and in children with phonological disorders (Panagos & Prelock, 1982) when this confound has been controlled, indicating that linguistic factors are indeed conditioning speech production.

Chapters 6 and 8 discuss the speech–language connection in children who have limited-use speech, either as augmentative system users or as children with hearing impairments. Paul has argued that severe speech impairments arising from physical disabilities, even in the absence of more general cognitive deficits, can have an impact on language acquisition. This position is analogous to the model of cognitive development proposed by Vygotsky (1962), who argued that language acquisition supports the organization of thought during child development. Paul has argued that speech acquisition may in some ways serve an organizational function during language development. Further support for this model can be seen in the transactional view of language growth described in Chapter 8 and in Yoder and Warren (1992). This transactional perspective includes the child's productions as a trigger for teaching responses (such as those described in the section on tricky mixes in Chapter 8) from the adult (see Figure 4, this chapter). Production of intelligible messages becomes extremely important in this model (see Camarata, 1996), because speech becomes the focus of the parent's response and the learning transaction is disrupted when the adult cannot understand the child's communicative act. Thus, as Paul (Chapter 6) and Nelson and Welsh (Chapter 8) have argued, the impact of speech impairments, either because of physical impairments or because of hearing impairments, should be examined beyond simple effects in the speech and phonology domain. The linguistic ramifications of these speech limitations should be examined as well.

CONCLUSIONS

This chapter has discussed the clinical implications of the speech–language connection. It is clear that all models of language, despite an often autonomous view of speech and language, either explicitly or implicitly are affected by the speech–language connection. This connection can have very important clinical ramifications: Effective case management, evaluation, goal selection, and intervention activities can be improved if speech–language integration effects are taken into account. The state of the art consists of a series of reports on potential speech–language integration effects that may be extremely important for individual cases but have yet to be examined systematically in larger clinical trials. Despite this potential limitation in the research literature, the speech–language connection should be included in clinical practice and can be particularly useful when the child demonstrates apparent plateaus or even regressions in one language level (this may be associated with advances in a related speech or language level) and to maximize clinical effectiveness by controlling associated speech and/or language contexts to ensure that the most supportive, linguistically simple contexts are used to facilitate production. As Crystal (1987) recognized, in many cases, the speech–language connection may be the most important consideration in the management of many children with speech and/or language disorders.

REFERENCES

Aram, D., & Kamhi, A. (1982). Perspectives on the relationship between phonological and language disorders. *Seminars in Speech, Language, and Hearing, 3*, 101–114.

Bernthal, J., & Bankson, N. (1988). *Articulation disorders.* Englewood Cliffs, NJ: Prentice-Hall.

Bloom, L., & Lahey, M. (1978). *Language development and language disorders.* New York: John Wiley & Sons.

Bloom, L., Lifter, K., & Hafitz, J. (1980). Semantics of verbs and the development of verb inflection in child language. *Language, 56,* 386–412.

Bloomfield, L. (1933). *Language.* New York: Holt, Rinehart & Winston.

Bock, J.K. (1982). Toward a cognitive psychology of syntax: Information processing contributions to sentence formulation. *Psychological Review, 89,* 1–47.

Brown, R. (1973). *A first language: The early stages.* Cambridge, MA: Harvard University Press.

Camarata, S.M. (1990). Semantic iconicity in plural acquisition: Extending the argument to include normal children. *Clinical Linguistics and Phonetics, 4,* 319–325.

Camarata, S.M. (1991). Assessment of oral language. In J. Salvia & J. Ysseldyke (Eds.), *Assessment in special and remedial education* (pp. 263–301). Boston: Houghton Mifflin.

Camarata, S.M. (1993). The application of naturalistic conversation training to speech production in children with speech disabilities. *Journal of Applied Behavior Analysis, 26,* 173–182.

Camarata, S.M. (1995). A rationale for naturalistic speech intelligibility intervention. In M. Fey, J. Windsor, & S. Warren (Eds.), *Communication and language intervention series: Vol. 5. Language intervention: Preschool through the elementary years* (pp. 63–84). Baltimore: Paul H. Brookes Publishing Co.

Camarata, S.M. (1996). On the importance of integrating naturalistic language, social intervention, and speech-intelligibility training. In L.K. Koegel, R.L. Koegel, & G. Dunlap (Eds.), *Positive behavioral support: Including people with difficult behavior in the community* (pp. 333–351). Baltimore: Paul H. Brookes Publishing Co.

Camarata, S.M. (in press). Assessment of oral language. In J. Salvia & J. Ysseldyke (Eds.), *Assessment.* Boston: Houghton Mifflin.

Camarata, S.M., & Erwin, L. (1988). Rule invention in the acquisition of morphology revisited: A case of transparent semantic mapping. *Journal of Speech and Hearing Research, 31,* 425–431.

Camarata, S.M., & Gandour, J. (1985). Rule invention in the acquisition of morphology by a language impaired child. *Journal of Speech and Hearing Disorders, 50,* 40–45.

Camarata, S.M., & Leonard, L. (1986). Young children produce object words more accurately than action words. *Journal of Child Language, 13,* 51–65.

Camarata, S.M., Nelson, K.E., & Camarata, M. (1994). A comparison of conversation based to imitation based procedures for training grammatical structures in specifically language impaired children. *Journal of Speech and Hearing Research, 37,* 1414–1423.

Camarata, S.M., & Schwartz, R. (1985). Production of action words and object words: Evidence for a relationship between semantics and phonology. *Journal of Speech and Hearing Research, 28,* 323–330.

Campbell, T., & Shriberg, L. (1982). Associations among pragmatic functions, linguistic stress, and natural phonological processes in speech delayed children. *Journal of Speech and Hearing Research, 25,* 547–553.

Carrow-Woolfolk, E. (1985). *Test of Auditory Comprehension of Language–Revised (TACL–R)*. Allen, TX: Developmental Learning Materials.

Chomsky, N. (1957). *Syntactic structures*. The Hague, Netherlands: Mouton.

Chomsky, N., & Halle, M. (1968). *The sound patterns of English*. New York: Harper & Row.

Crystal, D. (1987). Towards a bucket theory of language disability: Taking account of interaction between linguistic levels. *Clinical Linguistics and Phonetics, 1,* 7–21.

Fey, M. (1986). *Language intervention with young children*. San Diego: College-Hill.

Folkins, J., & Bleile, K. (1990). Taxonomies in biology, phonetics, phonology, and speech motor control. *Journal of Speech and Hearing Disorders, 55,* 596–611.

Gallagher, T. (1977). Revision behaviors in the speech of normal children developing speech. *Journal of Speech and Hearing Research, 20,* 303–318.

Hammill, D., & Newcomer, P. (1988). *Test of Language Development–2: Primary (TOLD–2)*. Austin, TX: PRO-ED.

Ingram, D. (1976). *Phonological disability in children*. New York: Elsevier.

Jakobson, R. (Ed.). (1980). *The framework of language*. Ann Arbor: University of Michigan Press.

Kirk, S.A., & Kirk, W.D. (1971). *Psycholinguistic learning disabilities: Diagnosis and remediation*. Urbana: University of Illinois Press.

Lahey, M. (1988). *Language development and language disorders*. New York: Macmillan.

Leonard, L. (1992). Specific language impairment in three languages. In P. Fletcher & D. Hall (Eds.), *Specific speech and language disorders in children: Correlates, characteristics and outcomes* (pp. 118–126). San Diego: Singular Publishing Group.

Leonard, L. (in press). *Specific language impairment in children*. New York: Cambridge University Press.

Leonard, L., Newhoff, M., & Mesalam, K. (1981). Factors influencing early lexical acquisition: Lexical orientation and phonological composition. *Child Development, 52,* 882–887.

Leonard, L., Schwartz, R., Terrell, B., Prelock, P., Rowan, L., Chapman, K., Weis, A., & Messick, C. (1982). Early lexical acquisition in children with specific language impairment. *Journal of Speech and Hearing Research, 25,* 554–559.

Leopold, W. (1947). *Speech development of a bilingual child: A linguist's record: Volume II. Sound learning in the first two years*. Evanston, IL: Northwestern University Press.

Merzenich, M., Jenkins, W., Johnston, P., Schreiner, C., Miller, S., & Tallal, P. (1996). Temporal processing deficits of language-learning impaired children ameliorated by training. *Science, 271,* 77–80.

Miller, J. (1981). *Assessing language production in children*. Austin, TX: PRO-ED.

Osgood, C. (1971). Where do sentences come from? In D. Steinberg & L. Jakobovits (Eds.), *Semantics, an interdisciplinary reader in philosophy, linguistics, and psychology* (pp. 497–552). Cambridge, England: Cambridge University Press.

Panagos, J. (1974). String complexity increases phonemic interference. *Perceptual and Motor Skills, 38,* 1219–1222.

Panagos, J., & Prelock, P. (1982). Phonological constraints on the sentence productions of language disordered children. *Journal of Speech and Hearing Research, 25,* 171–176.

Panagos, J., Quine, M., & Klich, R. (1979). Syntactic and phonological influences on children's articulation. *Journal of Speech and Hearing Research, 22,* 841–848.

Paul, R. (1995). *Language disorders: Early childhood through adolescence*. St. Louis: Mosby–Year Book.

Paul, R., & Shriberg, L. (1982). Associations between phonology and syntax in speech delayed children. *Journal of Speech and Hearing Research, 25,* 536–546.

Schwartz, R., & Leonard, L. (1982). Do children pick and choose? Phonological selection and avoidance in early lexical acquisition. *Journal of Child Language, 9,* 319–336.

Schwartz, R., Leonard, L., Folger, K., & Wilcox, M. (1980). Evidence for a synergistic view of language disorders. *Journal of Speech and Hearing Disorders, 45,* 357–377.

Shriberg, L. (1993). Four new speech and prosody-voice measures for genetics research and other studies in developmental phonological disorders. *Journal of Speech and Hearing Research, 36,* 105–140.

Skinner, B.F. (1957). *Verbal behavior.* New York: Appleton-Century-Crofts.

Slobin, D. (1973). Cognitive prerequisites for the acquisition of grammar. In C. Ferguson & D. Slobin (Eds.), *Studies of child language development* (pp. 175–208). New York: Holt, Rinehart, & Winston.

Stoel-Gammon, C., & Dunn, C. (1986). *Normal and disordered phonology in children.* Austin, TX: PRO-ED.

Thal, D., Oroz, M., & McCaw, V. (1995). Phonological and lexical development in normal and late-talking toddlers. *Applied Psycholinguistics, 16,* 407–424.

Vygotsky, L. (1962). *Thought and language.* Cambridge, MA: MIT Press.

Yoder, P., & Warren, S. (1992). Can developmentally delayed children's language development be enhanced through prelinguistic intervention? In A.P. Kaiser & D.B. Gray (Eds.), *Communication and language intervention series: Vol. 2. Enhancing children's communication: Research foundations for intervention* (pp. 35–61). Baltimore: Paul H. Brookes Publishing Co.

Author Index

Subject Index

Page numbers followed by "t" denote tables, those followed by "f" denote figures, and those followed by "n" denote footnotes.